# Health
# and Medicine
# in the Evangelical
# Tradition

# Health/Medicine and the Faith Traditions

Edited by James P. Wind and Martin E. Marty

The Health/Medicine and the Faith Traditions series
explores the ways in which major religions
relate to the questions of human well-being.
It issues from Project Ten, an interfaith program
of the Park Ridge Center for the Study of
Health, Faith, and Ethics.

Barbara Hofmaier, Publications Coordinator

The Park Ridge Center
is a corporation of the Lutheran General HealthSystem.

The Park Ridge Center
211 East Ontario, Suite 800
Chicago, IL 60611

# Health
# and Medicine
# in the Evangelical
# Tradition

## "NOT BY MIGHT NOR POWER"

## Leonard I. Sweet

TRINITY PRESS INTERNATIONAL
Valley Forge, Pennsylvania

Trinity Press International, P.O. Box 851, Valley Forge, PA 19482-0851

**Library of Congress Cataloging-in-Publication Data**

Sweet, Leonard I.
    Health and medicine in the Evangelical tradition : "Not by might
nor power" / Leonard I. Sweet.—1st ed.
      p.  cm. — (Health/medicine and the faith traditions)
    Includes bibliographical references and index.
    ISBN 1-56338-097-8 :
    1. Health—Religious aspects—Christianity—History of doctrines.
  2. Medicine—Religious aspects—Christianity—History of doctrines.
  3. Evangelicalism—United States—History.  I. Title.  II. Series.
BT732.S93   1994
261.5'61–dc20                                 94-8603
                                                      CIP

Printed in the United States of America

94    95    96    97    98    99        10   9   8   7   6   5   4   3   2   1

# Contents

# Foreword

Because the word *evangelical* comes from the Greek word for gospel, and because the Christian gospel has so much to do with healing and health, this book in a series on health and religious traditions should need no explaining or defending. All one expects Leonard Sweet to have to do is expound the evangelical tradition. It's as simple as that.

Of course, it is not simple at all. The issue of what evangelicalism is, who evangelicals are, and what evangelicalism has to do with health and medicine has grown as complex as have all the other connections made by authors of books in this series. While Sweet is perfectly capable of elaborating on the meanings of the tradition, this foreword by a bystander should locate evangelicals so that they can see how others see them and so that others can begin to see them. It should also locate evangelicalism so that readers can be prepared to let Sweet do the precise defining and the elaborating and applying of the tradition to matters of health.

*Evangelical:* the word has to be put in context and seen with its connections if the author who uses it wants to be intelligible. I am on occasion invited to participate in, observe, or report on conferences convoked by intellectuals and leaders in what we might call the orbit of Billy Graham, by far the best-known evangelical figure of our time. Their welcome is most cordial, but I usually get introduced as the invited "*non*-evangelical." Such references are ironic and mildly infuriating. (Evangelicals do not encourage intense infuriations.) Why? First, because I would make as much claim on receiving and holding the Christian gospel as evangelicals do, though in a slightly different way. Second, because, as I like to point out, I am the only person in the room who belongs to a church body — the *Evangelical* Lutheran Church in America — that has the word in its title. Do we get no credit for that? All anyone notices is that, yes, the Continental European Lutheran and Reformed churches were historically called evangelical, but the meaning there is different from the meaning here. The main difference, by the way, has

vii

to do with the concept of being "born again" and with the literalism these evangelicals tend to associate with biblical interpretation.

A second cast of people called evangelical are, after Lutherans, the world's second-largest Protestant (or, sometimes, "evangelical catholic") tradition, Anglicanism or Episcopalianism. Evangelicals in the Anglican communion were and often remain a mainstream part of that mainstream body. They positioned themselves over against what they saw as formalistic "High Church" or liberally compromising traditions on right and left. They favored revivals and sent missionaries into all the world. To them goes much of the credit for the abolition of slavery in England in 1829 and for many reforms since. But they, too, are not "born again" in the ways of modern evangelicalism, and they get written off as unscrupulously liberal on the matter of the Scriptures.

By now it is clear that claiming the word *evangelical* does not assure that other Christians will concede the claimants' primary right to that identification. It does mean that the claimants have to set aside the prior claims of two huge international Christian communions. It is also clear by now that the first three uses of the term in most English dictionaries will be of little help in identifying Leonard Sweet's evangelicals.

While the evangelicals of this book title are increasingly self-conscious of their internationalism and while they are actively forming new organizations in the name of what is evangelical, it will be most helpful if we locate their United States partisans, leaving to the reader the task of making his or her way through the thicket of denominations and emphases beyond this continent. Who are the American evangelicals, who are presumably one of two main readerships for this book? (The other readership, my fellow "nonevangelical" believers and unbelievers, are those who want to, *need* to make sense of this powerful, assertive, expanding group.)

Sweet sends out the right signals and sets up the helpful markers about how they see themselves, but that does not help us position them. For starters, picture who turns up in their camp in the polls. Ask one hundred Americans "What is your religion?" or "What is your religious preference?" and you will find fifteen to twenty of them identifying themselves as "conservative Protestant." (No longer can one use the pollster's question "Are you born again?" as a guide. *Born again* has entered the vocabulary so congenially in recent decades that Roman Catholics and New Age advocates may readily adopt the concept and identify with it.) Not all will actually say "conservative Protestant," but they will mention denominations regarded as being of that stripe. Most of these would call themselves "evangelical," though some would prefer "Pentecostal" or "fundamentalist," which are on the one hand more exuberant and on the other more hard-line than most self-described evangelicals.

One-fourth of the poll respondents will be classified as "moderate Protestants," or members of moderate denominations. Very many of these moderates identify with the evangelicals who tend to be seen to their right. Add to them not a few of the 8 percent who identify with "African-American Protestantism." It becomes clear that perhaps one-fourth of America has a claim on the word *evangelical* as Sweet uses it.

From all this gerrymandering of traditions, identifications, and polls it ought to be clear that finding and defining the evangelical place is a controversial endeavor. Its controversialism is evident at times in the chapters that follow. Not everyone liked it when around mid-century one Protestant party started claiming the word *evangelical* all for itself. In fact, at first, after a minority of its partisans organized a National Association of Evangelicals in 1942, or when a majority started linking with Billy Graham, or when leaders formed magazines like *Christianity Today* after mid-century, they often were described and self-described as "neoevangelical." Those were the days of neoorthodoxies and neoscholasticisms. But the "neo-" was cumbersome and gradually everyone dropped it, to the chagrin of those who had favored its use for their own creeds and causes.

In the nineteenth century, almost all American Protestants were simply called evangelical. The first good book on *Religion in the United States of America*, Robert Baird's work of 1844, uncontroversially linked as evangelical churches the Episcopal, Congregational, Baptist, Presbyterian, Methodist, Moravian, Presbyterian, Reformed, Lutheran, "smaller German sects," and Quakers. (Baird ended this section defensively, treating the "Alleged Want of Harmony among the Evangelical Christians of the United States.") Unevangelical Protestants were the few Unitarians, Christ-ian Connectionists, Universalists, Swedenborgians, and Dunkers. Baird's widely accepted classifications would help few today.

One set of American evangelicals sees itself as perpetuating the grasp of the gospel and the churchly style of nineteenth-century evangelicals. Another set got to its present state more controversially. In the 1920s American Protestantism was shaken to its core in a controversy labeled "Fundamentalist versus Modernist." (Most members were somewhere between the poles, but everyone was challenged and disturbed by the tensions and schisms.) The fundamentalist party, which lost in denominational warfare to the group that later came to be called mainstream or mainline Protestantism, went its own way, starting new denominations, ministries, seminaries, publishing and broadcasting ventures, and missionary and humanitarian agencies. But many of them found the fundamentalist label too constricting, the fundamentalist manners and modes too harsh. Hence the National Association of Evangelicals and the definings of the second half of this century.

Evangelicalism today, then, includes heirs of nineteenth-century Protestantism, offspring of the fundamentalists, and millions who have little historical sense and do not care where the tradition came from. They simply had the born-again experience, would like to convert you, are highly devoted to the Bible as they interpret it (usually but not always quite literally), and would adopt a certain Christian style.

This book is mainly about that style, and how it is trying to recover the concepts of illness and health, ill-being and well-being, that should go with the evangelical profession. That the tradition has much to say to its newcomers and neighbors, much that has been overlooked or not known in our time, is clear from the pages that follow.

I will resist here the temptation to say anything about the substance of the argument, which I find to be accurate, fair-minded, and eloquently, even elegantly, presented. Only a word about Sweet's evangelical style, chosen in his effort to have the medium match the message. Professor Sweet has all the conventional scholarly credentials; in fact, in addition to carrying out his research he is the chancellor of a flourishing United Methodist (and ecumenical) theological school and publishes a journal for preachers.* Presumably, he can write in stuffy academese for the more lugubrious journals, but for this book he has chosen to employ a rhetorical style that preserves the flavor of evangelicalism and echoes of pastors past.

The evangelical style is therefore not only argumentative but anecdotal. Evangelicals testify, and some of Sweet's most convincing sections are based on his autobiographical references to a childhood shaped by a more conservative evangelicalism than that which lures him now. (I do not even know if he would say "we evangelicals" in all evangelical company today.) He is never embarrassed to link heart-language with head-language, as evangelicals are allowed to do. At times the book has a folksy character, with light-hearted passages that antievangelicals, of whom there are not a few, would call corny or at least folkloric. Evangelicals never merely expound; they commend, at least implicitly, and Sweet does not always hide his sense that readers, be they evangelical or other, might be better off if they reclaimed their neglected tradition of health-seeking and interpreting illness, suffering, and death. Evangelicals can be contentious; Sweet's long section on evangelicals' opposition to most abortions of human fetuses will alienate some and force all who stay with him to examine their own assumptions and positions. Such

---

*For increased awareness and knowledge of evangelicalism, see "The Evangelical Tradition in America," a bibliographical essay by Leonard I. Sweet in *The Evangelical Tradition in America*, ed. Leonard I. Sweet (Macon, Ga.: Mercer University Press, 1984), pp. 1–86. Significantly, Sweet is chancellor of United Theological Seminary in Dayton, Ohio, which is always classified as "mainstream" Protestant, an identification that shows how for scholars and others the mainstream/evangelical boundary is blurred.

sections seem to be departures from the moderate or liberal outlook that characterizes Sweet most of the time. He sees them as consistent with the evangelical whole.

It is this evangelical whole, so often broken into denominations, forgotten by antihistorical born-again types, despised by antiintellectuals of the tradition, overlooked or unknown by the rest of America's believing communities, that comes through with such clarity and, yes, memorability in the evangelical-styled offering that Leonard I. Sweet presents. In *The Vindication of Tradition* historian Jaroslav Pelikan tells why choreographer Jerome Robbins was asked to stage *Fiddler on the Roof,* a play about a tradition: "If it's a show about tradition and its dissolution, then the audience should be told what that tradition is." Sweet stages the views of health and medicine in the evangelical tradition. He shows what it is and does, and he exemplifies it on every page.

Martin E. Marty

# Grace

The French composer and virtuoso pianist Charles Valentin Morhange, alias Alkan, was killed in 1888 as he reached for the Talmud, pulling a bookcase on top of his frail body. Many times during the preparation of this volume I feared a similar fate. It might have happened had it not been for Betty O'Brien, librarian, research assistant, and friend. She sleuthed for sources, checked references, and supplemented my own work with important original research on communion practices; her contribution was critical to the completion of this project.*

Patrick White, the Australian novelist, talked about his books as "a series of caesareans without an anesthetic." There are certain people who made this birth-process less painful than it generally is. Just as the swing (or slam) of a door can move ministers from death to birth, so the ring of the phone can move a seminary president from research and writing or teaching to fund raising or student recruitment or trustee cultivation. I could not have made these transitions without my assistant Thelma Monbarren, whose good humor, abilities, and sensitivities astound me more each day. Editor James P. Wind (now with the Lilly Endowment) gave the entire manuscript the kind of critical reading that leaves a book bloodied and battered, and healed of numerous diseases and defects. And I would never have attempted this book without the challenge thrown down by Martin E. Marty. His personal example of producing scholarship that is deeply intelligent without being too "intellectual" in the academic, Rip Van Winkle sense while being truly "intellectual" in the French sense of the term — a literary person or scholar who is unabashedly concerned with public affairs — is one that continually inspires.

In her disdain for authors who write with their hands, less with their heart, conservationist and ecologist Marie Aull kept this historian's feet to the fire of both the arts and sciences. The many dinner discussions in front

---

*Betty A. O'Brien, "The Lord's Supper: Fruit of the Vine or Cup of Devils?" *Methodist History* 31 (1993): 203–23, and O'Brien, "The Lord's Supper: Traditional Cup of Unity or Innovative Cups of Individuality," *Methodist History* 32 (1994): 79–98.

xiii

of the roaring "Great Fireplace" of Aullwood, where much of what follows (including this "Grace") was written, gave this study much of what snap-crackle-and-pop of life it may have. So too did Marie's modeling of learning that seems to be always looking, and always capable of seeing more.

This book was written at a time in my life as a parent when I felt most in danger of losing touch with my sons, Leonard and Justin. Many of their generation boast a past, but not a history. One of the gifts I thought I could give them, whether they wanted it or not, was this, their history. As I explain in the introduction, this book is really a greeting card to my ancestors in the form of a report card on how well I have mastered what they have taught me, how well I have utilized what they have left me. It is for this reason I dedicate this book to their great-grandfather, my grandfather and namesake, Ira Lucius Sweet (1879–1942), a man whom I never met but whose presence I always felt.

Leonard, Jr.'s, and Justin's gifts to me, it turned out, were and are much greater. I am from the early "Baby Boomer," late "Cold War" generation. They are part of the early "Buster," late "Thaw" generation that is engaged in the sweeping deconstruction of conventional old-paradigm assumptions, arguments, and arrangements. They have helped me understand why the gray suit of pious tradition no longer arouses great emotion, and why so many sacred cows are ending up in the stockyard. Even more, for someone who tries to make every word written the only word possible, the joy of their presence in my life is a constant reminder of how love throws language to the wind.

# Introduction:
# "There Is a Balm in Gilead"

A man will give all he has for his own life.

— Satan (Job 2:4)

Waterman Sweet, Bonesetter, hopes to meet the applause of all who may be under the necessity of employing him. He may be found at the Market Cellar, where he has a lot of good butter fit for table use.

— *Providence Journal* (1830)

Hel shines in the very word *Health*
as Ill in the Divine Will shines.

— Robert Duncan

In the very beginnings of Rhode Island's history, a pious Welsh-English artisan family known as the Bonesetter Sweets settled in the Narragansett Bay region and practiced the art of natural bonesetting. Not until the mid-nineteenth century did physicians routinely treat fractured legs, dislocated thumbs, or the like. That was the calling of the healer known as the bonesetter. Each generation of Bonesetter Sweets quietly passed on to succeeding generations a knowledge of natural remedies derived from plants, nature's healing powers to treat fractures, sprains, and dislocations.

The tradition can be seen most clearly in the 1843 publication of Waterman Sweet's *Views of Anatomy and Practice of Natural Bonesetting by Mechanical Process, Different from All Book Knowledge.*[1] By this time the Sweets enjoyed more than a regional reputation for their mysterious skill in natural healing, their sacrificial dedication to their patients, and their secret formulas for liniments using herbs, oils, and skunk grease. Maintaining

1

the artisan traditions of their ancestry, the Bonesetter Sweets conducted their healing practices as an avocation alongside extensive involvement in evangelical movements and activities. They became celebrated for their evangelical piety and, later, for their bibliographic mastery of evangelical theology, with a special concentration on holiness thought.

This tradition was handed down to me primarily in two forms. I inherited from my namesake, Ira Lucius Sweet, a marvelous library of books, notes, and manuscripts on evangelical theology and history — one that over the past hundred years was used privately by many bishops and holiness leaders who traveled to the Adirondack foothills to discuss finer points of doctrine with my lay-theologian, antiquarian, glove-cutting grandfather.

As part of this collection came a plain pine chair, old enough to be an antique but undistinguished in every way, its bottom rung almost worn away in two spots. Worthless to collectors, this chair is one of my most prized possessions. It is the chair on which my grandfather sat and studied church history and theology after a long day as factory fodder for the industrial age. The bottom rung is worn where he rested his feet while pouring over his beloved books, sometimes gently rocking and gradually rubbing down the wood to a ribbon-thin strip.

I also inherited a secret recipe for the making of "Sweet's Liniment." According to both written and oral tradition, Sweet's Liniment is a natural medicine one can swear by for the treatment of sore limbs, joints, bruises, and backaches. It also makes a wonderful local antiseptic and massaging ointment. In fact, the family oral tradition claims that the formula for the ointment Jack Cardiff and Albert Peterson used on revivalist Billy Sunday for his daily rubdowns was based on that of Sweet's Liniment (they added camphor and other ingredients).

I have broken with my tradition in a couple of respects. No longer is skunk grease used in Sweet's Liniment. Upon the ordination of three members of my generation (my brother, my cousin, and myself), no longer is the Sweet pedigree characterized by lay theologians and tent-making preachers. And at a time when politicizing forces have shred labels like "evangelical," one searches for new anagrams of faith by which to identify oneself. No longer would I simply say that I am an "evangelical student of history and theology" like my ancestors before me. It would be more accurate to say that I am a liberal-evangelical, charismatic-postmodernist student of history and eco-theology.

There is an old Welsh joke that one's conclusion is one's introduction in reverse. Let me honor my ancestors without becoming part of their joke by an advance summary of the most basic evangelical stance on health and medicine offered in this book. I learned it from my forebears while cutting the secret ingredients for Sweet's Liniment. I also learned that it is the real secret of healing that cuts closest to the core of the gospel. The words are inscribed over the entrance to one of the hospitals evangelicals helped build, Columbia-Presbyterian Medical Center in New York City: "Healing Comes from the Most High."[2]

It is the healing balm of Gilead — helped along of course by Salk's vaccine, Fleming's penicillin, and Sweet's Liniment — that makes the wounded whole.


## I

I am a firm believer that subject ought to shape, if not dictate, style. Accordingly, I have purposely written this book in an evangelical style. What is an evangelical style?

In keeping with Søren Kierkegaard's adage that one cannot sew without a knot in the thread, it is important first to define an evangelical.[3] Alas, the thread one has to work with does not form a neat line but a vast linen. To be American was almost to be evangelical in spirit, if not in substance, at least until the 1870s and perhaps as late as 1920. A master at mustering guises, evangelicalism's ambition to penetrate and conquer American culture led to a ventriloquizing of voices and actions that frustrates, even mangles analytic tidiness. Part of the challenge of writing this book has been to keep faithful to a changing, clamorous tradition as it moves from focal to fringe consciousness in American culture.

Because the evangelical empire is so vast, one can find almost any phenomenon one looks for within its orbit. We cannot safely generalize about a spiritual tradition in which at least forty-five million people in North America locate themselves, most of them coming out of the major Reformation churches that feed the evangelical stream of American spirituality. When any concept is blown too large it can burst.

Some scholars have isolated as many as fourteen distinctive kinds of evangelicalism in America, making any map of this theological universe dangerously reminiscent of the *New Yorker's* map of the world — I can't find my place in it. My favorite taxonomy of the nine major evangelical traditions includes the Anabaptist (for example, Mennonite, Brethren, and Evangelical Friends Alliance), African-American (such as National Baptist, Progressive National Baptist, Christian Methodist Episcopal, African Methodist Episcopal, and African Methodist Episcopal Zion), Charismatic-Pentecostal (nondenominational congregations and parachurch agencies as well as Assemblies of God, Full Gospel Church Association, Church of God [Cleveland, Tennessee]), Wesleyan-Holiness (Free Methodist, Wesleyan, Nazarene, Salvation Army, Church of God [Anderson, Indiana], Christian

Missionary Alliance), Reformed-Confessional (Christian Reformed Church, Orthodox Presbyterian Church, Presbyterian Church in America, Lutheran Church–Missouri Synod), Baptist (Southern Baptist Convention, Disciples of Christ, Plymouth Brethren, General Association of Regular Baptists, Seventh-day Adventists), progressive (represented by Wheaton College and Fuller Theological Seminary), radical (as expressed by *Sojourners, The Other Side, Wittenburg Door*), and mainline (those evangelical movements flourishing within major establishment denominations such as United Methodist, Presbyterian, Lutheran, United Church of Christ, Episcopal, American Baptist, and so forth). Trying to bring coherence and order to such a knockabout arena is enough to make a boxer throw in the towel, an archaeologist throw in the trowel, a historian throw in the note cards.

What makes speech possible is that evangelicalism, much like Puritanism before it, was at heart a movement, a shifting and multiform coalition of traditions that coalesced around a coherent worldview and spirituality. More a spirit or mood that swept American religious life, dominating Protestantism until the twentieth century as well as influencing other faith traditions, it is that evangelical whole, that evangelical worldview, that cohesive spiritual thrust that enables such a study as this even to be contemplated, as well as guides its trudge down the past's tracks. I have resisted more denominational taxonomies and analyses that, at least in the hands of this writer, would compromise the search for identity and wholeness.

Evangelicalism is *first* and foremost a biblical faith, a belief in the binding, bonding authority of the Bible. The evangelical journey is a dialogic process in which believers work on biblical texts in the expectation that these biblical texts will work on them, sticking to them like burrs on the soul.

Evangelicals like to tell the story of the little boy whose parents got him a new Bible to present to his grandmother on her birthday. Since he had seen other people write something on the front page when presenting a book as a gift, he wanted to do the same. Not knowing what to write, he copied an inscription from a book in the bookcase. When she opened her brand new Bible, the boy's grandmother was quite surprised to read the inscription: "To Grandmother, with the compliments of the author." Evangelicals spend their time discussing not who wrote the Bible but what in the Bible is being written in their hearts; not whether the Bible is true, but whether they are true to the Bible.

*Second*, evangelicals stress a personal relationship with God through faith in the atoning death and resurrection of Jesus Christ. This does not mean that evangelicals are doctrinaire, although some have been more doctrinal than others. It is simply not in the evangelical spirit, as J. Harry Cotton, onetime president of McCormick Seminary, used to chide liturgical churches, to use their complex doctrines and creedal declarations as a theological pistol, which demands assent down to the last fine point and proclaims anyone a heretic who falters at any point.

Evangelicals live lives that are theologically clarified. But their doctrines have usually been ones in which believers could move with some degree of freedom. God's touch works on each one of us in mysterious, individuating ways. Evangelicals trust that many people's hearts are nearer right than their heads.

*Third,* evangelicals are heavily conversionist, with evangelization of the gospel a high priority. *Gospel* is a distinctively Christian word, one of the Apostle Paul's favorite terms, and one of the most important words in the history of evangelicalism. It means literally "good news" — the usual translation of the Greek *euangelion* — about Jesus, who came to show us the kingdom of God, and it occurs more than seventy-five times in the Second Testament.

Conversion, an experience of the engrossing power of God's presence in one's life (also known as being born again), constitutes a rich and distinctive part of evangelicals' theological experience and a factor that can trump a lot of doctrinal and other considerations. For most of evangelical history, conversion was a spiritual decision to "follow Jesus" that had strong vocational components. Whether it went by the name of sanctification (in the Eastern Orthodox tradition it is called "divinization," in others "christification" or "celestification"), or tracking "in his steps," or simply praying "thy kingdom come...on earth as it is in heaven," evangelicals believed that they were to participate in the *missio Dei,* as many of them put it, the mission of God in the world. This opened up evangelicalism to a larger social canvas, and it created an enterprise culture of holy disquiet that gave evangelicals a rarin'-to-go impatience and rambunctiousness of spirit. Evangelicals have been uneasy pilgrims on the path of least resistance.

*Fourth,* evangelicals are strong believers that moral absolutes exist and that truth holds more than private meaning. One way evangelicals pay their respects to truth is by helping truth hold public importance: important moral issues must be recognized as public matters. Hence the willingness in the evangelical tradition to enter the public arena in support of a clash of clamoring causes, even to the point of "legislating morality." What evangelicals have not always appreciated, especially in the case of abortion, is that the principle that "hard cases make bad laws" applies to the general principle of legislating morality as well as to the specific moral principles themselves. Evangelical impatience with any lack of public moral stature or at least moral standpoint no doubt can sound moralizing to outsiders. But when this spiritual energy and stamina were put to work in the millennial ambition to build God's kingdom on earth, as we shall see, a host of social left-outs, left-overs, least-last-lost people and causes benefited greatly.

Health is not an end in itself among evangelicals, nor is ill health always to be avoided or ashamed of. In the words of one evangelical publication in the mid-nineteenth century, "Health is a glorious thing, but, like money, not so much for itself, as to be spent. — Squander it not, for you know not what moment you may need it to lay upon the altar of love, or friendship, or duty — to yield it up for the sake of its Great Giver, and of your fellow men."[4]

What happened in the evangelical tradition when spiritual push, in the cause of "spend and be spent" (as the Horatius Bonar hymn puts it), came to social shove? A variety of shoves and stances ensued, making evangelicalism one of the most aggressive social movements in American history. A revealing essay could be written on this simple definition: an evangelical is a Christian who overdoes overdoing it. Indeed, for this very reason the evangelical tradition had a dramatic, some would say decisive, impact on the course of American culture, including the history of health and medicine. A single uniform evangelical shove simply does not exist in this culture of overdoers overdoing it. But evangelicals are of single and uniform mind that personal and social ethics, private and public morality, should not be disjoined. They are also one in their conviction that the worst that can happen is when spiritual push never comes to social shove.

## II

What is an evangelical style? First, an evangelical style is a biblical style that moves from biblical material to present experience with great ease and economy. The importance of the Scriptures and biblical reasoning to the evangelical tradition would be hard to overstate. Evangelicals built a biblical culture in nineteenth-century America, successfully creating a scriptural consensus around most of life's ethical matters. Even today, evangelicals settle life-issues on the basis of biblical teaching. Evangelicals resist separating theology from ethics, and they especially insist on integrating biblical studies and ethics.

Because biblical background is of such great consequence in formulating positions on health and medicine, the reader can expect to confront in the course of this book many biblical references and arguments from what I choose to call, for more than idiosyncratic reasons, the First Testament and the Second Testament (traditionally known as "Old" and "New" Testaments). For the evangelical Christian, the Bible of Jesus, the apostles, and the early church is no less inspired or authoritarian than the "new" Bible.

The label "old" suggests something outmoded, passé, and inferior. Hence the alternative formulation "First" and "Second" Testament.

The unresolved problem for the historical theologian is the same as that for the evangelical: from the biblical sea can be, and has been, fished out whatever suits any angler's purpose on any given fishing expedition. The best in the evangelical tradition has picked passages without "passage picking." In one way, however, the evangelical tradition is vulnerable to the charge that it has not been biblical enough. When it elevates and absolutizes the Bible above Christ, the word above the Word, a condition known technically as bibliolatry, evangelicalism ignores the Bible's own witness that everything has been relativized by Christ (Philippians 2:9–10). Resistance to bibliolatry, and restraint in the use of texts, has been a goal of this book.

Second, evangelicals are great storytellers — or in words my mountain relatives used to say when they punctuated worship with their stories, "I feel a testimony coming on." There seems to be almost a genetic predisposition to organize experience through stories; as author Isak Dinesen noted, "Any sorrow can be borne if a story can be told about it."

Evangelicals have borne their sorrows by telling stories and giving testimonials. They have learned to interpret the language of pain, the language of need, by telling stories about the land of pits, the wilderness of thirst, the valley of the shadow. In so doing they have found there is a strength and inspiration to be drawn from every experience in life, no matter how "troublous." I have tried to honor this unblushingly anecdotal tradition by doing what is the evangelical thing to do — combining the analytical with the anecdotal, turning to my own experiences of growing up in the evangelical tradition and relaying stories I have heard around platforms, pulpits, pews, camp fires, and family altars.

Third, an evangelical style is an allusive style. Often the best followers of the Jesuit maxim for spiritual soldiers, as taught by St. Ignatius of Loyola — "Know your enemy's arguments better than he knows them himself" — evangelicals know far more about other members of the Christian and human community than is known about them. Indeed, some evangelical theologians seem to operate on the premise that they have no right to argue with anyone until they can state that person's position to their satisfaction. This gives evangelical literature a range of reference and breadth of compass that sometimes startles. In the words of someone who taught evangelicals so much in the first half of the nineteenth century, Samuel Taylor Coleridge, "Until I understand a man's ignorance, I must announce myself ignorant of his understanding."

Fourth, an evangelical style exhibits an apologetic rationality that marshals both theological and historical forces and sources. It readily and freely ransacks resources within the tradition and beyond it. Richard Mouw, president of Fuller Theological Seminary, admits that in his own life "I borrow unashamedly from the teachings of the Roman Catholics and Eastern Orthodoxy in my attempts to grow in holiness."[5] Such "borrowing" often gives evangelical writings an eclectic character, even making the evangelical community seem less a menage, more a menagerie. As a theologian, at times I shall be hollering "Come over" to those who, when it comes to evangelicals, usually pass by on the other side. But at times I shall be defending evangelicals from some of their advocates as well. As a historian, I shall attempt not to intrude into the text those aspects of the evangelical tradition to which I take theological and ethical exception.

I shall often be found rolling back the history of evangelicalism to its origins in eighteenth-century transatlantic culture and to its formative period in nineteenth-century America. This helps to explain the book's persistent digging around, and sometimes up, the Wesleyan root system of evangelicalism. This also accounts for the wisdom of the series' editors in commissioning a separate volume on Methodists, a field expertly mapped already by E. Brooks Holifield. The Wesleyan emphasis functions partly as a corrective to contemporary historiography, which starts too much of the story of evangelicalism with the heavily Calvinist-influenced fundamentalism of the twentieth century; partly as a reflection of the reality that it was primarily Wesleyan modes of thinking and modalities of action that shaped the bulk of this tradition.

Two great American presidents, Theodore Roosevelt and Woodrow Wilson, gave extraordinary witness to why historians have called the nineteenth century in American history "the Methodist Age." In 1905 Theodore Roosevelt stood before a Chautauqua Institution crowd and announced that he would rather speak to this audience than any other. Chautauqua, with its Methodist roots, represented what is truest Americanism, he said, and embodied in its origins, outlook, and outreach what is best about this great country.[6] Not long before this Woodrow Wilson had delivered an address on the occasion of the bicentennial of John Wesley's birthday, part of a study which he later published as a book entitled *John Wesley's Place in History* (1915). Both these presidents struggled to keep faith with evangelical values as they came to terms with evangelicalism through its distinctively Methodist cadences.

## III

In the last epigraph to this introduction, the poet Robert Duncan uses Miltonic spelling to capture a couple of the giddy paradoxes of health and healing, medicine and morality that appear throughout this volume on the evangelical tradition in America. There are some important background paradoxes to American religious history, however, that do not make their appearance but need to be given at least a cameo role at the very outset.

Paradox one: There is increasing awareness of health factors at the same time that health itself is diminishing. Americans are among the least healthy people of the industrialized world. And no matter how well we are, we are more worried about our health than ever before. Goethe liked to tell the story about a friend of his who wrote a book about the future and sent it to him for critique and comment: Goethe wrote back that the new world described in the book sounded like a fine place, but if its logic were realized, the whole world would end up being one great hospital, with all the people in it attendants ministering to one another. As medicalized and medicated as we are a mediatized and mediated people, it seems at times almost as if the prime aim of human existence has become health.[7] More than a nation of healthy hypochondriacs, Americans have come to see health as a basic human right.

Americans also spend billions each year in pursuit of their rights. Over 11 percent of the Gross National Product is spent on health. But where is that money going? Ninety-seven cents of every dollar spent pays for treatment, 2.5 cents pays for disease prevention, and .5 cents pays for teaching people how to stay healthy. It has been as hard for Americans to let go of treating diseases as it was for Sigmund Freud, whose collected works contain over four hundred references to neuroses but none to health.

Yet coincident with this hyperquest for health, infant mortality claims 1 percent of America's live births (1.8 percent among blacks). There are 7.7 fetal deaths per one thousand births. Cancer today kills one American a minute, a statistic more than doubled by deaths from cardiovascular diseases. Approximately three times as much is spent per capita on health care in the United States as in Great Britain, "without much in the way of improved health to show for it" in the words of one critic.[8]

Paradox two: A community of healing is the church's forte, its lack of healing spirit its foible. The church is willy-nilly in the health business, yet resists seeing itself as a "health club." It is more prone to offer "sickness care" than health care. Or in the words of a veteran medical missionary to central Africa, the church "concentrates on diseases — how to cure them — not on how to promote health."[9]

Health is not a social service issue, or even a medical issue alone. It is fundamentally a religious issue. Historian Mark Noll, a sensitive interpreter of the evangelical mind, observes that "the web of relationships between religion and medicine, between faith and bodily well-being, is thus extraordinarily dense."[10]

In the evangelical tradition, issues of health, disease, and healing have been tied to issues of salvation, thereby helping evangelical circles recognize health and medicine as subjects of great theological importance and historical interest. The linkage of health and salvation is etymological as well as theological. Theologically, when evangelicals sing the Christmas carol "Hark! the Herald Angels Sing," announcing the coming of the Savior, they also sing praises for what that advent brings: "Risen with healing in his wings." Psalm 103:2–3 (New International Version, hereafter NIV) makes the connection explicit: "Praise the Lord, O my soul, / and forget not all his benefits. / He forgives all my sins — / and heals all my diseases."

This fundamental, so-called material principle of evangelicalism, the doctrine of salvation or justification by faith, is etymologically hitched to health in English, German, Hebrew, and Greek. The word *salvation* comes from the root *salve*, which means something that heals or makes whole. To be saved is to be made whole, complete, well. In German the principal word for salvation, *Heil*, is derived from the word for "welfare" and "well-being."

The word for salvation in Hebrew — *yeshuwah* — means to save, heal, make whole. The word for save in Greek — *sodzo* — means to save, heal, and make whole. Indeed, in Jesus' miracles of healing, the Greek word meaning "to save" is used.[11] The first printed English edition of the New Testament appeared in 1526. It was immediately burned by the bishop of London, and its translator William Tyndale was executed in 1536 at the behest of the pope. When Tyndale first translated the Greek New Testament into English (1524), he chose as the word to translate the good news offered by the gospel, which evangelicals know today as "salvation," the English word *health*. Here are verses 69 and 77 of Luke 1 in the original Tyndale version, followed by their current translation in the New International Version:

> And hath reysed uppe the horne off health unto us
> in the housse of his servaunt David. (v. 69, Tyndale)

> He has raised up a horn of salvation for us
> in the house of his servant David. (v. 69, NIV)

> And to geve knowlege off health unto hys people
> for the remission of sinnes. (v. 77, Tyndale)

> to give his people the knowledge of salvation
> through the forgiveness of their sins. (v. 77, NIV)

On this basis the church built hospitals. But what kind of hospitals did it build? Russell L. Dicks, who looked back in the mid-1950s at the first fifty years of the churches' hospital building in this century, described church hospitals constructed with no chapels, hospital staffs assembled with no chaplains, and medical schools endowed with no ethicists or instructors in the philosophy of healing.[12] Many evangelicals would say that this reflects the twentieth-century influence of the social gospel movement, not the evangelical movement, on hospital building. That may be, and Dicks's statistics are not refined enough to probe further.

But what is certain is that in a large portion of the contemporary evangelical community and in almost the whole of establishment religion in America, issues of health and healing are not center stage. In the absence of the church's leadership as a healing community, however, there has suddenly appeared, like mushrooms on the landscape of religion in America, a host of college-educated, middle-class practitioners of nonmedical religious healing — psychic healers, reflexologists, pain therapists, Therapeutic Touch practitioners, charismatic prayer groups, to name but a few of the most obvious.[13] A populist counterculture distrusting "experts" and disdaining "professionalism" has exerted its authority, which is proving to be considerable. As one of American society's primary health-producing institutions, the church is losing out to a loose amalgam of faith healers, holistic and home remedies, and quack cures.

Paradox three is a paradox and irony put together: the more a "new medical priesthood" has replaced the old religious priesthood in American culture, the more likely health issues are to be discussed, and thus shaped, in evangelicalism's popular literature than in its scholarly studies. Again in Mark Noll's words, some of evangelicalism's "first-rank intellects devote a disproportionate share of their energies to itinerant preaching and the writing of popular books."[14] After someone dubbed the American Medical Association (AMA) the "American Meatcutters' Association," the response was something like this: "to talk like that about a minister is bad enough, but to talk like that about a surgeon is to know there's no religion left in the country."

Columnist Ellen Goodman analyzes in illuminating fashion the "religious intensity" with which Americans now deal with medical issues: "The old taboos were religious. Ours are medical. Our ancestors talked about risks to the soul, and we talk about risks to our bodies. They kept faith with tradition; we put faith in 'the best scientific evidence.'" Whereas in the past we memorized Scriptures, the catechism, or the names of the saints, today "we learn by rote the ingredients that will lower and reduce the chances of heart disease or cancer." The scientific priesthood "argues over interpretations the way medieval rabbis argued over the Talmud....As lay people we worry about these arguments between scientific sects the way our ancestors worried about the struggles of the Reformation."[15]

Unfortunately, not enough of these worries and arguments have as yet taken place in evangelicalism's scholarly publications and intellectual life. Too much of its constituency has allowed Christian aerobics, Christian nutrition, and the Christian Yellow Pages to define its positions and perspectives.

The three gifts offered by the Magi to the Christ child may have been gold, frankincense, and myrrh, the three most valuable commodities of their time. They were such priceless gifts in part because of their medicinal values. Gold, frankincense, and myrrh were among the first medicines, recorded as early as 1500 B.C.E. in the Egyptian Papyrus Ebers, the oldest known list of prescriptions.

The gifts of the Magi to the Christ child, the Savior of the world, were gifts of health and medicine. This book aims to explore to what extent the gifts of health and medicine were part of evangelicalism's contribution to the wider Christian tradition.

# ·1·

# Fearing and Believing: "Lead, Kindly Light"

The world's objection is that of all kind of men in the world, those that profess religion are the most melancholy....But if that be so, it is because they are not religious enough.
—Sir Richard Sibbes (1577–1635)

Here lies one who feared God so much that he never feared the face of any man.
—Words spoken at the burial of John Knox

One day a little girl from the city visited her grandmother on the farm. They spent a wonderful morning riding horses and enjoyed a picnic lunch together by the river. In the afternoon they went on a hike through the woods, and they ate fresh country cooking for supper. At night the little girl was told stories by the crackling fire, followed by more stories after she was tucked into bed. Just when the lights of the house were put out, and everyone ensconced in bed, hard rains began pouring down and a crash of thunder jolted the house. Out of the darkness came the cry: "Grandma, I'm scared. Can I sleep with you?" Snuggling in under the covers, the little girl asked one last question out of the darkness: "Grandma, is your face turned toward me?"

"Over the river and through the woods to grandmother's house we go": the traditional Thanksgiving song presents a picturesque image, especially if one imagines an aproned grandmother, cookie jar full of homemade goodies behind her, and grandfather stomping into the kitchen on his way to the wood stove, his arms full of firewood he has just cut from his own timber. Alas, this idealized image no longer comes close to the reality of family life for most Americans. Grandparents most often live in urban communities or

13

retirement centers away from their children, with whom they spend less and less time.

This chapter is about the personal storms that roll across our life and the social storms gathering strength on the horizon of our world. This chapter is about the ways evangelicals have connected mind and body, emotions and health, internal and external environments, somatic and psychological factors in the etiology of sickness. It is also about the evangelical belief that our only safety, our only sanity, is in knowing that God's face is turned toward us.

## I

If God is love, how can Christians not be emotional? We are emotional creatures because God has emotions and we are created in God's image. Evangelical faith comes fully alive to the emotions and seeks to make the right emotions come fully alive. In fact, Anglo-American evangelicalism pioneered in the study of emotion, long before the advent of modern psychology's heightened attention to the emotions. It has done this through the development of methodologies to awaken emotions through the medium of the intellect (as well as the other way around), and its expectation that true religion issues in a culture of emotionality as well as rationality.

John Wesley and Jonathan Edwards, whose *Treatise on Religious Affection* (1746) Wesley abridged in 1773, are evangelicalism's greatest theologians of the affections. The evangelical tradition claims to understand emotional factors, to distinguish between God-honoring or God-defiling emotions, and to follow Jesus' guidelines for expressions that channel emotional energies rather than deny them. Evangelical theologians also insist that the emotional life of believers is different from that of nonbelievers.

Habitually pointing to the intricate connections between the mind and the body, evangelical awareness has been high that a healthy religious faith affects our physical well-being as well as our mental health.[1] No evangelical worth his or her weight in theological salt has missed many chances to argue that faith in God is chemically true. Faith releases good hormones — literally. It is a prerequisite to mental and physical health. One cannot be healthy, physically or emotionally, without being spiritual.

The "pressure of psychology on physiology," as Episcopalian Phillips Brooks put it in the 1890s, means that "there is no true care for the body which forgets the soul" just as "there is no true care for the soul which is not mindful of the body."[2] The condition of one's psyche determines to a large degree the condition of one's soma. Meditate on the good, the true, and the beautiful, and good, true, and beautiful things happen in one's body. Faith is a real factor in keeping and making people well, as recent studies demonstrate in their discovery that mentally ill people are "significantly less religious than the general population."[3]

Serious psychic snags develop when one follows the French philosopher René Descartes in segregating the mind and the body into two separate branches of worldly existence. The human being is "two-sided," one evangelical editor argued, "and the whole man can be approached and affected from either side."[4] If the mind is the cause, the body can be the effect, and vice versa; evangelicals learned this emotional calculus from reading their Bibles. "The lamp of the body is the eye. Therefore, when your eye is good, your whole body also is full of light. But when your eye is bad, your body also, is full of darkness....Foolish ones! Did not He who made the outside make the inside also?" (Luke 11:34–36, 40, New King James Version, hereafter NKJV).

A rich and distinctive part of evangelicals' theological experience was the interconnectedness of physical and emotional health. If the mind suffers, William Andrus Alcott lectured, the body suffers with it, "and often in a corresponding degree."[5] Evangelicals warned of perilous theological waters for those who made rock-hard distinctions between body and mind. A nineteenth-century evangelical physician and minister argued that the human connections between the physical and spiritual, the mental and emotional, create a nature "like a harp of many strings exquisitely attuned."[6] Unbalanced emotions produced unbalanced mental states and all manner of physiological dysfunctions. Evangelicals predicted pendulum swings in the rhythms of the spiritual life — it was the soul's nature to be moody — because of these psychosomatic connections between mind and body.

How interconnected are mind and body? "Just as there are causes for heart trouble," theologian Harold John Ockenga wrote when he was pastor of Park Street Congregational Church, "there are also causes of the troubled heart."[7] They are often the same. When we meet somebody we like, our eyes brighten and our eyebrows fly up. The connections between mind and body are that simple and that powerful. Every thought vibrates in our bodies. Every thought carries with it a physiological effect.

Some evangelicals have even denied that there is any such thing, technically speaking, as mental illness or a diseased mind since "all mental aberration, however slight it may be, results from the connection of the mind with the body, and would not occur without this connection."[8] Mental and emotional troubles are "the most sharp and bitter" precisely because of the embeddedness of this connectedness.

Evangelicals have been as open as any major religious body to viewing disease in relation to social and personal stress. Evangelical preaching has also been among the first to disseminate the results of studies that indicate persons who experience a prolonged grief are highly susceptible to diabetes;

that repressed anger can generate ulcers and high blood pressure; that ob-
sessive/compulsive behavior patterns are breeding grounds for arthritis; that
Type-A personalities are prone to heart disease. Some studies even suggest
that the majority of illnesses are psychosomatic in origin. Of course, not until the last third of the nineteenth century were emotional ills and deviant
mental states recognized as legitimate diseases in and of themselves.[9]

It is crucial for those studying issues of religion and health to understand
the emotional values, or emotionology, prized by evangelical theology and
the emotional ties to one another fostered by the tradition.[10] Suffice it to say
that in the midst of medicine's traditional separation of the central nervous
system from the endocrine system from the immune system, evangelicals
tended to tear down barriers separating the mind and the body in many
of the same ways that those working at the convergence of molecular biology, immunology, and neuroscience ("psychoneuroimmunologists") are doing
today.[11]

The psychosomatic context of evangelical experience has been an important one, and the emotional component a controversial one, for several
reasons. First, evangelicalism is a person-centered faith, and the person on
whom evangelical faith centers is one with a rich and diverse emotional life.
Christians have been left with virtually no descriptions of Jesus' physical
being. But Jesus' soul had an unforgettable motion. The direction of these
motions, or Jesus' emotions, is well attested and chronicled.

A Jesus of agile emotions is only slightly less surprising than the Bible's
presentation of Jesus' emotional nakedness. Jesus cried over Jerusalem's fate
(John 11:35). He exulted over Peter's faith (Matthew 16:17–18). He anguished
over doing his Father's will (Mark 14:35–36). He sometimes erupted in rough
and blunt language, calling one group of religious leaders, "You snakes!" and a
"brood of vipers." Another time a group got called a " 'whitewashed tomb' full
of putrid and decaying flesh" (Matthew 3:7 and 23:27, 33). Jesus' emotional
side stormed impatiently at his friends, "I can't stand you any longer" (see
Matthew 17:17). Jesus expressed blazing anger by flinging church furniture
down the front steps of the church (Luke 19:45–46). He frequently hung out
with people of shady character (Matthew 11:19), and he was criticized for
eating and drinking too much (Luke 5:33). A man who teased and joked with
his friends, he was known and respected for his wit. Jesus experienced the
entire spectrum of emotions — fear, grief, compassion, joy, love, anger — that
we experience.

Second, evangelicals have historic sensitivity to the all-pervading connection between the mind and body because of their biblical reading, especially
of the Psalms. Every time someone blushes, there is graphic evidence of the
power of the emotions to create chemical changes in the body; the Near East-

ern authors sensed this from an early date and gave testimony in the Bible to physiological reactions to emotional states. "My heart [liver] is poured out on the ground" (Lamentations 2:11). "My heart [kidneys] failed me" (Job 19:27, New English Bible, hereafter NEB). "My flesh and my heart may fail" (Psalm 73:26). Medieval physiology took one step further and located emotions in various organs. The seat of laughter, for example, was the spleen. The center of one's life and personality was the heart. Just as Joseph's "bowels" longed for his brothers (Genesis 43:30), so were Christians expected to have functioning within them "bowels of mercy" (Colossians 3:12) and to put on "bowels of compassion" (1 John 3:17).

Evangelicals never went so far as the medieval Christians who replaced the signs of the zodiac with patron saints for various parts of the human body: St. Blaisius for throat and lungs, St. Erasmus for the abdomen, St. Apollonia for the teeth, St. Lucia for the eyes, with certain saints specializing in the cure and treatment of various diseases — St. Vitus for chorea ("St. Vitus's dance"), St. Anthony for erysipelas ("St. Anthony's fire"), for example. All the same, evangelicals have found their own ways of expressing and expanding the interrelationships of emotions and health, spirit and body that say the same thing as Wittgenstein's much-quoted remark, "the human body is the best picture of the human soul."[12]

Not too long ago a friend gazed into my sunken, cavernous eyes and quoted Scripture: "You look exhausted; your eyes are as black as burnt holes in bed sheets." The Bible knows how emotions can wear out various parts of the body: "For this our heart has become sick, for these things our eyes have grown dim" (Lamentations 5:17, Revised Standard Version, hereafter RSV). The Scriptures are remarkably candid about emotional responses, even of its heroes: Noah becomes a drunken fool; David lusts after a woman and commits homicide; Jacob emerges as a polygamous cheat.

Third, evangelicals have not esteemed all emotions as a faithful reflection of God's will. To what emotions are Christians entitled? This question has been an absorbing one throughout the evangelical tradition. Little emotional tidiness comes naturally, necessitating the sorting and selecting of human emotions, picking out those that honor God and are led by the Spirit. Evangelicals have worked hard to discern for themselves the emotions of spiritual things and to make people responsible for the totality of their emotions. Choice and responsibility have retained a central place in evangelicalism's moral assumptions and etiological frameworks. Choose the wrong life-style (as we might call it today) and one can expect to face health consequences: licentious living exposes one to venereal disease; tobacco and alcohol put one at risk of lung cancer, liver disease, and other maladies; and so forth. In varying degrees, evangelicals have steadfastly insisted that one is personally responsible for one's own clinical history. How well we live shapes how well we will be.

Emotions are only part of the soul, evangelicals insist. Volition and cognition are as important dimensions of the soul as emotion. True religion, nineteenth-century Reformed theologian Charles Hodge contended, does not nurture faith by feel. Faith is not merely "a fitful ebullition of feeling."[13] Even the charismatic or Pentecostal wings of evangelicalism have declaimed against those who would show thought the door. They have strained to surrender subjective emotions to the objective work of grace through the word of God.

Wednesday night prayer meeting is where I got a "gospel education." Part of that education warned against the gods of good feelings that teach one to exegete Scripture only after having exegeted experience. These old words of unknown origin I heard quoted many times:

> Feelings come and feelings go,
> And feelings are deceiving.
> Our warrant is the Word of God,
> None else is worth believing.

Prayer must gush forth unceasingly "with or without joy, with or without fast flowing words, with or without spontaneity," because "prayers are not answered according to feeling, or nimbleness of mind, or facility of expression."[14] Early evangelicals moved to govern and check the natural passions while gardening and cultivating the spiritual passions and moral emotions.

The evangelical tradition has even established an elaborate, volitional hierarchy of emotions where the "holy tempers" (John Wesley's phrase) reign paramount: humility, gentleness, forgiveness, and so forth (Galatians 5:22–23). These are opposed to what E. Stanley Jones liked to call the twelve emotional apostles of ill health: "anger, resentments, fear, worry, desire to dominate, self-preoccupation, guilts, sexual impurity, jealousy, a lack of creative activity, inferiorities, and a lack of love."[15] Evangelicals discipline themselves primarily to satisfy the right human passions, to submit to emotions that would glorify God, promote health, and advance Christ's kingdom.[16] What appears at times as unseemly preoccupation with the emotions' measurements, the rigorous tracing of every tiny tendril of emotionality that evangelicals learned from Puritans, is precisely this pursed-lips, steely character of the disciplining exercise.

The mind, when emotion is steamed out of it, becomes hard and impermeable. But evangelicals equally believe that the mind struggles under powerful emotional impulses that can lead it astray, natural emotions both good and bad which in heated, foamy form become no respecters of rationality. For this reason nineteenth-century evangelicals believed the natural passion of joy had to be treated as well as the natural passion of anger — the latter by drinking cold water and repeating the Lord's Prayer, the former by drinking cold water and applying slight pain to some part of the body.[17]

For evangelicals putting on the mind of Christ does not mean putting one's heart on hold. It does not mean holding one's heart in one's hands, either, or going around with heart stuck in throat. It means renewing the divine image in human hearts — heart transplants from the very being of God. Evangelicals kept alive the Augustinian vision of *theologia pectoria* — a theology of and for the heart, or what Count Nikolaus von Zinzendorf, the founder of the Moravians, called *Herzenreligion* (heart religion). But when early-twentieth-century evangelicals sang "Let Jesus Come into Your Heart" (Mrs. C. H. Morris, 1898) or "Since Jesus Came into My Heart" (Rufus H. Mc-Daniel, 1914), most were less concerned about what they do and experience than about what God does in and through them. It was the theological content of the emotion — the so-called material principle of evangelical theology, justification by faith — that had central significance.

This explains why many evangelicals, especially out of the Reformed and Wesleyan traditions, have led the charge against America's twentieth-century "cult of feeling," which has turned so many into a quivering mass of religious Jell-O. Assigning reason a higher plane than emotion and realizing that how we think affects and infects how we feel, evangelicals have been inclined to raise their guard at displays of education by feel, morality by feel, salvation by feel, even therapy by feel.[18] Contemporary evangelicals are more prone to stress the objective reality of the gospel, presenting Christianity as a deeply historical religion, based on objective facts, not inward, subjective experiences. To those in every era who court mystical religious experiences, such as New Agers today, evangelicals propose a twin agenda: the critical task of "testing of the spirits" (1 John 4:1) and the constructive cognitive task of "giving reason for the hope that you have" (1 Peter 3:5).

In fact, evangelicals present to the world three life-style strategies by which one can live, or what one might call three kinds of emotion management: paranoia, euphoria, metanoia. Only the last of these, evangelicals believe, brings life.

## II

The first level of mindbody experience on which one can seek emotional satisfaction is that of paranoia. *Paranoia* literally means "beside the mind" or "out of one's mind." This was the scuttlebutt about Jesus in Mark 3:21 — he was out of his mind. Many "normal" people live every day "beside themselves," "out of it," living in a state of "ego chill" (Erik Erikson) and "ontological anxiety" (Ludwig Binswanger). The best description of the paranoid mind is this one from Leviticus 26:36–37:

> As for those of you who are left, I will make their hearts so fearful in the lands of their enemies that the sound of a wind-blown leaf will put them to flight. They will run as though fleeing from the sword, and they will fall, even though no one is pursuing them. They will stumble over one another as though fleeing from the sword, even though no one is pursuing them. So you will not be able to stand before your enemies.

In short, the chief emotion excavated from the depths of paranoia is fear. Philosopher Bertrand Russell once said that if he had only one lecture to leave with the world, its subject would be humanity's worst evil, fear. Journalist Gilbert K. Chesterton, asked by a British publisher to write for a series entitled "If I Could Preach Only Once," responded: "If I had only one sermon to preach, it would be a sermon against fear."

Evangelicals have not been above using the moral emotion of fear — at least enough for poet Edgar Lee Masters to cast evangelicals as fearmongering fanatics:

> preachers
> Of the Baptist, Methodist, Presbyterian, Campbellite, and other denominations,
> Who live in ease off the money gathered by fear,
> While scarcely any of them are enlightened or worth anything to civilization.[19]

Ambrose Bierce called religion "the daughter of fear." But evangelicals distinguish between the moral emotion of fear and fear's natural passions. As the twentieth-century French novelist Régis Debray has pointed out, "In this new world tell me what you fear the least and I'll tell you what will harm you the most."[20]

The word *paranoia* denotes the fear of something that is not there. Evangelicals believe that life's greatest dangers, however, come from not fearing something that is there: God and hell. "The fear of the Lord is the beginning of wisdom," the Bible says (Psalm 111:10). There comes a time for fear and trembling. It is possible to be too ignorant, too cowardly, to be afraid. There is no word in English for this lack of fear of something that is there. The fear that destroys fear is as important to faith as the love that casts out fear.

From an evangelical perspective, Masters's harsh poetic caricature is but another tired version of modernity's stubborn failure to make this distinction between the moral emotions and natural passions. Evangelicals have not been averse to employing scared-saved evangelism.[21] But they have done so worryingly, aware of the danger that the emotions aroused would be more unregenerate than moral.

Evangelicalism's two greatest theorists, Jonathan Edwards and John Wesley, were both accused of fearmongering. Yet any serious reading of revivalistic sermons (starting with the best known but least read sermon in American history, Jonathan Edwards's "Sinners in the Hands of an Angry God"), with their emphasis on God's love, disputes this simple antimony between a "city of gold" and a "lake of fire." In the very beginnings of the evangelical revival in eighteenth-century England, the minutes from the second Methodist Conference (1745) reveal the ultimate verdict on what to do about scaremongering sermons:

Q.17 Do not some of our assistants preach too much of the wrath and too little of the love of God?

A. We fear that they have leaned to that extreme; and hence some of their hearers may have lost the joy of faith.

Q.18 Need we ever preach the terrors of the Lord to those who know they are accepted of him?

A. No; it is folly so to do; for love is to them the strongest of all motives.[22]

Revivals in the early nineteenth century were criticized for playing on people's fear and releasing passions until they caused mental derangement, even to the point of suicide.[23] Ronald and Janet Numbers have shown how "the American religious revivals of the early nineteenth century coincided with — and directly encouraged — a boom in asylum building that saw the opening of about two dozen new asylums in America between 1810 and 1850."[24] Antebellum physicians admitted more patients to mental institutions because of religious excitement than were admitted to hospitals because of ill health. This was especially pronounced in the 1840s, when fear of growing insanity in American culture reached levels of feverish proportions and "religion-related insanity," allegedly caused by revivals, seemed to reach a high.

It was a universal assumption in antebellum America that religious emotions could at least impair personal contentment if not cause insanity. Two causes of mental illness were isolated by the 1830s — biological (insanity as a disease) and emotional (insanity as a moral struggle). Whereas from the mid-seventeenth to the mid-eighteenth century religious madnesses were seen as the products either of supernatural causes (for example, fighting with the Devil) or "melancholic vapors" created by an uncontrollable psychophysiological disorder induced by an excess of bile,[25] religious insanity in the first half of the nineteenth century was seen most often as the product of thought disorders or a violation of nature's laws (for example, the strain of excess passions released from wrestling with religious emotions). Insanity was still interpreted within a supernatural context, but it was not attributed to a supernatural cause. Even the nineteenth-century Millerites and Adventists, who were members of the evangelical tradition in every way except their distinctive premillennial belief in the personal, imminent advent of Christ, "adopted the prevailing view that undue religious excitement might be harmful to a person's mental health," the Numberses have observed.[26]

A Connecticut physician, Amariah Brigham, who at one time headed the Utica State Lunatic Asylum in the heart of the "burned-over district," wrote an 1835 study on the connections between religious emotions and mental health in which he argued that overstimulated nerves more than outpourings of the Holy Spirit were responsible for the "outward signs" of revivals. (The "burned-over district" in western New York State was so named because it was frequently set aflame during the nineteenth century by religious enthusiasm and evangelical revivals.) Brigham ranked the premillennial Millerites, those who embraced the predictions of Baptist teacher William Miller that Jesus would return in 1843 (then 1844, then "soon"), above yellow fever and cholera as public health enemies.[27] In his famous fifth chapter, Brigham argued that a "hundred times" more damage is done to the nervous system of women by revivalism's "night meetings" and "protracted meetings" than by balls, theaters, and fashionable dissipations.[28]

The linkage of natural passions and mental illness bound together Brigham's supporters and detractors. The only question was how much natural passion was required to cause insanity. The question of "whether a delicate female, in hysterical paroxysms, is really a subject of disease or of grace" should not be dismissed, one evangelical writer argued in reviewing Brigham's book. Religious excitements *alone* cannot create mental illness, but when they are coupled with long-standing predispositions they can lead "more likely, by universal consent, among competent judges, than any other one thing, permanently to disorder the mind."[29]

Whereas Hippocrates, the founder of medicine, believed that all wrongdoing springs from some sort of mental disorder, Charles G. Finney, the founder of modern revivalism, believed in the moral basis of mental illness. In his classic *Lectures on Revivals*, Finney admits that religious "excitements are liable to injure the health. Our nervous system is so strung that any powerful excitement, if long continued, injures our health, and unfits us for duty."[30] Finney recommended doing away with "spasmodic religion." But he agreed with George Campbell and other scholars of rhetoric that "in order to persuade, it is always necessary to move the passions."[31] Or in Finney's words, "to expect to promote religion without excitements is unphilosophical and absurd."[32] Barbara Sicherman has found that "the older view that religious revivals themselves caused insanity had generally declined by 1880," at which time "religious agitation" was now viewed as a "*symptom* of *dementia praecox* (schizophrenia) or some other disease, and the term *religious insanity* gradually disappeared from the vocabulary of medicine."[33]

The issue of the relationship between religion and mental health is almost as controversial today as it was in the 1840s. In *The Religious Experience* social psychologists Daniel Batson and Larry Ventis summarize the current state of research into the religion–mental health link, finding both positive relationships (absence of symptoms of mental illness), negative relationships (positive feelings about oneself), and no correlations (freedom from guilt and worry).[34] Evangelicals are not unduly concerned about the findings of such studies, partly given the medical professions' changing perception of mental health and the unbiblical definitions of what is sane and what is not.

But mostly, when the charge that religious faith induces madness is finally wheeled out, evangelicals use it to good effect by making everyone sit up and take notice of the kernel of truth contained in the accusation. A favorite biblical story that illustrates this is the account of the man possessed of demons (Mark 5:1ff.). The people there could learn to accept the insane man, but they would not live with the sane visitor, whom they drove out of town. His name was Jesus. "Some people will say you are mad," evangelicals warn new converts. God preserve you from sanity.

It is not news to evangelicals that fear can produce a genuine disease. The epidemics of plague and cholera had often been attributed to fear. This belief in a fear-inducing disease was, in fact, the precise spot within evangelicalism that incubated some of the impulses giving rise to "water cure" sanitariums and "mind-cure" theologies, the latter the preferred name among evangelicals for Christian Science and New Thought. In fact, the proliferation of faith-healing movements in the last third of the nineteenth century was an almost predictable manifestation of evangelicalism's mindbody emphasis on moral responsibility and self-control.

The evangelical belief in the power of fear to predispose one to illness, even cholera,[35] is perhaps nowhere better tested than in exploring the spiritual therapies offered by evangelical faith in treating the common cold of mental illness, depression. The ensuing exploration of evangelical approaches to this mental difficulty serves as a case study on how evangelicals deal with a variety of mental illnesses and paranoias that plague people.

This is the "Age of Melancholy," announced America's highest-ranking mental health officer, Dr. Gerald L. Klerman, in 1979.[36] If so, the estimated 10 percent of the American population who suffer from serious depression can thank evangelicalism for not hiding the commonness of this social disease and emotional disorder and for providing some important guidance on how to convert the stones of depression and darkness into bread, and even "angel's food." In contrast to the extensive history of emotional dishonesty that characterizes the treatment of depression by other groups in American culture, evangelicals have been remarkably frank and forthcoming in their discussions of depression, nervousness, melancholia, or, earliest of all, "Satan's bath."[37] They have also been some of the least likely to fear depression's stigma of mental deficiency or emotional flabbiness, and the least likely to recommend psychotropic drugs and chemical cures for mental problems.[38]

In medieval art the saints were often portrayed with a nimbus, what we now call a halo. But *nimbus* today is a weather word for a dark cloud. Key architects of evangelical theology like Martin Luther, John Calvin, and John Wesley testified quite openly to depression's haze of fear and tortured faith.[39] Some of the world's greatest political leaders influenced by evangelical faith have also been left flat on their faces by depression — Abraham Lincoln, Woodrow Wilson, and Martin Luther King, Jr. — although their falls have been more muffled.

Evangelicals have approached the clinical category of depression from three distinct standpoints: first, as a spiritual condition; second, as an emotional, later psychological, state; third, as a medical problem. The best of the evangelical tradition has blended all three understandings into an overarching approach to depression that accents identifying causes as the key to cures.

### Depression as a spiritual condition

David Hume once remarked that he had never met a pious person who wasn't melancholy. Evangelicals have been among the first to admit their depressions, the last to deny that being close to God means being far from a downcast spirit. They know their Bible only too well: "Kill me, I pray thee, out of hand" (Numbers 11:15); "O Lord, take away my life" (1 Kings 19:4); "O Lord, take…my life from me" (Jonah 4:3). Depression as a problem of the mind and spirit warrants an entire chapter in J. Oswald Sanders's classic *Spiritual Clinic* (1958).[40]

But evangelicals have also been adamant that depression is not a natural, customary consequence of piety. Upbraiding feelings of unworthiness and reprobation are normal, night phases of the spiritual cycle, often treated by evangelicalism's seemingly favorite antidepressant: do-good activism.

To be sure, some suffer from religious despondency occasioned by morbid obsession with sin, especially those secret little "housekeeping sins" or the big "unpardonable sin." But evangelicals deem these "satanic buffetings" a perversion of piety, not a perfection of it. The early-eighteenth-century English evangelical Hester Anne Rogers had one foot in the Puritan era, the other in the evangelical era. Like a good Puritan she resisted her fits of depression as "satanic," the invasion of her mind with Satan's evil thoughts. But like a good evangelical responsible for her every thought and emotion, she believed the roots of her depressions lay in her theological confusion over what is a temptation and what is a sin, and her consequent misnaming as "sin" what was really the frustrations of a "corruptible body."[41]

The notion that if one were truly spiritual, one would not get depressed is refuted by a host of biblical characters — King Saul (1 Samuel 16:14, 23), Nebuchadnezzar (Daniel 4:33–34), Elijah (1 Kings 19), the Apostle Paul (Romans 7:15, 18–19; 2 Corinthians 12:11), even Jesus himself, who experienced depression firsthand (Matthew 26:38). Perhaps the respected evangelical counselor Walter Trobisch put it best and most bluntly: "We do not need to be ashamed of [feelings of depression]. They are no flaw in our makeup or a discredit to the name 'Christian.' On the other hand, however, we should not sit on the pity pot and mope the whole day."[42] Besides, one mid-nineteenth-century evangelical observed from personal experience, "much of the spiritual darkness of which pious souls complain comes from the shadows which the body casts upon the mind." A lot of people foolishly think that they can achieve "unclouded mental serenity" through religious exercises while at the same time "violating the commonest laws of health, whose penalty often is depression of spirits."[43]

The biblical account of Elijah's post-achievement syndrome and symptomology (the loss of a challenge or struggle can precipitate depression as readily as the loss of a loved one) has almost become the generic prescription given by pulpit pharmacists in their pastoral care of depression. It is an evangelical cliché worth repeating. After Elijah was informed of Queen Jezebel's vow of vengeance, the one who would never see death began calling on God to let him die. The ordinary steps that God instructed Elijah to take, lifting him from his depression and freeing him from fear for his life, are paradigmatic for the spiritual repair of damaged minds.

Step one. Since frayed nerves often attend fatigued bodies, Elijah was told to get a good night's rest. Much depression stems from sheer exhaustion, especially among perfectionists and high achievers. A sound mind and sound body go together.

Step two. God then directed Elijah to "Get up," to stop wallowing in self-pity. It is therapeutic to make an effort on one's own behalf, even if it is simply getting one's body in motion. Rather than being told to "hang in there," hands tied and head dangling in the noose of helplessness, Elijah is counseled to "stand in there" and take an active role in resolving the situation. Elijah was an early example of the James-Lange theory of psychology: we feel like doing things after we start doing things.

Step three. After a refreshing night's sleep and after rousing himself from his torpor, Elijah is told to eat some breakfast. The change of appetite that usually attends depression (usually a loss of appetite, although sometimes the reverse occurs) further exacerbates the biological basis of depression and conflicts with a healing life-style.

Step four. His body strengthened through sleep, exercise, and food, Elijah is commanded to look up: "Go forth, and stand upon the mount before the Lord." When depression descends, it is not enough merely to feed the body and flog the will. The mind must be fed and fixed on God if the spirits are to be lifted. A characteristic way evangelicals have of putting the self on the shelf and orienting themselves to God, especially during the numbing, deadening periods of depressions, is through song — choruses and "praise songs" such as this one: "Turn your eyes upon Jesus, / Look full in his wonderful face, / And the things of earth will grow strangely dim / In the light of his glory and grace."[44] Music, through its immediate effect on the emotions and nervous system, plays a significant therapeutic role for evangelicals in re-membering and re-turning the mind toward the God who knows our every "downsitting and uprising" (Psalm 139:2).

Step five. The last step takes Elijah from preoccupation with self to self-forgetting associations of ministry among new friends, new sights, new fields of service. An Elijah who has obediently gotten up, eaten up, and looked up is finally told to link up: "Go, return on your way to the wilderness of Damascus," where new challenges await him. Depression as a spiritual condition is often best addressed by feeding the body with a good night's rest and morning's breakfast, feeding the mind by looking around to see God at work in creation and life, and feeding the spirit and soul by linking up with people in need and with challenges awaiting leadership.

### Depression as a psychological state

Evangelicals also recognize that depression is a psychological state, also known as "reactive depression." Psychiatrist Emil A. Gutheil defines depression as D=S+P: Depression=Sadness+Pessimism.[45] This depression is a temporary condition precipitated by bereavement, loss, disappointment, uprootedness, or a disturbing event. Clergy in the Ohio and Mississippi valleys early in the last century told of the severe depressions endured by settlers from New England who had left everything and migrated to an inhospitable environment.[46]

This too is normal and is to be anticipated, as Jonathan Edwards wrote to his daughter Esther Burr after her husband's death in 1757: "Don't be surprised, or think some strange thing has happened to you, if after this Light, clouds of Darkness should return. Perpetual sunshine is not usual in this world, even to God's true saints....If God should hide his Face in some respect, even this will be in Faithfulness to you, to purify you, & fit you for yet further & better light."[47] Severe life dissatisfaction can be a normal reaction to overwhelming life crises and to feelings of hopelessness, defeat, and despair.

The number of clergy who have waged a lifelong battle with depression — people as diverse as seventeenth-century Puritan Richard Baxter, eighteenth-century Evangelical Association founder Jacob Albright and Lutheran Henry Melchior Muhlenberg, and nineteenth-century Methodist John Lee — has prompted suggestions that some professionals, like the clergy, are more prone to prostrations of despair, anxiety, and depressions than others.[48] Charles H. Spurgeon warned his students about "The Minister's Fainting Fits": "Most of us are in some way or other unsound physically....The great mass of us labour under some form or other of infirmity, either in body or mind....As to mental maladies, is any one altogether sane? Are we not all a little off the balance?"[49] In such cases the medicinal properties of faith, hope, and love far outweigh chemical antidepressants. Indeed, evangelicals are averse to mood elevators, which obstruct opportunities to find and face the anxieties underlying the emotional upset itself, anxieties which cause us to do things we normally would not do. Grudge-holding, anger-nursing, guilt-bearing attitudes bring on depressions. Covering them up with chemicals only makes the depression more cocooned and repeatable. We all have to learn how to take a fall.

A divinity student once made an appointment with the Boston preacher Phillips Brooks to seek counsel about some emotional problems and difficulties that were troubling him. After having spent a considerable amount of time with this great preacher, the seminarian left, joyful and full of strength, only to remember his unasked list of questions and forgotten problems. Reflecting upon the unexpected escape from his emotional furnace, the student realized that what he had needed was not the solution to his specific problems but the contagion of a triumphant spirit. Evangelical prayers do not plead "God, save me from this trouble" but rather "God, strengthen me for this trouble." We cannot live without stress and anxiety, but we can meet our anxieties bravely and creatively, and we can refuse to allow the normal stresses of life to become distress.

*Depression as a medical problem*

Finally, evangelicals recognize that depression can physically disable people as badly as high blood pressure, diabetes, and other ailments treated by primary care physicians. In fact, one recent study found that only patients with angina or coronary artery disease were more limited in routine daily activities than were depression sufferers; only patients with arthritis reported more bodily pain; and only coronary disease patients reported more days in bed.[50]

Also known as endogenous depression, depression can be a true disease, the product of a chemical imbalance that often requires medication. Missionary David Livingstone was afflicted with cyclothymia (manic-depressive syndrome) before treatments were available, and he suffered his entire life from onrushing bouts with this disease.[51] This also seems to be the case with Charles Spurgeon, who confessed from the pulpit, "I am the subject of depressions of the spirit so fearful that I hope none of you ever get to such extremes of wretchedness as I go to." An evangelical physician and preacher in the mid-nineteenth century contended that "the physicians' knowledge is often of far more account to the melancholy soul than religious counsel or Christian sympathy can be, because the source of the trouble is corporeal, and not spiritual."[52]

"The person who fears suffering," Montaigne wrote centuries ago, "is already suffering from what he fears." What are evangelical fears, those peculiar fears that nip at evangelical heels and assail their minds and emotions? Is it fear of failure that throttles? Then that fear is coming true. Is it fear of risking that controls? Then one is leading a high-risk life.

It is amazing what the human body and mind can take. "I praise you because I am fearfully and wonderfully made," exclaimed the writer of the 139th Psalm. Our bodies often absorb cruel and unusual punishment: sleepless nights, nutritionless days, backbreaking jobs, and brutalizing schedules. Burning the candle at both ends is the worst way of making ends meet, but our bodies often withstand the heat. Our minds are equally durable: they absorb numbing news that no one could have imagined; they bear up under heavy strain, they often survive earthquaking personal loss, waterfalls of grief, volcanic explosions of dreams.

There is one blow, however, that can fatally maim this being that is so fearfully and wonderfully made. It is the hardest blow of all to take. It is the final blow: rejection. Few words are freighted with heavier pain, says theologian David Allan Hubbard. Few experiences in life cut us more sharply. Few memories are as deeply etched in our minds as when we were turned aside or turned down by someone or something important to us.[53]

I remember the fear of rejection I felt as a high school student. I still can feel the fear clutching my heart when I opened one of the "slam books" that were in fashion to see what people were saying about me. The only worse fear, and feeling, was not to be in the slam book at all. A reject. A total reject. No one alive does not know the reality of William James's words:

> No more fiendish punishment could be devised...than that one should be turned loose in society and remain absolutely unnoticed by all the members thereof. If no one turned round when we entered, answered when we spoke, or minded what we did, but if every person we met "cut us dead," and acted as if we were non-existing things, a kind of rage and impotent despair would ere long well up in us, from which the cruellest bodily tortures would be a relief; for these would make us feel that, however bad might be our plight, we had not sunk to such a depth as to be unworthy of attention at all.[54]

Evangelicals often quote the story of the blind man in John 9:32–38 to prove that an encounter with Christ does not insure an end of rejection. Before he met Jesus, the blind man was rejected because he could not see. After he met Jesus, the blind man was rejected because he could see — rejected in order by his neighbors, by the Pharisees, by his parents (the worst hurt of all), and by the synagogue.

The fear of rejection is mitigated for evangelicals because Jesus, as the suffering servant, "was despised and rejected" (Isaiah 53:3). Jesus was unwanted by the church, by the government, by the society in which he lived. At his birth, there was no room at the inn for him (Luke 2:7). When he came to his own, "his own did not receive him" (John 1:11). They laughed at his mission — "Nazareth! Can anything good come from there?" — and his own people threw him out of his hometown (Luke 4:29). Even after he healed the sick, the people begged him to leave their neighborhood (Mark 5:17), until Jesus had no place to lay his head (Matthew 8:20). His best friends rejected him. Even his disciples deserted him (John 6:66). Suspended between heaven and earth, as if wanted by neither, he was crucified on a cross outside the city walls, double symbols of his rejection and outsiderhood. No wonder Jesus cried out, "My God, my God, why have you forsaken me?" (Matthew 27:46). No wonder evangelicals have found tremendous release from fear of rejection in Jesus' outsiderhood. It makes their sense of insiderness and acceptance by God so strong.

### III

The second level of mindbody experience on which one can choose to live one's life is that of euphoria, or happiness. Evangelicals have sometimes fooled themselves into thinking that "sinners" aren't happy. The dictionary defines *happiness* as "a state of well-being and contentment." For some people, a trinity of idols — Mammon, Baal, and Molech — makes life worth living. In this life-style disorder of euphoria one can go contentedly through life in a hedonic state, getting turned on by shiny new cars and fat wallets. The problem is that every idol requires a victim, a sacrifice, a soul.

The first member of the trinity of idols is Mammon: the idolatry of money and prosperity. Ever watch people at an amusement park riding the bumper cars? You will never see a more enthralled, happy bunch than these driving dervishes who get high from banging each other and creating head-on collisions. This is the way many Mammon euphorics go through life. Indeed, America has raised a generation of Toys-R-Us kids who know only immediate gratification, who think they deserve everything they can get, and who believe that their deepest happiness can be found in material things. Even evangelicalism itself raised a generation of Christian leaders, both Anglo-American (led by Kenneth Copeland) and African-American (Kenneth Price), who left the tradition to tout a "prosperity evangelism" promising wealth and health.

The second member of the trinity of idols is Baal. Baal euphorics find happiness in more obviously destructive patterns of free-lance living. One does not have to have been born within sight of Times Square to appreciate the ways in which the idol of Baal deifies pleasure, sex, and self. In a strained attempt at an ethical prime rate, many evangelicals have argued that rates of drinking, gambling, and illicit sex (some have added dancing) rise and fall together.

Novelist Philip Roth has paid satiric tribute to America as the country where "everything goes and nothing matters."[55] The prophet Jeremiah graphically portrayed one feature of an "anything goes" society when he described the men of his day as "well-fed lusty stallions, each neighing for his neighbor's wife" (Jeremiah 5:7–9, New Revised Standard Version, hereafter NRSV). Evangelicals decry a world where these two conditions — love and marriage — increasingly don't coincide.

One of the characters created by comedienne Lily Tomlin says that reality is a crutch for people who can't cope with drugs. Drugs come in various dress, in various dosages. They are not all the celebrated nostrums, narcotics, and nicotine with such innocent names and such evil effects — angel dust, ice, crack, slims, and so forth. Over fifty million people in this country take legal drugs, and twenty million take them daily. Some find validation in valium, or energy in chocolate and caffeine. Some smoke themselves into lung cancer, while others drink themselves into liver failure. In the words of poet Vernon Scannell's boozer's lament, Baal euphorics often spend their lives "drinking up time, as we have always done."[56]

Evangelicals have played crucial roles in countering the addictive behaviors of Baal euphorics. "Addictions" have replaced "neuroses," which replaced "neurasthenia" as the diagnosis of choice in the mental ache and pain field. Psychological "addictions," according to one recent listing, include

| | | | |
|---|---|---|---|
| alcohol | tobacco | sex | money |
| health | food | drugs | TV |
| pets | decorating | cars | danger |
| fashion | news | recognition | gambling |
| power | work | dieting | romance |
| religion | children | sports | computers |
| gossip | crime | jogging | |

Those affected by someone else's addictions are now called codependents, especially when the addict's behavior impinges on the codependent's ability to live fully and freely. Codependency has been designated a medical illness, and its "victims" treated by family therapy and counseling.

Such formulations are no master key to the problems of Baal euphorics, many evangelicals argue. Herbert Fingarette's book *Heavy Drinking: The Myth of Alcoholism as a Disease* (1988) adds corroboration from the medical and social sciences to arguments some evangelicals have been making against the notion of alcoholism as a disease ever since the disease concept was first proposed, ironically, by evangelicals themselves in the 1890s, when Frances Willard and other leaders of the Women's Christian Temperance Union (WCTU) broke with their own evangelical colleagues like Methodist Annie Wittenmyer and defined alcoholism as both an environmental illness and a sin.[57]

The temperance movement, one of the greatest reform movements in American history, was an important manifestation of the evangelical tradition's ability to exert strong leadership in the arena of drugs and addiction. Founded in 1874, the WCTU, the first nondenominational mass women's organization, stood for the "reign of a religion of the body," in Willard's words, which would work and witness alongside evangelicalism's "blessedly spiritual religion of the soul."[58] Through temperance camp meetings, temperance hospitals (the first one opened in Chicago in 1886 with a nursing school attached), tracts and books (three-quarters of which women had written by 1875), rescue homes, day-care centers, low-cost restaurants, and much more, Americans began to see alcoholism as a serious health problem.

Since women, defenders of the home and domestic values, were particularly vulnerable to alcohol abuse and were themselves particularly susceptible to prescriptions laced with alcohol, opium, cocaine, or morphine, evangelical women claimed the right to lead the profamily, prowomen temperance crusade. Their success was so remarkable that by the early 1880s (1882 and 1883 to be exact), both Vermont and Michigan had enacted legislation requiring the public school systems to instruct "all pupils in every school in physiology and hygiene, with special reference to the effects of alcoholic drinks, stimulants, and narcotics generally upon the human system."[59]

The nineteenth-century evangelical dispute whether drinking was an issue of physiology or moral character — whether they were crusading against the evils of a disease or the evils of sin — still rages. The Southern Baptist television evangelist who blasts "those liberals who have taken the sin of alcoholism and called it the disease of alcoholism" speaks for a large number of evangelicals who are pleased that science may be proving them right in their suspicions. In Fingarette's words, "No leading research authorities accept the classic disease concept."[60] Once alcoholism is defined as "a biochemical genetic disease...in the form of addiction-prone body chemistry," as the American Medical Association has defined it, its treatment is no longer a matter of changing the will, convincing the mind, or moderating behavior patterns. By this definition the alcoholic is a victim of circumstance, powerless to control his or her problem, not someone who can choose to change or stop. This violates the volitional character of moral accountability as well as the evangelical principle always to be satisfied with life but never to be satisfied with oneself.

The third member of the trinity of idols is Molech and the idolatry of power, armament, security, and national survival. Nations as well as emperors like Domitian can demand to be addressed as "my Lord and my God." Molech strives to be first in terms of military hardware, whereas the best of the evangelical tradition has counseled giving pride of place to spiritual hardware.[61] But too often to tell here, William Blake's lines have proved their accuracy in the evangelical experience: "the strongest poisons / Come from Caesar's laurel crown."

The problem comes after the vintage wine is drunk, the new sexual partner asleep, and the patriotic song finished. What do we then call ourselves to ourselves? An overwhelming emptiness creeps in, and with it a new refrain: "Is that all there is?" Emotional flatness is the inevitable by-product of living the life of Mammon, Molech, and Baal. More and more Americans are outwardly in a state of prosperity, happiness, sunniness, and security — and inwardly sick of being so well.

A young man, successful by every social measurement, stunned everyone who knew him when he committed suicide. His simple note read: "I am tired of being so damned happy." With only "me" to live for, there is laughter without joy, sex without love, fruit without juice, fun without fulfillment, pleasure without serenity, religion without meaning. Elton Trueblood has observed that our lucrative entertainment business is an accurate measurement not of our happiness but of our sadness and boredom. Self-seeking is self-consuming. The self burns up in the flames of euphoria's futility. In turning from paranoia to euphoria, one can turn one's life around. But one goes from being depressed and miserable to being miserable and depressed.

The value of a temperate life in an intemperate age is a common topic whatever page one turns to in the memoirs of evangelicalism. In fact, Dwight L. Moody's temperance sermons came back to haunt him on a trip to Italy in 1892. During a conversation with a local resident, the subject of wine came up and Moody announced that he was a teetotaler. The Italian responded with obvious disbelief. Moody insisted it was true. The Italian looked at Moody's 280 pounds, pulled a loaf of bread from beneath his coat, and said laughingly: "You may be a teetotaler in drink, but you are no teetotaler in eating."[62]

To be an evangelical Christian and not to give up anything is simply not to be an evangelical Christian. Long before the best scientific evidence pointed to diet, viruses, sexual practices, alcohol, and above all tobacco as factors in nearly 92 percent of all cancer deaths (the remaining 8 percent are allegedly caused by carcinogenic substances in the environment, workplace, food additives, and industrial products), evangelicalism encouraged its constituency to discipline itself into temperance if not total abstinence in most of these areas. Evangelicals have been some of the most outspoken on issues of nonprescription drugs — chemical (diazepam, quaaludes, amphetamines), plant (cocaine, marijuana, tobacco, alcohol), food (chocolate, caffeine), technological ("the great technological nipple," TV), pornography (movies, videos, magazines, adult book stores), and gambling (bingo, lotteries, casinos). The pursuit of pleasure can kill — both you and those closest to you. An undisciplined life can lead to suicide and murder at the same time.

Evangelicals have come down the hardest against the emotions of "happiness" because the evangelical perspective acknowledges that the Bible never promised the believer dictionary happiness. *Happify* was a popular Shaker folk term picked up from evangelicals. But even here it describes a grace through which a believer is "happified" into a higher level of spiritual being. The blind mid-nineteenth-century evangelist G. W. Henry defined true happiness as that outpouring of God's spirit that one received while attending camp meetings, where "I had been about as happy...as I could be and live on earth."[63] What the Bible does promise is not happiness but the "holy temper" or moral emotion of joy. The dictionary defines *joy* as a "condition of delight, gladness, exultation of spirit, beatitude of heaven." Joy comes from the third emotional context in which one can live one's life: metanoia.

## IV

Jesus turns our minds, lost in the forest of fear and deserts of despair after the mirage of euphoria, to their lost home, the third and biblical level of mindbody experience. Kicking both the fear habit and the high habit, we come to our senses, following the new and living way of metanoia, an about-face that turns us around and restores our mind.

The word *metanoia* is the converse of *paranoia* and the obverse of *euphoria*. He "came to his senses" Luke says about the prodigal son (Luke 15:17) in evangelicalism's favorite gospel story. Metanoia makes evangelicals conversionist, as the tendrils of the wounded heart, torn, trembling, and twisted in fear, become entwined around the most powerful healing force in the universe: love.

Psychologist Fritz Perls made into an adage the need to lose one's mind before one can come to one's senses. Metanoia is facing the profound half-truths of paranoia (there are things to fear) and euphoria (there are erotics to celebrate). Metanoia is facing and outfacing those innermost fears that haunt us — Paul's "thorn in the flesh," Moses' stammering tongue, Jeremiah's massive inferiority complex, Elijah's mental depressions, Jesus' fear of rejection. Metanoia is a new rationality and emotionology, a new standard of mental and emotional values that fundamentally alters our thinking and feeling. This new evangelical anthropology is best understood by a phenomenon that has a checkered career throughout religious history and that is primarily identified in modern times with the evangelical wing of Protestantism: conversion.

Conversion is the evangelical word for metanoia. The most influential evangelical of the nineteenth century defined conversion in this way: "Conversion to God is becoming morally sane. It consists in restoring the will and the affections to the just control of the intelligence, the reason, and the conscience, so as to put the man once more in harmony with himself — all his faculties adjusted to their true positions and proper functions."[64]

Conversion means literally a profound, self-conscious, paradigmatic shift from an old worldview of beliefs, habits, and orientation to a new, life-satisfying structure of belief and action. In his classic book *Conversion* (1933), Arthur Darby Nock argues that until Judaism and Christianity, "adhesion" rather than "conversion" had been the keynote of Hellenistic religious life.[65] Adhesion meant adding a new cult on to one's religious repertoire. Conversion meant a turning from one commitment to another.

In a famous sermon of the nineteenth century, the British evangelical Thomas Chalmers pointed out that sometimes the dead leaves of a tree refuse to fall to the ground during the winter. They cling to the branches and are only discarded as the new life of the sap rising in the spring replaces them with new leaves. Chalmers went on to suggest that the dead and sinful parts of the human soul can only be expelled and conquered when something new and powerful and alive takes possession of that soul. The title of this masterful sermon was "The Expulsive Power of a New Affection."[66] Conversion is the flow of God's grace, working from within to produce new leaves, the dried up, dead ones dropping off, blowing away, never to be a factor again.

Since the turn of the twentieth century, over five hundred publications dealing with the psychological dynamics of conversion have appeared. Five distinct issues reappear in most of the discussions. First, there is the definitional issue of whether conversions, to be called conversions, must be sudden or developmental and whether a process of change must be religious for it to be called religious. The consensus is that even though a sudden change of heart is what people usually mean by conversion, either developmental or sudden changes can legitimately be called conversions, and that there are political and ideological conversions as well as religious ones. Indeed, some from outside the evangelical tradition have argued that both psychotherapy and brainwashing are similar to conversion, with one author finding striking similarities between Chinese brainwashing and the eighteenth-century evangelical revival. From within evangelicalism, conversion is seen as a "complex process" that defies stereotyping but that entails "thinking and rethinking; doubting and overcoming doubts; soul-searching and self-admonition; struggle against feelings of guilt and shame, and concern as to what a realistic following of Christ might mean."[67]

Second is the issue of whether conversion is pathological — abnormal, regressive, a sign of emotional instability — or a constructive, healthy pattern of behavior leading to "true" maturity. Once again, the consensus depends on what psychologists mean by "mental health." Many psychologists have an image of mental health as the self-sufficient individual who stands on his or her own two feet and does not burden others (including the fiction of God). Conversion thus appears as a turning from independence to immature dependence.

Evangelicals initially rejected the authority of psychotherapy as a theory of the meaning of human behavior, even while using it as a perspective of analysis and sometimes referring people with mental problems to psychiatrists, in part because of the Freudian bias against dependence on God.[68] It was mainly in reaction to Freud that evangelicals, until about thirty years ago, exhibited their notoriously smug "shirk-the-shrink" attitude. Indeed, evangelicals did not resist Jungian analysis as much as Freudian theory because Jung, the principal dissident from Freudian orthodoxy, was hospitable to religious concerns. He was known to send patients he could no longer help to their priests and ministers, and he has been credited with believing that psychoneurosis must ultimately be understood as the suffering of a soul that has not discovered its meaning.

Freud believed the basic dynamic in conversion was related to the Oedipus complex, a regressive defense against repressed hostility toward authority, specifically hatred toward the father. Conversion, with its talk of the sin problem and gospel cure-all, thus was seen as a pathological way of dealing with deep psychological problems treated best by psychoanalysis. The fact that it was not until 1990 that the American Psychiatric Association issued guidelines reminding its members that they were to respect and to reference their patients' religious beliefs, not ignore or belittle them, says a great deal both about the stranglehold Freud's mistaken views on religion had on therapists and about the new day of cooperation that is dawning.

Evangelicals themselves did not embrace the language and techniques of psychotherapy until the post-Freudian era of psychotherapy, when a variety of therapeutic approaches appeared on the scene, when respected Christian psychologists and counselors like Clyde Narramore, Paul Tournier, Frank Minirth, and Paul Meier honored the marriage of psychology and religion, and psychologists of the stature of Gordon W. Allport supported the validity of conversion and its utility in authentic character formation.[69] Evangelical colleges such as Fuller, Rosemead, Wheaton, Regent, Houghton, and Denver have been training psychologists and therapists for two decades. Today, 29 percent of *Christianity Today*'s readership and 38 percent of *Today's Christian Woman* readership have sought counseling for themselves or a close family member within the past three years.[70]

Evangelicals are also more likely to seek help from "Christian therapists" than from other skilled professionals. As the *Christian Yellow Pages* reveals, filled as it is with listings of physicians, psychologists, and dentists, evangelicals have been more likely than their religious colleagues from other traditions to see themselves professionally, and to want others to see them, as "Christian dentists" or "Christian psychiatrists," or "Christian nurses." The very names Rapha, Minirth-Meier, New Life, and Kairos have become synonymous with "Christian" psychiatric care and inpatient centers of the highest professional caliber. Brethren theologian Vernard Eller is one of the few evangelicals who questions whether there really is such a thing as *Christian* therapy.[71]

Third, there has been extensive discussion over convertible types. Is there a typology of personality of those who are convertible and those who are resistant to conversion? The consensus regarding differences between once- and twice-born people is that conversion is culturally relative. Some have found "converted" students to be more extroverted, more emotionally stable, and more dogmatic; they come from less religious homes than non-conversionists. In one of the earliest studies of conversion Edwin Diller Starbuck compared those who had cataclysmic conversions with those who professed gradual growth in grace. What he found was that "the conversion group approach religion more from the subjective, emotional standpoint... and are more suggestible, more impressionable, and, accordingly, more liable to undergo mental crises."[72] John P. Kildahl found that sudden converts were less intelligent than persons of gradual religious development, that they register higher on the hysteria scale of the Minnesota Multiphase Personality Inventory, but that they were not less humanitarian.[73]

Fourth is the question of whether conversion is more likely to occur at a certain age than at others. Most scholars, historians, and psychologists are unanimous in interpreting conversion as a rite of passage for children of American evangelicals. The later a conversion comes, the more likely it is to be intense and revolutionary. In terms of Erik Erikson's theories, the identity crisis in adolescence and integrity crisis in middle years are ripe moments for conversion.[74]

The final question has revolved around whether conversion is voluntary and conscious or involuntary. If involuntary, is conversion manipulated by others or is it caused by unconscious forces? Although the weight of psychological opinion falls with those psychologists who agree with Freud that forces beyond one's conscious control are decisive, Allport, Maslow, Rogers, and others stress the role of conscious decision making.

In the darkest days of World War II the theologian Karl Barth was asked "What should we do?" What can ordinary people do to make a difference in these perilous times? Barth's answer: "We shouldn't worry so much." If deep mental relaxation is as essential to our survival today as were quick wits and reflexes earlier in our history, then Jesus' words "Be not anxious" carry both urgency and unguency.

"God blessed the seventh day and hallowed it, because on it God rested from all his work." God did not bless the day on which the beasts of the earth were created, or the birds of the air, or the fish of the sea, or "every creeping thing that crawls upon the earth." God did not even bless the day humans were created, "male and female." Rather, God blessed the day on which God did nothing. The Sabbath is a symbol for evangelicals of more than a day of rest. When the Bible says "and God rested," the meaning is not that God got tired from the hard work of creation and needed some time to take it easy.

It means rather that God must rest because God is free and fully God only when God has ceased to work.

We too are free and fully who we are when we are not at work but at peace with nature and neighbor. Sabbathness symbolizes a state of complete harmony between humans and nature and between neighbor and neighbor. By not working — by not participating in the process of natural and social change — humans are united to nature and to time by being free from the chains of nature and of time.

Sabbathness is God's way of turning our heads to face the morning.

# ·2·

# Sinning and Suffering: "Ours the Cross, the Grave, the Skies"

> Soar we now where
> Christ has led
> Following our exalted Head;
> Made like him, like him we rise,
> Ours the Cross, the Grave, the Skies.
>
> —Charles Wesley,
> "Christ the Lord Is Risen Today"
> (1739)

Almighty, everliving God, maker of mankind, who dost correct those whom thou dost love, and chastise every one whom thou dost receive; we beseech thee to have mercy upon this thy servant visited with thine hand; and to grant that *he* may take *his* sickness patiently, and recover *his* bodily health, if it be thy gracious will; and whensoever *his* soul shall depart from the body, it may be without spot presented unto thee, through Jesus Christ our Lord. Amen.

> —Collect for "The Communion of
> the Sick" (1784)

> For I will be with thee
> thy troubles to bless,
> And sanctify to thee
> thy deepest distress.
>
> —"How Firm a Foundation" (1787)

> Give us this day our daily bread,
> And pies and cakes besides,

39

To load the stomach, pain the head,
And choke the vital tides.
And if so soon a friend decays,
Or dies in agony —
We'll talk of "God's mysterious ways,"
And lay it all to thee.

. . . . . . . . . . . . . .

And if defying nature's laws,
Dyspeptic we must be —
We scorn to search for human cause,
But lay it all to thee.

—Joel Shew,
"Fashionable Lady's Prayer" (1847)

In the spring and summer of 1832, major American cities were surprised by an incurable and irresistible visitor, a disease that "walked in darkness," leaving as suddenly as it arrived. Methodist itinerant George W. Walker had just been appointed to Cincinnati, a city particularly ravaged by the march of this "angel of death." He immediately began ministering to those who had not fled the city, comforting families with a member alive and well one evening, dead the next morning; many died only a few hours after they were "visited." In the words of an unknown nineteenth-century poet, victims were taken "In the wink of an eye, / In the draught of a breath, / From the blossom of health, / To the paleness of death." Nothing, not medicine, garlic, amulets, or the magic word *abracadabra* left over from Black Death days, warded off the killing fever.

Along with the rest of America, Walker called the dreaded visitor Asiatic cholera. In Britain it was known as Indian cholera. Every culture has a knack for finding some group to blame, a scapegoating escape from responsibility. Almost a hundred years later another worldwide visitor would be called by Germans the Chinese flu, by Russians the Kirghiz flu, by Argentineans the Spanish flu, and by Americans the German flu or, in words that testified to fears of the kaiser's secret weapons, "the plague of the Spanish lady."

Walker's wife and family wondered why a stranger to the city would hazard placing himself in a situation that others were clogging the roads and rivers trying to leave. Walker wondered aloud as well. "Notwithstanding the violence of the scourge, the daily evidences of mortality around, and the possibility that I may fall next, yet I do not feel at *liberty to leave my post.*" In some inscrutable way, Walker sensed that his presence was not coincidental: "MY COMING IS UNDER THE SPECIAL DIRECTION OF MY HEAVENLY FATHER." And even if the disease had not appeared to defy all quarantines, protections, and sanitary defenses, making flight of little avail, his choice would have been the same, for "the path of duty is the path of safety."[1]

Walker's faith ground its teeth at the suggestion that the epidemic was none other than the visitation of Jehovah's awful voice of justice, God's punishing hand of judgment against the dissolute, the intemperate, the profligate.[2] "Such statements libel the dead," he retorted indignantly. "Some of the most temperate and pious persons in this city have died of the epidemic."[3] It may be that the pestilence taught the American people habits of holiness they might not otherwise have learned so readily — "the value of cleanliness, of ventilation, of pure air, and the imminent and certain danger of overcrowding," not to mention the safeguard of "a calm, quiet, cheerful mind."[4] It may even have taught "moderation in eating" and "total abstinence in drinking ardent spirits."[5] But the plague of 1832 was no manifestation of the wrath-of-God syndrome.

## I

The unruly realities of this chapter are among the greatest temptations of the faithful, the greatest challenges to religious experience. In our time, sinning and suffering have become the greatest challenges to Christian apologists. Only in the twentieth century has there been talk about the problem of evil, as if there were political and scientific solutions to sickness, suffering, and death.

> Man has been pondering the origin of evil at least since the days of the Sumerians some five thousand years ago, and probably a lot longer than that. Medicine men and high priests have ascribed it to witches and demons, theologians to original sin or the devil. More recently, psychoanalysts have linked man's inhumanity to man with the unresolved Oedipus complex, psychologists with the wrong kind of reinforcement, neurologists with imbalances in the humors that bathe our brain cells. Historians have chalked it up to history, sociologists to society.[6]

Evangelicals have not traditionally exhibited a chivalrous attitude toward God — defending God against those who would use against God the perennial question of the human species, *unde malum* (why evil)? Indeed, evangelicals rebel against a religion that is painless and without struggle. Evangelical literature comes alive with Luther flinging ink pots at the devil, Paul fighting wild beasts at Ephesus, and Jesus struggling with Satan in the wilderness. There is no cloudless communion with God.

For evangelicals, life reveals clearly the ineradicable, irreducible component of evil. In fact, *live* is evil reversed, as the Welsh poet Dylan Thomas discovered. When the fact of evil is faced, God turns evil inside out, enabling us to live. God turns the world upside down, bringing strength out of weakness, wholeness out of brokenness, gaining out of giving, finding oneself out of losing oneself, life out of death. Evangelicals espouse an upside-down, inside-out, topsy-turvy spirituality that wrenches good out of bad.

Evil is bred in the bones of every fallen human being. Evangelicals have denounced as philosophical sleight of hand the Platonic conception of evil as merely some sort of hypostatized abstraction. Similarly, the notion that evil is nothing more than the absence of good violates direct experience of the psychological as well as the historical reality of evil. Sickness then can best be defined as a power hostile to God that destroys life.

Some contemporary evangelicals are moving away from dualism's affirmation of opposing forces locked in a static, satanic struggle, with the competitor devil-god having as large a following as Yahweh-God's, if not larger. But most evangelicals have nevertheless resisted the interiorization of evil. They have sensed, as Carl Jung argued, that we have no choice but to take the devil inside of us if we have no doctrine of Satan.

The explanation for evil provided in a world driven by nothing more than fate is chillingly impersonal. It serves only to confuse. Evangelicals have been dissatisfied with viewing health and disease as matters of chance or fortune separable from their lives. This is due in part to the evangelical understanding of the Holy Spirit, who does not appear in our lives vagrantly, randomly, without purpose or reason.

For evangelicals, evil's brutish existence begins in sin, what Billy Graham has called "man's fatal disease."[7] Evangelicals have never been known for their perky assessments of human nature, no matter how badly the Calvinist doctrine of human depravity has been disregarded or brought into disrepute. "Sin is the great fact in human experience," J. H. Fairchild, president of Oberlin College, announced in 1868.[8] America's greatest evangelists, such as Charles G. Finney, Dwight L. Moody, Billy Sunday, and Billy Graham, spent their entire ministries unveiling the soul's hidden defilement as the first step in bringing people to salvation. Moody summed up his theology by the "three R's in the Bible: Ruin by sin, Redemption by Christ, and Regeneration by the Holy Ghost."[9]

Evangelical theologian Bernard Ramm is alarmed by contemporary religion's tendency to wink at sin, wave as it passes by, or waive its penalties. Evangelicals have not quite known how to handle their success at convincing psychotherapists like M. Scott Peck (*People of the Lie: The Hope for Healing Human Evil*, 1983), Karl Menninger (*Whatever Became of Sin?* 1973), and earliest of all, O. Hobart Mowrer (*The Crisis in Psychiatry and Religion*, 1961) to agree with their position on the importance of sin. The question of sin is both urgent and timeless: "Can there be a more important topic for human discussion?"[10]

My parents embodied the traditional evangelical understanding of sin. They taught my brothers and me that a trinity of evils — the world, the flesh, the devil — were lurking everywhere, ready to devour innocent young victims who ventured too close. If the devil gets all the good tunes, as both Luther and Wesley argued, the devil usually plays them masterfully and voluptuously. There are 786 different sins listed in the Bible. Sometimes it seemed as if my brothers and I heard "no" said to each one of them. Sometimes it seemed that sins were all there were in life. As early as 1893, someone satirized evangelicalism's development of a new "Pentalogue": "Thou shalt not smoke. Thou shalt not drink. Thou shalt not play cards. Thou shalt not dance. Thou shalt not go to the theatre. On these five commandments hang all the law and the prophets."

Some members of an evangelical church in the late nineteenth century, for example, were expelled simply because they were sighted on a steamboat where there was a dance band (but no dancing). Baptists have been the strictest about dancing. Ever since "John the Baptist lost his head by reason of dancing," one early evangelical reasoned, "the Baptists have never been fond of dancing from that day to this."[11] Reformed and Confessional evangelicals have shown more reserve and restraint than Baptists and Methodists in exercising church discipline for offenses involving "worldly amusements."[12]

As recently as the early 1950s my mother, Mabel Boggs Sweet, an ordained minister in good standing in the Pilgrim Holiness Church of America, was defrocked by her peers because she "bobbed" her hair and wore lipstick and a wedding band. A few years later, our family was "disciplined" by removal from the membership rolls of a Free Methodist Church in Gloversville, New York, because my father allowed into the sanctity of the home "the devil's blinking box" (a television set).

Evangelical life-styles are now less preoccupied with fire-breathing, soul-killing laws against worldly amusements and more sensitive to the fact that the first recorded sins in the universe were not on account of the flesh or the vitiosity of matter but on account of the spirit — Luciferic pride and arrogance, Adamic greed and disobedience. For most of its history evangelicalism has been dead serious about sin's deadly seriousness.

What is sin? Sin is not ignorance. Evangelicals admit that ignorance often begets sin and ignorance can be a by-product of sin. But ignorance is not sin. Ignorance is cured by knowledge; sin is cured by repentance and forgiveness. "Sin is any want of conformity unto or transgression of the law of God," states the *Westminster Shorter Catechism*.[13]

Sin is a violation of God's law, pure and simple. When evangelicals talk of God's law, they mean both physical laws, the laws of our material state that preserve life and health, and moral laws, the laws of our spiritual state that preserve faith and community. The connection between the moral and the physical is undisputed. A healthy body presupposes a healthy soul, and vice versa. Henry Hayman says "there may be as real a connection between pain...and moral corruption...as there is between the clouds and rain-fall on the one hand and the water-surfaces of this our earth on the other."[14]

We are sinners, evangelicals never tire of reminding the world, not because of moral peccadilloes, some secret ickiness, or spiritual slip-ups, or into-every-life-a-little-sin-must-fall fatalism. "For from within, out of men's hearts, come evil thoughts, sexual immorality, theft, murder, adultery, greed, malice, deceit, lewdness, envy, slander, arrogance and folly. All these evils come from inside" (Mark 7:21–22 NIV). We are sinners because evil leaks out from the inside until we yield to sin, with deep disagreement within the evangelical community over whether we have physical and metaphysical power to prevent or resist sin's seepage.[15]

At first existing happily alongside the notion of sin as seepage, then overshadowing it, was the understanding of sin as blockage. Sin as seepage meant willful transgressions of the law of God. Sin as blockage meant failure to love and be loved, to be what God had made one to be. From seepage to blockage spelled a major departure from evangelicalism's Puritan past. It signified an important shift in the evangelical mind.

By the middle of the nineteenth century, evangelicalism's favorite metaphor for the blockage of sin was disease. Evangelical theology came to be understood in this shorthand fashion: Christ came to diagnose and heal our illness. Our disease? Sin. Our symptoms? Suffering, pain, cruelty, violence, meaninglessness, and the like. Our prognosis? Despair unto death. Our salvation? The healing news of the gospel. And what is this good news? John 3:16: "For God so loved the world...that whosoever believeth...should...have eternal life." In the words of John Wesley's classic sermon entitled "Original Sin," "Know your disease; know your cure!"[16]

Evangelicals devised a language encompassing both the experience of salvation and the phenomenon of hygiene within the unified conceptual framework of "health." Sin became to the soul what disease was to the body. The soul is not made sinful any more than the body is made sick. The body is made for health, and the soul is made for virtue. Sin is a chronic condition that blocks the moral system, producing moral diseases that parallel physical diseases in almost every way: in disease's origin (innate liability is enhanced by civilization's artificial causes — modes of dress and of living, processes of cookery and distillation, and habits of mind, cares, anxieties, and sorrows that are superinduced by society); in disease's progress, often imperceptible, irregular, unpredictable; in disease's effects, often an offense against medicine and morality alike; and in disease's recovery — slow, disciplined, with moderation and restraint essential.

A study in the early 1980s revealed that 48 percent of people with lung cancer resume puffing on what early evangelicals called "the devil's kindling wood" after leaving their tumors at the hospital. In both moral and physical diseases, patients abhor the very thought of discipline and diet. Some would rather die than diet; and they will die both physically and spiritually without vigorous discipline and exercise.

Whether the disease be of the body or mind, bringing the body and mind under the subjection of the spirit — what nineteenth-century evangelicals called "keeping the body *under*" or what today's evangelicals are prone to call deferred gratification — is the only cure available. Observing health principles in body, mind, and spirit is a form of natural healing. And yet multitudes "will do anything — attend meetings, rush into excitements, make much ado, use prescriptions, seek counsel only to resist it, and after all, suffer tortures and vent groans of remorse — anything will they submit to but sober, strict, daily, hourly self-denial."[17]

In a study of "physical religion," historian Catherine Albanese analyzes the evangelical contribution to this emerging mentality in which a chain of cause and effect links disease to hygienic disobedience, in which medicine did not cure disease, as one nineteenth-century evangelical physician asserted, so much as "aid nature in her efforts to throw off morbific matter."[18]

> The gospel good news was *natural* sin and *natural* grace. The would-be convert had sinned against physiological nature. Violation of its immutable laws had brought its stern and debilitating judgment of disease. In like manner, health, when it came, was a work of harmony with the same immutable laws. Healing grace came in the nature of things when one cooperated with the decrees written into one's physical frame. The evangelical message had not stifled the Enlightenment: it had only recast it in a new form.[19]

Evangelical theodicies have always admitted the complicity of sin in the curse and calamity of pain, disease, suffering, and death. For example, Billy Graham once counseled those suffering from hypertension that their medical problems were likely related to their "alienation from God."[20] Sickness and affliction are often brought on oneself as a natural penalty for violating some fixed law of nature or God.

Yet at the same time evangelicals have insisted that pain and illness are also character builders for moral agents, elements of the world's moral education and renovation. There is no greater evidence of the draining of Puritanism out of evangelicalism, with only drops left by the Civil War, than what happened to the commonplace Puritan idea of an impassible, sovereign God dispensing suffering as a punishment for sin.

By the mid-nineteenth century, evangelical theologians like Andover's William G. T. Shedd rejected this idea by pointing to Job and Jesus, each encountering in his own day the view of suffering as a consequence of and punishment for sin and each repudiating it (John 9:2, 3).[21] Jesus used the word *sin* only nine times in the synoptic Gospels, the noun six times, the verb three.[22] By the late twentieth century, Daniel E. Fountain, a medical missionary in central Africa for over a quarter of a century, could state bluntly that "the God who created the morning star and the lily of the valley is not the God who dispatches cancer to this one, or a malaria-bearing anopheles mosquito to that one."[23]

There was a threefold problem with suffering as a retribution for and antidote to sinning, contended Henry Cowles, theologian, editor, and one of those responsible for siphoning Puritan residues out of evangelicalism. First, "judging from the limited efficiency of suffering to restrain from sinning, as things are and have been, how much of its influence could well be spared?" Second, in the case of infants, "suffering precedes sinning." Third, in the case of animals, suffering "falls upon the unsinning."[24]

Without sin, evangelicals have argued, there would be no suffering in the universe. But every instance of suffering is not singly or simply a penal consequence of sin. Nor is every violation of natural law something sinful, as parents attest who tend sick children, day after day, night after night, to the detriment of their own health. To attribute the wreck of well-being to a single cause — divine command or satanic powers or punishment for sin — simply allows people to avoid what nature, science, medicine, and religion offer for restoration.

God's chastening, correcting rod of the Puritan divines still lingers in modern evangelicalism. Increasingly, however, evangelicals have counseled sufferers to vent healthy expressions of anger toward God when faced with unspeakable suffering. Gone are the days when evangelicals obediently learned to "kiss the rod," however severe the blow, by submitting to suffering as retribution by a righteous God. Gone too are the days when evangelicals cited approvingly Protestant reformer Martin Bucer's estimation of the plague that visited Strasbourg in the first half of the sixteenth century (exterminating his wife and five children) as well-deserved punishment from the Almighty.

Two of evangelicalism's favorite-son writers, C. S. Lewis, who came into the evangelical fold, and Peter DeVries, who came out of it, exhibit the appropriateness of anger in suffering. In *A Grief Observed*, Lewis speaks to God and himself: "Already, month by month and week by week you broke her body on the wheel whilst she still wore it. Is it not yet enough? The terrible thing is that a perfectly good God is in this matter hardly less formidable than a Cosmic Sadist. The more we believe that God hurts only to heal, the less we can believe that there is any use in begging for tenderness."[25] DeVries ends *The Blood of the Lamb* with the father of an eight-year-old girl who just died of a rare blood disease hurling a cake at a stone carving of the crucified Christ. The chapter concludes with these words: "Thus Wanderhope was found at that place which for the diabolists of his literary youth, and for those with more modest spiritual histories too, was said to be the only alternate to the muzzle of a pistol: the foot of the Cross."[26]

But as soon as evangelicals loosen these connections between God's justice and Jesus' love, they start making them again. Suffering does not necessarily presuppose sin. But sin presupposes suffering. The notion of suffering as a necessary penalty of sin has never been dismissed entirely from evangelicalism. Retributive theology reminds evangelicals of the truths that disease has both a natural and supernatural cause, and that both God and creation pay a cost when love is violated.

The ratios of relationship between sin, evil, suffering, and pain have been connected for evangelicals less in the question "Why do I suffer?" than in the question "Why do I cause others to suffer?" The innocent suffer with the guilty. Even God. Moral defects and diseases are not unrelated to physical diseases and natural disasters.

## II

Whether suffering comes from happenstance, from the violation of the laws of heaven and health, or from hidden causes, it comes "by divine appointment" as early evangelicals liked to put it. Evangelicals often talk less about "second causes" or "nature's laws" than of divine providence, because the former "puts God at the distant end of the line" rather than "at the end of the line nearest us" where, and only where, there is comfort and hope and power of endurance.[27] The awkward question of the design of suffering and the "uses of pain" in the spiritual culture of evangelicalism still lurks.

Evangelicals have the temperament that makes a great hostage (although not from the captor's point of view). They are trained both in meeting suffering head-on and in finding meaning in suffering. They have also been taught "if the first mark of a true and living church is love, the second is suffering"; and again, "if we are true, we shall suffer. But let us be faithful and not fear."[28] What Abraham Maslow called the "Jonah complex" — running away from one's future and not facing pain and suffering — can seldom be attributed to the evangelical movement. Nor do evangelicals align themselves with English novelist W. Somerset Maugham, who denied that suffering ennobles people. Judging from his experience, Maugham said, suffering only embittered people and made them mean.[29]

Whatever happens can be either a blessing or a curse; the individual decides which it will be. Life is modulated by meaning. Evangelicals believe that there will be suffering in life but that if you let it, suffering has redemptive functions. One classic study compared pain intensities in postoperative hospital wards, as rated on the one hand by wounded soldiers and on the other by civilians. The amazing discovery was that, with nearly identical physical ailments, soldiers consistently reported less pain than did civilians. For civilians, sickness and surgery were invasive interruptions in a normal life. For soldiers, sickness and surgery constituted escape from the ravages of war and the possibility of an early homecoming. The deciding variable was the meaning assigned to suffering.[30]

Evangelicals identify two uses or positive purposes in pain: the preservative and the educative (didactic). The preservative use of pain is the body's physical response to stimuli, communicating messages about one's state of health that the organism ignores at its peril. The educative use of pain is the theological reflection on the whole pain experience that raises the question of pain's meaning and the purpose of suffering.

Turn-of-the-century Presbyterian minister E. R. Eschbach summarized the complexity of the classic evangelical position on pain and suffering with laconic lucidity. Pain is a warning, a distress signal, and a teacher. But it is also, and always, a "mystery." Pains are not "lawless" or "accidental" but stem from causes, whether physical or moral, and spawn purposes. "Sin is moral evil," and "an immense amount of physical suffering is due to moral evil." Pain does not come "without God's permission." If we greet pain's arrival as an "avenging messenger," inflicting punishments for sinning, we shall miss receiving the positive meanings and blessings that come from greeting pain as an "errand of love," come to "chasten us, perhaps to cure us of follies and sins, to lead us nearer to God, and to bring out of us more of the beauty of Christ."[31]

There are worse things in life than pain — for example, separation from God, alienation from truth. As Billy Graham said, "physical illness is not the worst thing that can happen to one. Some of the most twisted, miserable people I have ever met had no physical handicap."[32] Life's supreme success comes not in escaping pain but in glorifying God and laying hold of righteousness. Sometimes we glorify God with our bodies more in sickness than in health. Pain and suffering are not the greatest evils known on earth; and pleasure is not life's greatest good. As C. S. Lewis pointed out on a variety of occasions, the martyr slowly burning to death on a griddle may be said to be happy. But it would be crazy to say that he was having fun or experiencing pleasure.

Even when both the preservative and educative functions of pain are accounted for, evangelicals admit, there is still a surplus of suffering. Even if troublous times can make us more patient, more loving, more trusting, so much suffering seems awfully out of proportion to the disease. That is why suffering is fundamentally, as Eschbach insisted, a mystery. There are no easy explanations for suffering. Even the Book of Job is not an essay on suffering and pain, but a narrative commentary on whether it is possible to know God and be in relationship with God in the midst of unanswerable questions about suffering and pain. Job was one of those on the griddle, charred by burning questions about life and evil, but the most burning of all was this one about being in relationship with God.

Suffering has a proximal place in God's purposes, but not an ultimate place or purpose. Our inner distresses, our outer dissolutions, do not last forever. God does not wish that even "one of these little ones should perish." Yet look what happened to God's own son. The hands that healed were pierced with nails. The eyes that loved and lifted others toward God were strained with the pain of utter desolation. The tongue that blessed was swollen in fearful thirst. If even "God's son not sparing," how dare we place ourselves above "burden-bearing"?

## III

Consider the preservative uses of pain and suffering. Pain needs to be treated as an asset, an ally, even a friend, not for its own sake or as some means of grace, but as a monitory design in the economy of health. Since the 1950s, when mood and behavior technology began with tranquilizers, antidepressants, and sedatives, evangelicals have been nervous about these psychotropic drugs because they can prevent the body, spirit, and mind from receiving pain's warning signals. Since pain is for one's "safety and protection," it is worth the price of pain to protect oneself against the dangers of a pain-free existence. Being a Christian does not mean an end to pain and problems, Edna Hong lectures evangelicals.[33] God has not provided creation with a compulsory health system.

George I. Chace, a Brown University professor in the 1850s, lectured fellow evangelicals on the way pain protects us from the various dangers to which our bodies are exposed, alerts us to the existence of disease, warns us that some natural, hygienic, or "organic law" is being disregarded or violated, wards off danger, and serves as a "guide to the proper remedies."[34] "Pain is nature's splint," contended Buffalo physician Woods Hutchinson; another mid-nineteenth century evangelical, Benjamin W. Dwight, a physician from New York City, demonstrated medically how diseases can be "needful lessons to us of the evils of breaking or ignoring necessary laws."[35]

Pain preserves the body by shocking us into respecting the human form and returning us to the biblical principle of the body as a dwelling place of God. "No true Christian can treat his body as an encumbrance to his soul, which it were well to be rid of, without doing injury to one portion of his human nature," another evangelical wrote.[36] As much as evangelicals sought to bring the body under subjection to the spirit (1 Corinthians 9:27), they also sought to honor and consecrate it as God chose and consecrated it above all the created forms to reveal the divine nature. The health practices of clergymen in general, and itinerant preachers in particular, observed hygienic precepts mainly in the breach. Evangelical ministers took a perverse pride in having, as one circuit rider wrote in his journal, a "good constitution to wear out in [God's] service."[37] And wear out they did, with "bronchitis, nervous afflictions, liver complaints, consumption, and all the what-not's of disease, which assail and destroy the clerical portion of God's heritage."[38]

But even these clergy preached a different message from the Bible, one which teaches us to present our bodies as a "living sacrifice" unto God. Do I have the right to do as I please with my body? Preachers responded emphatically, No! My body does not belong to me. My body has been given me as a living sacrifice to God to be the temple and worship of God's spirit (Romans 12:1; 1 Corinthians 3:16). It is a sin to defile one's body. Or, as one evangelical put it, "the sacrifice is not to be a dead, but a living sacrifice."[39]

By defying known laws of health, one is "criminally" inducing disease and denying God a "living sacrifice." Considering the health-defying habits of Christians, physician Larkin B. Coles wrote in his book *Philosophy of Health* (first published in the 1840s), "if the bodies offered upon Christ's altar were examined by the scrutiny to which Jewish sacrifices were subjected...how many would be left upon the altar accepted?"[40] Everyone has the power to choose his or her state of health in the same way everyone chooses a level of education or moral condition, argued Coles. "As surely as you can be wise, or good, just so truly can you be healthy," William A. Alcott lectured young evangelical men and women in the last half of the nineteenth century. God has placed one's health in one's own hands. Sickness and disease can be transformed by God into sanctifying influences for human advancement, but there is nothing about sickness itself that is good for spiritual growth and moral development. God wants us to choose health.[41]

Nineteenth-century evangelical periodicals headlined some of the earliest announcements that cigarette smoking is dangerous, denouncing tobacco as the "twin sister" of that other deadly stimulant, alcohol.[42] U.S. Surgeon General C. Everett Koop's May 1988 declaration of war against cigarettes, citing them as substances as addictive and almost as abusive as cocaine and heroin, was nothing more than his evangelical forebears had been saying since the 1830s. "Does [one] love his neighbor, who gradually, though it may be very slowly, poisons him" through the pollution of tobacco smoke, William Alcott asked. "And do they love their families as they ought, who poison them by inches?"[43]

Unable to garner full endorsement of either the medical establishment or the evangelical establishment itself, some health reform evangelicals like the Sabbatarian Adventists established their own denominations to insure, when Christ returned, they could stand before him blameless as habitats of God's spirit, having prepared their bodies for his coming by healthful living and abstaining from tobacco, tea, coffee, alcohol, and other injurious substances.[44] Other reform-minded evangelicals picked up allies wherever they could find them as their campaign gathered momentum in the 1880s with the mechanization of cigarette manufacture implemented so successfully by James B. Duke and his American Tobacco Company. Eventually fourteen states passed cigarette prohibition laws, starting with Washington in 1893. "Stimulants" and "narcotics" may "exalt nervous action temporarily and compel the wheels to revolve rapidly," one column in the "Health and Disease" section of an evangelical periodical put it, but they "soon or later break the shuttle."[45]

Until recently, evangelicals were conspicuous in not coming when called by Horace's classic summons *nunc est bibendum* ("it's time for cocktails"), not because of moral starchiness but because the body is the temple of the Holy Spirit and must not be defiled by drugs. The biblical basis of this belief in the accountability of the creaturely body to the creator was made by Ralph Barns Grindrod in his popular temperance tract *Bacchus* (1839),[46] dedicated to the American Temperance Society. Temperance reformer Frances E. Willard made what she called a "religion of the body" central to the mission of the Women's Christian Temperance Union, even providing women with their own "Decalogue of Natural Law," which Willard brought down "from the ever-radiant Sinai of physiology and hygiene."[47]

The link between food and religion has been a strong one in the evangelical tradition. Because what one puts into one's body is a theological issue, food is a moral matter.[48] Nineteenth-century evangelical preacher Peter Akers symbolized the interconnectedness of divinity and diet in picturesque terms. He selected as a fitting oblation to the devil "a hog stuffed with tobacco in an alcohol gravy." Frances Willard, who used the Akers quote prophetically, testified how in her own life "pastries, cakes, hot bread, rich gravies, pickles, pepper-sauces, salads, tea and coffee are discarded from my bill of fare, and I firmly believe they will be from the recipes of the twentieth century," when they will be replaced with "entire wheat flour bread, vegetables, fruit, fowl, fish, with a little beef and mutton and water as the chief drink."[49] This was a far stricter regimen than the cultural nutritional ideal of the time: "A regular, systematically served diet of a mixed character, embracing both animal and vegetable materials, proportioned agreeably to the taste of an individual, secures the highest condition of mind." Evangelicals did, however, agree with the rest of the cultural critique from this *Harper's Weekly* article: "Neither savages, barbarians, mendicants in search of dinner, nor gourmands write books or contribute to the progress of mankind."[50]

As we have seen, evangelicals deny an ontological dichotomy between body and soul or spirit. The body is quite capable of taking out its abuse and frustrations on the mind and the soul. One nineteenth-century evangelical testified to the body's revenge on the soul and mind as experienced by the laity. "Many a sermon, breathing the threatenings of the law instead of the gentle pleadings of the gospel, has been occasioned by a fit of indigestion, which soured the speaker at the whole world around him."[51] The linkage of the body and spirit is such that spiritual health depends on being in good physical condition. It is our spiritual duty, evangelicals announced, to "cultivate high health."

## IV

Evangelicals believe that the more one obeys nature's laws, the less pain one experiences. What then prevents them from giving birth to or becoming partners in what Donald De Marco has tagged "the anesthetic society"?[52] The belief that suffering is somehow not to be an accepted part of life has become increasingly present in American culture, as the German preacher and theologian Helmut Thielicke observed in 1963 while visiting the United States. Thielicke said he got the feeling that in America "suffering is regarded as something which is fundamentally inadmissible, disturbing, embarrassing and not to be endured."[53]

The sense that suffering can be annihilated by medical advances and technological progress or that, in Christopher Lasch's words, "hardship and suffering…are no longer accepted as part of the natural order of things" has achieved orthodox standing in many cultural quarters.[54] Cultural pressures have even led evangelicals to be more accepting of the "count-your-blessings" school of therapy, health-and-wealth prosperity evangelism, and even a variety of popular theological equivalents of poet Walt Whitman's "religion of healthy-mindedness," philosopher William James's phrase for "the tendency which looks on all things and sees that they are good."

Evangelicalism may have been the nest in which healthism was hatched, but it quickly got booted out. Evangelicals have resisted healthism's pressures in large measure because of the second use of pain — its educative, didactic purpose. More than he would have liked, Gordon Allport stated the evangelical orientation succinctly: "The main purpose of religion, I repeat, is not to make people healthy, but to help them fit themselves into the Creator's context for them."[55] Pain has meaning. Pain has providence. Thus suffering can be embraced and endured. Without meaning, pain cannot be tolerated. Hence our culture's low pain threshold, its diminishing pain tolerance, and its remaking of physicians into pain removal experts.

A favorite story in evangelical circles concerns an emperor moth struggling to get out of its cocoon. A man watching the moth struggle feels sorry for its plight, so he takes out his pocketknife and slits the opening in the cocoon just a mite wider to spare the poor creature some of the effort. His attempt to help the moth actually ruins it. The pressing and squeezing were necessary because the pressure pushed blood and body fluids into the wings. Without that struggle, the moth could never develop its wings, and it could never fly.

Just as muscles need exercise such as stretching and bending if they are not to atrophy, so too does spiritual maturity need the twisting and stretching of pain. "The discipline of sorrow is to moral improvement what exercise is to muscle" testified one of evangelicalism's sufferers.[56] Pain, someone has said, is "the keen and biting chisel under whose edge alone can the figure of the perfect human be hewn out of the lifeless marble." Or, in another evangelical adage, "the harsh grindstone makes the sharp axe." Evangelicals were interested in Italian artist Domenichino's late-nineteenth-century painting "Communion of St. Jerome" because it portrayed pain's purging and purifying powers.[57] Pain was a physical means to a spiritual end. Henry Ward Beecher likened affliction to the tempering of steel. The burning and hammering and filing not only do not weaken the metal; they are God's instrumentalities for giving it shape and strength and service. Without suffering, life's highest virtues of courage, endurance, trust, and compassion could not be developed. Pain is necessary to Christians' training and discipline. In one of the most moving passages in the Second Testament (Hebrews 2:10), the writer says that the most perfect man who ever lived was made perfect through suffering.

Early evangelicals called such suffering "afflictive providences,"[58] which they defined as sicknesses that lead us to God, a sickness that teaches us to kneel. Christ never explained suffering or glorified it. He only identified it as a vital ingredient in the making of ourselves. In the same fashion evangelicals cited suffering's providential purpose in making us into the likeness of Christ, producing in us perseverance, character, hope, and so forth (Romans 5:4–5), and making us dependent on God. Nineteenth-century Methodist bishop William Quayle once walked the floor far into the night, his spirit tormented by pain and anxiety, until he heard God speak to him: "Quayle, you go to bed. I'll sit up the rest of the night."

If pain is "God's megaphone to rouse a deaf world," as C. S. Lewis phrased it, then evangelicals have been riveted on those holding the megaphone. Evangelicalism's fixation on annals of suffering, its formation of a culture of invalidism, its formulation of sufferings' solitudes were propelled by this need for sublime assurance. Accounts of missionaries stricken by deadly diseases; saints bearing up under lifelong suffering with unbelievable patience; the handicapped bravely bracing against life's unfair onslaughts: all confirmed evangelicalism's belief that suffering could be a sanctifying experience. We can be "more than conquerors" (Romans 8; 2 Corinthians 7). Affliction, handicap, and persecution need not break the believer. The purest piety and highest possibilities for usefulness can be reached through the refinements of agony, hardship, and trial. Joy can be found in suffering. If we walk in the light, we can dance in the dark.

The relationship between joy and suffering has a complex history in Christianity. To the evangelical mind, joyless suffering betrays ugliness of spirit and willfulness of body. Each evangelical generation finds its own voice for suffering's sacrificial efficacy — like that of French philosopher and mystic Simone Weil, who eventually starved to death joyfully rather than touch one morsel of food more than the ration in Nazi-occupied France. In the four suffering-servant songs of Isaiah (42:1–4; 49:1–6; 50:4–9; 52:13–53) can be found perhaps the most profound passages of suffering in the First Testament. Here is suffering for the benefit of others, a ministry of suffering love that finds joy in the very heart of pain. There are biblical passages suggesting that we are to rejoice in suffering (John 21:19, "I cannot contain my happiness in the midst of all the trials of mine," is a typical verse, but see also Acts 5:41, Galatians 2:19, and Romans 5:3–5). Yet even Jesus and Paul did not always rejoice in suffering. In Mark 14:34 (compare Matthew 26:38), Jesus says, "My soul is ready to die with sorrow." At one point Paul's sufferings became so acute that he "despaired of life itself" (2 Corinthians 1:8).

Among the people evangelicals admire most are those sufferers who do not get healing but get something far better — grace. Individuals who rise above suffering, not allowing it to dull human sensibilities but instead even using pain to sharpen them, are among evangelicalism's greatest heroes. Some of these "wheelchair saints," for example, the blind composer Fanny

Crosby, stand firmly within the evangelical tradition, while others, like the writer Robert Louis Stevenson, stand without. Robert Louis Stevenson, who was sickly from childhood and in pain almost every day of his adult life, once described his sickbed with a sense of mission:

> For fourteen years I have not had a day's real health; I have wakened sick and gone to bed weary; and I have done my work unflinchingly. I have written in bed, and written out of it, written in hemorrhages, written in sickness, written torn by coughing, written when my head swam for weakness....I was made for a contest and the Powers have so willed that my battle-field should be this dingy, inglorious one of the bed and the physic bottle.[59]

One morning toward the end of his life, when he was hemorrhaging so badly that he could not even whisper, Stevenson wrote his wife and daughter a little note: "Mr. Dumbleigh presents his compliments and praises God that he is sick so he has to be cared for by two tender, loving fairies. Was ever a man so blest?" It was in those latter days of his life, too, that Stevenson wrote a prayer that has become a minor classic: "We thank thee for this place in which we dwell; for the love that unites us; for the peace accorded us this day; for the hope with which we expect the morrow; for the health, the work, the food and the bright skies that make our lives delightful....Give us courage, gaiety and the quiet mind."[60]

Paraplegic Joni Eareckson Tada's daily radio broadcasts, popular appearances, and best-selling books *Joni* (1976), *A Step Further* (1978), *All God's Children* (1981), *Choices, Changes* (1986), *Secret Strength* (1988), *Glorious Intruder* (1989), and *Seeking God* (1991) all feed the evangelical need for evidence that suffering can release tremendous creative powers. Evangelical appetites continue to be insatiable for accounts of the meaning of suffering and for firsthand discoveries of what Hosea and Jeremiah meant when they talked about the deeper knowledge of God that is possible through suffering. Southern Baptist pastoral theologian Wayne E. Oates has written about "the covenant of suffering" in his book *The Revelation of God in Human Suffering* (1959).[61]

A hundred years ago evangelicals were gripped by the tale of Ohioan Jennie Smith, bedridden at an early age after a typhoid-induced spinal disease. Smith's writings testify that the valley of Baca ("weeping") can become a vale of blessing, even opening to the plains of Beulah ("joy" and "intimacy"), both to the sufferer and to those willing to be educated in the suffering. Her name became a household word among evangelicals, and she supported herself almost totally from the sales of her books. *The Valley of Baca's* frontispiece is a picture of Smith in a bed resembling an altar, from which she presided as a pastor presided over a congregation. From her sickroom she held a catechism class, conducted a subscription school, witnessed to visitors, and led prayer meetings. When she was given a wheelcot, she worked for sixteen years among railroad workers and their families, and she was known at camp meetings as the invalid preacher. In the words of her pastor, Jennie's cot has been a "mount of blessing; her sick chamber, a Bethesda, indeed."[62]

The foundation of evangelicalism's educative use of suffering is the resurrection of Jesus Christ. Paul promises the Christian that life involves suffering (2 Corinthians 12:7–10). But through suffering we identify with Christ and realize Christ's victory over suffering. Pain rouses in us fight and opposition to pain and suffering. Healing relief, not masochistic relish, is the purpose of the educative function of pain.

Evangelicals like to talk and sing of each Christian's mission of "cross bearing." As theologian Charles Hodge put it, "Each man has his own cross. One has...sickness, feebleness of body; another, poverty; another, want of success; another, reproach; another, insignificance. In any case we must bear our burden cheerfully, looking unto Christ as our example, our helper and our reward."[63] One of the greatest sermons I have heard was given by Dr. Arthur P. Whitney, for many years deputy general secretary of the American Bible Society. I shall never forget his castigation of the way in which we identify our troubles with Jesus' sacrifice; we say "that's a cross I'll just have to bear" — about acne, gout, obesity, and all sorts of styrofoam crosses, easy and light to bear. These conditions are burdens but not crosses. True cross bearing comes only when we willingly take on the sufferings of others...that they may be healed.

The educative use of pain has been recognized in evangelical child-rearing practices as well. The Pentecostal emphasis on the laying on of hands was demonstrated in my evangelical childhood by a parental form of laying on of hands known as spanking, switching, and, most ominously, "the Four-Way." The correction of children by corporal punishment, or what evangelicals called "the disciplinal use of artificial pain," was justified only insofar as there was "defective reflection" and a dearth of experience. Once children amassed true experience, and "in proportion as that experience accrues and is turned to account, the resource of artificial pain is superseded."[64]

My parents' use of discipline on us children, as well as the church's use of discipline on my parents, was not so much to punish or purge as to restore to health and fellowship. Suffering's instructive rule is aimed to rouse our identification with others who suffer and are needy and to stir us to strive to eliminate suffering wherever it may be found. In his history of one of evangelicalism's greatest families, Lyman Beecher Stowe, grandson of Harriet Beecher Stowe, tells the story of Isabella Beecher. A few months before her death in 1907 she said to her granddaughter and namesake, Isabel, "I can't stand all the suffering in the world." Her granddaughter replied,

"Well, grandmother, you have the satisfaction of knowing you have always done more than your share to relieve it."

"That's the point," replied the grandmother. "As long as I could help, I could stand it, but now that I can no longer help, I can't stand it."[65]

The greatest challenge to evangelicalism's tradition of tenderness toward human wreckage, of true cross bearing, may be the current one of AIDS. Will evangelicals stay in there and minister faithfully, even after everyone else leaves in fear, as their ancestors did during the 1832 cholera plague? Will they live up to the standard of Christ invoked by the Christian Medical Dental Society in an 1988 resolution?[66] Will American evangelicals, like their African counterparts, come to see that "sick societies" create their own pathologies as a symptom and symbol of their sickness; and that AIDS victims are in some way enduring the burden of the diseases of that society, with healing possible only when the "community becomes a therapeutic one in which the members act as healers to each other"?[67]

Or will evangelicals be counted among those who dismissed Black Death victims as "wogs" (wrath-of-God syndrome); among those Christians who abandoned diseased relatives and neighbors, leaving the sick to die alone, the dead unburied; among those medieval bishops and monks who resisted using their churches and monasteries for hospitals and secluded themselves instead in communities where the frightened well banded together to isolate themselves from the "sentenced" sick?

The variety of evangelical responses to the December 1986 Surgeon General's report on AIDS gives one pause. The report called for monogamous sexual relationships, condoms for casual sex participants, and early sex education in America's public schools and families. With deep hurt and embarrassment C. Everett Koop had to admit that his strongest criticism and nastiest hate mail came from his own brothers and sisters across America — evangelical Christians.[68] "Choices in plague time," as an article in *Christianity Today* puts it, "are really as old as plague itself. They are the choices of the ancient plague doctor and the enraged and baffled medieval citizenry. When finally confronted by plague, we can each choose to desert, to persecute, or to care."[69]

It is encouraging to note that official public statements on AIDS issuing from evangelical bodies do not portray the disease as God's judgment on AIDS patients. To be sure, evangelicals have not been able to let the AIDS pandemic pass without underlining the morality of traditional sexual patterns and sermonizing about chastity in singleness and fidelity in marriage.

But through their official documents, evangelicals have also been in the forefront of calling for compassion and care and sacrificial service on behalf of those suffering with AIDS.[70]

The intricate, loose strands remaining in evangelicalism's theology of sinning and suffering are once again perhaps best brought together in one of the most remarkable of Wesley's hymns, blatant in its patripassionist portrait of a God who suffers along with the rest of us. Wesley wrote it "For a Sick Friend."

> See, gracious Lord, with pitying eyes,
> Beneath Thy hand a sufferer lies,
> Thy mercy not thine anger proves;
> And sick he is whom Jesus loves.
>
> His to thine own afflictions join,
> Accept, exalt, and count them Thine;
> Thy passion which remains fulfil,
> And suffer in Thy members still.
>
> His sickness feel, endure his pain,
> His burden bear, his cross sustain;
> Grieve in his griefs, and sigh his sighs,
> And breathe his wishes to the skies.
>
> Enter his heart, possess him whole,
> Inspire and actuate his soul;
> Himself no longer let it be
> That suffers, or that lives — but Thee.
>
> Thyself, through sufferings perfect made,
> Conform him thus to Thee his Head;
> Refine, and raise his virtue higher,
> When tried, and purified by fire.[71]

# ·3·

# Weeping and Laughing: "Fer Cryin' Out Loud!"

"You won't make yourself a bit realler by crying," Tweedledee remarked....
"If I wasn't real," Alice said,... "I shouldn't be able to cry."
"I hope you don't suppose those are real tears?" Tweedledum interrupted in a tone of great contempt.

—Lewis Carroll

Laughter and tears...I myself prefer to laugh, since there is less cleaning up to do afterward.

—Kurt Vonnegut

I'd rather be a Baptist and wear a smiling face
Than be a dirty Methodist and fall away from grace.
I'd rather be a Methodist and talk about free-grace
Than be a hard-shell Calvinist and damn near half the race.

—Kentucky mountain hymnbook

Evangelicals use curses as everybody else does. When hammer hits finger, mouth pops open. What evangelicals usually blurt out, however, is not at God's (or anyone's) expense. I learned my locker-room language from my Free Methodist father and Southern Methodist grandfather. "Fiddlesticks!" "Pshaw!" "Horsepuckey!" and "What'n tarnation!" were some of my grandfather's favorite curses. Once I heard my father catch himself with the words "Sometimes, young man, I feel like kicking the...stuffing out of you!" But number one in my father's list of expletives deleted was "Fer cryin' out loud."

Truly, I used to think, this was a Christian obscenity, a curse unbecoming to a believer. Christians are supposed to laugh out loud, not cry out loud. From the throne in heaven, the Lord laughs, Psalm 2:4 proclaims. We are much more comfortable with the notion "God has made me laugh" (Genesis 21:6 NKJV) than we are with the ways God makes us cry. We like the fact that the Scriptures include comic literature (Ruth, Jonah, Ecclesiastes). "Rejoice in the Lord always. I will say it again: Rejoice!" the Bible says in Philippians 4:4.

The Bible also teaches us to "lament in the Lord, sometimes; and again I say: Lament." The Book of Lamentations is in the Bible for a reason. Most evangelical churches have not preserved this lament tradition. It is primarily in the African-American church that the historic evangelical rhythm of weeping and laughing is most carefully safeguarded.

Good Friday and Easter freed a cry and a laugh for all eternity. Of all earthlings, humans are the only creatures that laugh and cry. Is it not conceivable that this ability to express ourselves in laughter and tears may be part of the divine image we carry with us? "Sorrowful, yet always rejoicing" is how Paul describes the state of the Christian (2 Corinthians 6:10). Evangelicals are in the midst of rediscovering their native theology of tears that says with the Psalmist, "My tears have been my food day and night" (42:3).[1]

The task of rediscovery will not be easy. For one thing, as William Blake said, tears are an "intellectual thing." For another, a tearless church reflects a modern tearlessness. The "cool look" of a David Salle postmodernist painting reproduces the stylishly icy and affectless ethos of yuppie culture. Movies are filled with macho displays of stoicism and indomitability. The word *wimp* is now back in circulation, as is what British psychologist Ian Suttie calls the male "taboo on tenderness."[2] Parents join peers in decrying a "cry-baby." Anger is acceptable in the workplace, but tears are not. Former president Ronald Reagan, whom the White House claimed cried only at funerals, denied the rumor that Supreme Court nominee Judge Robert Bork had tears in his eyes when he asked that his nomination be withdrawn. In the words of John Milton's poetic drama *Samson Agonistes*, "Nothing is here for tears."

The equation of tears with weakness is virtually as strong today as it was during the 1972 presidential campaign, when Senator Edmund Muskie lost the Democratic presidential nomination because he wept publicly while defending his wife against scurrilous attacks. It was also in 1972 that Senator Thomas Eagleton was dumped as George McGovern's running mate because the American people could not tolerate as vice president anyone who carried the stigmata of weakness. As recently as 1987, Representative Patricia Schroeder seriously undermined the confidence of the American people in her leadership, reduced her future chances for occupying the White House, provided the women's movement with its "most uncomfortable, embarrassing moment"[3] in years and set the movement back twenty years when she did not hold back the tears during her announcement declining to seek the 1988 Democratic presidential nomination.

At its worst, Americans have wrung their emotions dry, creating a culture of waterproof hearts — except, that is, when technology tosses in the eyewash, and water is wrung from our eyes artificially. At its best, America is a culture of "silent tears" — wanting to cry, needing to cry, but unable to squeeze out tears from eyes that have been dried once too often.

Churches also get embarrassed by the tearjerker. They often prefer the knee slapper and fist pounder. Or even the white knuckler. Alexander Cruden, still honored as the compiler of the standard concordance to the Bible ("Cruden's Concordance" became a household name among English-speaking evangelicals), wrote in 1769, "To laugh is to be merry in a sinful manner." No wonder he ended his life as a litigious, amorous madman.[4] A century later, physician, poet, and humorist Oliver Wendell Holmes admitted he probably would have become a member of the clergy had preachers of his day not looked and acted like undertakers. A century later still, a friend of mine, a retired preacher from the hills of West Virginia, was asked by an usher to leave an Indiana sanctuary when, in the midst of worshipping God, he was moved to tears. Again, except in the African-American religious community, there is a growing tendency for Christians to absent themselves from church the Sunday after a death in the family — for fear they will cry in church.

Evangelicals have found a passage in Augustine's *Confessions* especially helpful in handling their tears. Soon after Augustine's conversion (387 C.E.), the person who had played the most important role in his turning to Christianity — his mother, Monica — died. Yet he suppressed his grief and held back his tears — partly not to spoil his witness to unbelievers, and partly not to display "weakness." The result of Augustine's swallowing his true feelings was a severe depression from which only weeping released him.[5] Congregations have for too long been taught to believe, in the words of the popular gospel song, "Not a doubt nor a fear, / Not a sigh nor a tear / Can abide while we trust and obey" (James H. Sammis, "When We Walk with the Lord"). Criers have been made to feel as out of place as the proverbial "cowbell in a concert" alluded to by Alexander Campbell, founder of Disciples of Christ. What was said of one turn-of-the-century evangelical leader can now be said of too many Christians: "His lachrymal glands were cased in bone, and hard to reach, but God could touch them."[6]

# I

In the evangelical tradition, a tearless church is an unbiblical church. "The Lachrymal excites in us intense and peculiar interest," one evangelical wrote in the mid-nineteenth century, "as it is so intimately associated with the moral man." Tears symbolized for evangelicals the connection between the moral and physical nature. "Tis often said that the 'eye is the window of the soul,'" one evangelical observed in 1849, but "we would add that the tear was the *soul* at the window."[7] For this reason "Chapel of the Air" radio broadcaster David Mains registers his doubt about America being in the midst of a "great revival." If it is true, he asked participants in the annual meeting of the National Association of Evangelicals (NAE), "where are the tears?"[8]

Evangelicals make much of the fact that in the Bible, there is no shame or embarrassment in weeping. The voice of weeping is heard scripturally over and over again. In fact, the problem some Hebrews had with the "weeping prophet" Jeremiah, who wished that his head were an ocean and his eyes a fountain that he might weep night and day for the sins of his people (Jeremiah 9:1), was that they thought he was more concerned about tear ducts than truth. For biblical authors, crying is less a sign of sensitivity than a signature of greatness. Jacob wept and Esau wept. Joseph wept at Jacob's deathbed (Genesis 50:1). In fact, Canaanites observing Jacob's burial were so amazed by all this Israelite crying and their vigorous expression of emotion that they named a place after the event (Genesis 50:11). Jonathan and David wept with each other. David wept over Jonathan's death (2 Samuel 1:12). Saul wept when David did not kill him. Psalm 6:6 says that David flooded his bed with tears. Peter wept after denying Jesus (Matthew 26:75). Jesus found Mary weeping at his tomb (John 11:33). Hebrews 5:7 speaks of Jesus responding "with loud cries and tears." Even Paul, usually not thought of as a particularly sensitive soul, wept, enjoyed being wept over, and enjoined Christians to "weep with them that weep" (Romans 12:15, Authorized Version, hereafter AV). The Bible never says, "Don't weep." The Bible only says, don't "grieve like the rest of men who have no hope" (1 Thessalonians 4:13).

The evangelical tradition goes beyond the belief that crying is normal. It asserts that crying is good for us.[9] Science is now coming around to what evangelicals have always known and prescribed but are increasingly forgetting: the healing power of tears. Medicine as yet does not understand fully the dynamics of tears, but it does know some things. Humans secrete two kinds of tears: reflex tears and emotional tears.

Reflex tears are what we call onion tears, or crocodile tears. Reflex crying is what initiates the breathing process. At birth infants cannot weep emotional tears. This ability normally develops anywhere between the second and twelfth week of life (before laughter, which does not begin until about five months). Emotional tears, or what William Frey and other scientists call "psychogenic lacrimation," differ chemically from reflex tears in a couple of ways.[10] Emotional tears have more protein (no one knows why). Emotional tears also have more toxins — thereby, some have theorized without much clinical data, purging the body of toxins built up under stress. Recent studies have also shown that infants with illnesses that prevent them from shedding tears and relieving the body in this way have a higher death rate; they are unable to handle as much emotional stress as those who can "cry it out."

Crying is good for us. Tears heal. Presidential hopeful Patricia Schroeder's testimony in the *Washington Post* that the tears she shed were tears of "compassion, not weakness" — "No tears, no heart" — bears up under both scientific and theological scrutiny. Sometimes the best advice anyone can give is "cry it out." Weeping can be God's best medicine. Repressed grief is prolonged grief. A blockage of tears can create blockages of the heart, blockages of the intestines, blockages of the brain. Crying reduces stress, releases negative emotions, and removes harmful toxins from the system.

Evangelicals believe that the tears shed by Christians are different from the tears of non-Christians. The church has been given a third kind of tears. The tears of Mother Nature are reflex tears. The tears of human nature are emotional tears. But the tears of God's nature are the gift of tears given to the church. In the words of the eighteenth-century Baptist David Thomas, "lively Christians are apt to weep much."[11] Evangelical Christians historically cry more than others, one nineteenth-century evangelical minister and physician wrote, because "God formed us to weep....There is a blessedness in tears. They raise us nearer to the Divine."[12]

Ascription to the church of the "grace" and "gift" of tears arises not simply from the charismatic wing of evangelicalism but from the customs and culture of the whole evangelical tradition, as well as from the rich theological reflections of the Eastern Christian tradition. Since many of the "grace" and "gift" tear rituals have been lost or forgotten in contemporary evangelical experience, I shall attempt to add to the rediscovery movement by exploring the theological meaning behind what is called the tears of God's nature. I shall be drawing in tandem from sources within evangelicalism and without, especially from the non-Greek, non-Western form of Christian belief and practice known as the Syriac Orthodox tradition, a unique form of Semitic spirituality that bears some marked similarities to evangelical spirituality.

First, the tears of God's nature are the tears of seeing eyes. As long as the eyes are open, one is crying all the time. Tears are what keep the eyelids from turning to sandpaper, and the cornea from becoming raw meat. Water bathes the eyeball, which floats in tears. Tears that run down the cheek are simply tears of overabundance, tears that overflow the eye-sac and spill down the side of the face. The only time one can do without tears is when the eyes are closed. Once the eyes are open, one cries; we are, as the New Zealand poet and playwright James K. Baxter puts it, "Those who are lucky to be sad."[13] The unseeing and unfeeling are the earth's most unfortunate.

The tears of seeing eyes are the tears of repentance. Repentance so over-whelmed St. Paul, the Syrian tradition said, that he was not free from tears for three years because he was unable to suppress them. "I set free the tears...that they might flow at will, spreading them out as a pillow beneath my heart" is how Augustine, a beloved evangelical authority, expressed it in his *Confessions*.[14] Ever since the early nineteenth century this has been sym-bolized in the evangelical tradition by the "mourner's bench" and "altar call." Repentance is to open one's eyes.

Asked what he was doing in the desert, Patriarch Meletios of Antioch (d. 1906) replied, "I came here to weep for my sins." Repentance is to see how far one has fallen from the divine image. "Repentance is to know that there is a lie in your heart," wrote Orthodox priest John of Kronstadt (1829–1908). Opening one's eyes brings the sorrow of repentance. Without sorrow, there can be no salvation. The Syriac Christian tradition speaks of repen-tance as the "baptism of tears," the tears of penitents as "the wine of angels," and the tears of insight into the goodness of God and the rottenness of the human heart as "baptism of the eyes."[15] Even though there is one baptism, St. Ephrem the Syrian wrote, "yet there are two eyes which, when filled with tears, provide a baptismal font for the limbs." Later writers called the tears of repentance that flowed from these two fonts "a second baptism" or a "baptism after the baptism."[16]

A favorite evangelical illustration of the tears of seeing eyes, or the tears of repentance, concerns a backsliding believer expelled from heaven. The only way he could get back in would be to return with a gift God valued most highly. He tried a dog-eared, marked-up, battered old Bible used for many years by a great evangelical pulpiteer. He tried the sandals of a missionary martyred in some foreign field. He tried drops of blood from a dying pa-triot. He tried a widow's mite. He tried many objects of devotion, but each time he was turned away. One day, as he watched a child playing by a foun-tain, he saw a man ride up on horseback and dismount to take a drink. The man's gaze fastened on the child, and suddenly he remembered his boyhood innocence; then he looked into the fountain and saw the reflection of his hardened face. Conscious as never before of the mess he had made of his life, tears of repentance welled up in his eyes and began to trickle down his cheeks. The backslider took one of these tears back to heaven, and the gates of eternity opened wide to reveal God's loving and tender welcome home.

Second, the tears of God's nature are the tears of washing feet. Evangel-icals often link two passages of Scripture: Psalm 56:8, where the psalmist reveals that God collects our tears in a bottle, and Luke 7:37–38, where the woman (a streetwalker) scandalized the disciples by pouring the cruse of precious ointment upon the head of Jesus and by washing Jesus' feet with her tears. Those tears, offered to God in wonder and praise for the gift of the Messiah, were as sweet-smelling a perfume to God as any collected in a bottle.

Many evangelical sermons have been preached on the "tear cup" or "lachrymatory," a long-necked vase found in ancient Roman tombs that was supposedly used by the ancients for depositing mourners' tears at the graveside or by pious Jews symbolically to collect their lifetime release of tears. I remember holding back my own tears as an evangelist described the woman washing Jesus' feet with the tears of her life. All the collected pain of her existence, he said, she poured out at his feet. I shall never forget his suggestion that Jesus may have been referring to his own tear cup when he prayed in Gethsemane that the cup might pass from him, implying that Jesus not only observed this custom but shed a lot of tears.

Actually, evangelical scholars knew as early as the mid-nineteenth century that these so-called tear bottles were really perfume jars or flower vases. Even evangelical reference dictionaries stated that the Psalmist's petition to "Put thou my tears in thy bottle" (Psalm 56:8 AV) was more figurative than anything else. But the sermons kept coming, as the homiletic temptation to turn true stories into tall ones proved irresistible. The popular fiction even showed up in church architecture. I have a photograph of a church rooftop shaped like a tear cup, built to commemorate Jesus weeping over the city.

The tears of washing feet are the tears of worship. Indeed, one reason evangelicals go to church (and some *don't* go) is that church is, or should be, a safe place to have a good cry, to be moved to tears. Tears are as accepted a part of evangelical worship as singing, praying, and laughing. Movie theaters and music halls should not be the only sanctuaries for tears. Just as newborn children weep as they are born into the world, evangelicals have anticipated newborn Christians weeping as they are being reborn into the world to come.

The tears of worship can be prompted by a brief tour of the evangelical gallery of saints. We see there

Thomas, discovering a God who honors doubt in the wounds of Jesus;

Peter, dying from the "Parrot's Perch" torture — upside down, with his whole body weighing on his arms — because he did not feel worthy to be crucified like his Savior;

St. Augustine (354–430), peeling away the gloom of doubt as the light of full certainty infused his heart;

George Whitefield (1714–70), praying in his closing years the constant refrain, "O Lord, grant me a warm heart";

William Wilberforce (1759–1833), pouring out his life for fifty years in the British
    Parliament fighting against the slave traffic, and dying shortly after he saw
    victory assured;

Charlotte Elliott (1789–1871), composing "Just as I Am, without One Plea" after many
    long years of struggle with her physical handicap;

Sojourner Truth (1797?–1883), enraptured by a vision of the "altogether lovely" filling
    her heart with joy and gladness.


In the Bible the tears of worship were most fully expressed by the father of the epileptic boy who cried out "with tears": "Lord, I believe, help
thou mine unbelief" (Mark 9:24 AV). In my own life I have seen the tears
of worship most fully expressed in the experience of seven-year-old Peter
Hodgins (1975–82). No matter how racked with pain from the ravages of
bone cancer and radiation/chemotherapy treatments, he would prop up his
minister-father and family with cheer and courage, praying every night the
prayer he got from some mysterious source: "Lord, camp your angels around
our house, and on our lawn, and on everything that is yours. In Jesus' name."
Just before Peter died, the daughter of a family friend asked me through her
tears what she could do to help. "Why don't you pray for him?" I asked. "But
I *can't* pray for him. I'm too busy crying." She didn't know it, but she already
*was* praying for him. Peter's prayer, and that little girl's crying, prove that
instead of the world being a "vale of tears," as the poet John Keats put it, it
can be a vale of soul-making.

Third, the tears of God's nature are the tears of bloody souls. Gregory
of Nyssa once said that tears are "blood from the wounds of our souls." The
truly wounded people are only those who have, as Welsh poet Dylan Thomas
said of artists and lovers, "their arms / Round the griefs of the ages."[17] And
wounds of love bleed tears.

The tears of bloody souls are the tears of service. One prominent evangelical understanding of the church, in fact, sees the church as the tear in
the eye of culture. In his farewell to the Ephesians (Acts 20:31), Paul testified
to having served them with tears for years. Disciples of Christ, evangelicals
believe, are never without the nimbus of servanthood. A life dedicated to service does not always bring the cup of blessing. Sometimes it brings the bitter
cup; in the words of British poet and novelist W. H. Davies, "Time never
turns a thought to gold, / Unless a tear has made it wet."[18] Luke, chapter 22,
records how angels ministered to Jesus in the Garden of Gethsemane. One
can hardly imagine any higher pastoral care and healing than that. But Jesus'
spirit was still so anguished by the pain of servanthood that he sweat blood.
Hebrews, chapter 5, reveals that in the agony of Gethsemane Jesus offered
prayers with loud cries and tears to the God who could deliver him from the

bitter cup of death. The toll exacted by true servanthood can be measured in beakers of blood and sweat and tears.

Claudia Cassidy was a young doctor, who after submitting her life to Christ, felt the tug of the poor and forgotten of Chile. For treating the medical needs of a Chilean revolutionary leader she was thrown into prison. In her prison cell she wrote this dialogue with herself in which she discovered that the tears of bloody souls are really the tears of the cross:

> You offered yourself freely, did you not? No one forced you?
>
> *Of course!*
>
> Well then? Now your offer's been accepted.
>
> *But I didn't think it would mean this.*
>
> What did you think, then?
>
> *I don't know. I thought it might mean being a famous missionary doctor.*
>
> Perhaps Christ doesn't want you to be a missionary. Not yet, anyway.
>
> *But why?*
>
> Who knows! Perhaps He wants you here among these prisoners. To be a presence, to be a Christ for them.
>
> *But for five years?*
>
> So what. You offered yourself. Was it only a short-term offer?
>
> *No, no! It was for always, anywhere!*
>
> Well, what are you worried about, then...?[19]

Fourth, the tears of God's nature are the tears of shaking heads. The emotional life of Jesus — his anger, joy, humor, depression — is one of the most neglected areas of biblical study. Some biblical writers like Matthew were reluctant to attribute emotions to Jesus. But the gospel records two occasions when Jesus wept. The first was at Bethany, where Jesus' friend Lazarus was buried and "Jesus wept" (John 11:35). The second was on Palm Sunday. "As he approached Jerusalem and saw the city, he wept over it" (Luke 19:41). What caused the tears of Christ as he stood on Mount Olivet and looked out on Jerusalem?

Jesus wept over Jerusalem because he saw a people who needed and wanted God's love but would not receive it at the time it was offered to them. When Jesus looked over the city he did not see men and women in their sins. Jesus saw men and women through their sins. Jesus always saw potential, not actual; destiny in people, not pedigree. He did not see the past of saints, but the future of sinners. Jesus wept, not because of the violence committed by that city in stoning and killing God's prophets, but because that city could not see those things that would bring it peace: "If you, even you, had only known...what would bring you peace" (Luke 19:42). Jesus wept, not for where Jerusalem had been, but for where it was going. Evangelicals' tears of shaking heads are Christ bearing our sins and taking our tears, our sorrows, our pains, our sadness.

Jesus' tears of sadness always turned to tears of joy. So did Peter's tears. And Mary's tears. And the streetwalker's tears. Evangelicals shed tears of sadness so that they may shed tears of joy. It is a "joy-creating sorrow," as St. John Climacus, the seventh-century ascetic from the desert of Sinai, puts it, that not only laughs so hard until it cries, but cries so hard until it laughs.

> Those who sow in tears
>     will reap with songs of joy.
> He who goes out weeping,
>     carrying seed to sow,
> will return with songs of joy,
>     carrying sheaves with him.
>
> (Psalm 126:5–6)

As grace is wrenched from tragedy, as order is created from chaos, as music is conceived from pain, so laughter is harvested from weeping. It is the Gethsemane weepings and the Cana weddings that can teach us to cry, and laugh.

## II

Shortly after Andover Theological Seminary was founded in 1807, the faculty set up a series of evening conferences for the spiritual benefit of the students. At one session Dr. Edwin Dorr Griffin, professor of rhetoric, informed the students he was worried about their thinness and sullenness. Many of them might be a joy to their parents, but they had become a downright despair to their friends and faculty. He attributed the sad state of affairs to the students' neglect of a Christian theology of laughter and proceeded to put them through some hearty calisthenics. Laughter, they were told, was indispensable to a Christian's health.[20]

Many scholars have portrayed both Puritans and evangelicals as people of lemon-sour dispositions and prune-wrinkled personalities who looked like they had been born in crab-apple season. Friedrich Nietzsche, looking at a gloom-bitten portrait of John Calvin, is supposed to have said that God's people should look more redeemed.[21] Charles Dickens, who paid his last visit to America in 1868 at the height of the evangelical era, was asked by reporters what struck him most about the American people; Dickens commented that Americans are not a humorous people. Henry Fielding's widely known jibe at English Methodism in *Tom Jones* (1749) is partly responsible for the image of the evangelical church as, in the words of Evangelical Covenant theologian Karl A. Olsson, "not a party at all, but a drill hall where hilarity is occasional and accidental and where the purpose is to fashion well-disciplined soldiers for the holy war."[22]

The depiction of evangelicals as somber strivers, leery of laughter and jittery at overt expressions of joy in their lives, is, ironically, as wrong as one can get about a tradition that began in protest against fifteenth-century spiritual uptightness and a tradition that to this day loves to sing "Him serve with mirth, / His praise forthtell" ("Old Hundredth"). Jonathan Edwards's father celebrated his son's 1694 ordination into the ministry by hosting a dance as part of the festivities. The problem with the piety of Thomas à Kempis, John Wesley wrote to his mother, was that he had the mistaken notion that mirthfulness was either wanton or wicked. "I can't think that when God sent us into the world he had irreversibly decreed that we should be perpetually miserable in it....Another of his [à Kempis's] tenets, which is indeed a natural consequence of this, is that all mirth is vain and useless, if not sinful. But why then, does the Psalmist so often exhort us to rejoice in the Lord, and tell us that it becomes the just to be joyful?"[23]

Hatred of laughter is not hard to find in the Christian tradition, especially in the early church where "the hilarity of the saints" (Tertullian's phrase) was mainly observed in the breach. To be sure, evangelicalism has drawn its share of people who like their religion strong and bitter, like oversteeped tea. Evangelicals can be found who believe that every word out of the mouth of God was, is, and always shall be deadly serious. How many "celebrants" at the communion table ever truly celebrate?

But it is harder to find a laughterless spirituality in the evangelical tradition than in most other branches of the Christian faith. In fact, evangelicals enjoy quoting Søren Kierkegaard's *Journal* where he calls Christianity "the most humorous view of life in world-history."[24] It is no accident that *The Door*, the radical evangelical journal of religious humor and satire, is without peer or even counterpart in Christianity today. If one does not laugh or at least smile when reading Scripture fairly regularly, most evangelicals have come to believe, one is missing the point.

No one has a greater right to a faith of humor and play than the Christian. Evangelicals have been among the first to see that Christ rebuked the notion that religion, to be genuine, has to be characterized by a morbid or pestilential sadness. The evangelical author Sherwood Eliot Wirt wrote a book designed to straighten the tilted picture of Jesus as a "man of sorrows,

acquainted with grief"; Jesus was just as importantly a *Man of Joy* (1991), acquainted with celebration and jubilation. Wirt calls the unbalanced portrait
"the heresy of the serious."

The Bible suggests that joy may be the only unmistakable, the one in-
fallible sign of the presence of God. "Do not be grieved," reads one of
evangelicalism's all-time favorite Bible verses, "for the joy of the Lord is
your strength" (Nehemiah 8:10). Jesus drenched his disciples in joy: "Be of
good cheer," the first-century version of "Be happy" (John 16:33). "Do not
look somber," Jesus ordered in Matthew 6:16. Then he added the punch line:
"They have received their reward." In other words, some people, Jesus said
playfully, try to look dismal. They then get their reward. They succeed. They
become dull and dismal. The last entry in English novelist and critic George
Orwell's diary reads: "At 50, every man has the face he deserves."

The miscasting of evangelicals centers in the widespread confusion over
what one understands by laughter. Evangelicals have never been inclined to
view laughter as a form of faith. It has been up to others to argue that since
Abraham was the first link in the chain of faith, the second link in that chain,
Abraham's son, is laughter (the meaning of "Isaac"). Not until recently would
evangelicals have fully comprehended the combination in chapter 50 of Carl
Sandburg's biography of Abraham Lincoln, "Lincoln's Laughter — and His
Religion."

Nor have evangelicals been likely to view laughter as a foyer to faith or, in
Kierkegaard's words, the antechamber of faith. In fact, evangelicals are more
likely to point to the paradox of a society more lavishly entertained than ever
before while at the same time more anxious, more depressed, and more suicidal than ever before. Modern society pays premium prices for its humor, the
spiritual sedative of a market economy. Some of the most highly paid persons
in Western culture today are entertainers. The entertainers in the medieval
period were called court jesters. They were brought in after royal meals
to induce laughter among the diners, because it was believed that laughter
aided digestion. But these medieval jesters were not elevated to the highest social positions — they resided within the servants' quarters. The power
of the technomythic industry and the commercialization of laughter is such
that entertainers today are the idols of a culture requiring the ministrations
of a commercial priesthood of professional jokesters and entertainers.

This kind of laughter still aids digestion, evangelicals believe, but it di-
gests the believer into a demeaning if not demonic world of compliance and
consumption that one is to be in but not of. It was this principle that caused
my parents to prohibit any of us from participating in school activities that
smacked of worldliness. I shall never forget the embarrassment of having
to obtain written permission from a physician to be excused from square-

dancing classes in grade school. Part of evangelicalism's pugilistic stance toward the entertainment industry — at various points in its history taking swipes at worldly amusements like dancing,[25] card playing, even novel reading, and giving nasty chops at movies, television, and theater — was that these were seen as ersatz excitements. The soul would become unsettled with counterfeit pleasures — the stimulus of materialism, softness, hedonism, hypocrisy — instead of the stimulation of honesty, discipline, worship, and work. Merchandised laughter is slaughter to a spirit of holiness "unto the Lord" and a mind "set on things above."

Not surprisingly, evangelicals have been the last to see Jesus as a jokester himself or to confuse, as one church bulletin board did with a sermon title, "The Divine Comedown" with "The Divine Comedian." The biblical outlook has sensitized evangelicals to laughter as one of the most potent of all social forces and as something not to be sought for its own sake. Jesus began his ministry as the brunt of jokes (Luke 4:22–24). Jesus ended his ministry as a laughingstock — first to the Roman soldiers, symbols of political power; then to the common folk, seed of God's chosen people who deserted Jesus and retaliated in face-saving taunts; then to the religious establishment, who jabbed Jesus with jokes and stabbed him with derision; and finally even to the bandits who were crucified with him (Matthew 27:27–44).

But evangelicals have also been the first to appreciate what theologian Conrad Hyers calls the "grand parenthesis" of Jesus' earthly ministry: he began it all at the party in Cana, and he ended it all at the festivals of Easter and Pentecost. For evangelicals laughter is not a product one pays for like everything else. It is rather a by-product of a life freed from the shackles of sin and selfishness and guilt, a function of faith that soothes the spirit, stimulates the mind, activates the hands, and maybe even settles the stomach. Elton Trueblood used to say over dinner with friends, "Isn't it fun to be a Christian!"[26]

In the prologue to his 1525 English translation of the Second Testament, William Tyndale defined the Greek word for "Gospell" or "Good News": "Evangelion (that we call the gospel) is a Greek word; and signifieth good, merry, glad and joyfull tydinge, that maketh a manness hert glad, and maketh him synge, dance, and leepe for joye."[27] Laughter is a by-product of the joy of living the abundant life, the fruit of faith. Or in the poet Isaac Watts's words that evangelicals love to sing each Christmas, Jesus brought "Joy to the World" and caused all of creation to "repeat the sounding joy."

It often strikes people oddly that evangelicals will laugh in situations that others find too tragic or terrible for laughter. The degree to which evangelicals are able to laugh and keep a sense of humor, even in times of immense suffering and pain, comes as a surprise to health-care professionals. Indeed, the density of darkness in the world today is almost enough to make one a principled pessimist, or at least to agree with the playwright Bertolt Brecht that the person who is still laughing has simply not yet heard the terrible news.

Evangelical cheerfulness, however, is more than a chirpy, chin-up attitude in the face of adversity. It is more than being trained in the art of concealing one's feelings, of maintaining composure even under trying circumstances. How could Jesus endure the cross? Hebrews 12 gives the answer: "because of the joy that was set before him." The gospel remakes a person into a joyful being and a thorough optimist.

This theme of optimism was set by an evangelical editor who wrote in 1899 a column entitled "Should a Christian Ever Laugh?" While "earnestness" and "serious business" properly characterize the Christian's approach to life, the fact that "God lives" and "All is for the best" means that a grim, gloomy faith is an affront against God, especially in times of crisis. "Who knows whether Christ ever laughed?" the author concluded. But "if he did not, he is not necessarily an example unto us in that particular."[28] (Comedian Robin Williams reaches the same conclusion about how hope and humor go together — comedy is "acting out optimism.")

Evangelicals are more likely to agree with Quaker theologian Elton Trueblood's popular book *The Humor of Christ* (1964), which isolates thirty-one instances where Christ used humor, than they are to agree with Anthony M. Ludovicki, who speaks for many readers of Scripture when he insists that "there is not a joke in the whole of the New Testament."[29] Psychologist Robert C. Roberts has argued that God's omniscience is not incompatible with a divine sense of humor, a sense of humor that confronts evil with satire, sarcasm, irony, and derisive laughter.[30] Evangelicals have also done the most to preserve the medieval notion, perpetuated by Protestant reformers such as Martin Luther, that the devil cannot tolerate being laughed at or mocked, for laughter exposes the devil's weakness.[31] Love and laughter: two ways to conquer evil.

The role of humor as a hormone that has both psychological and physiological effects was not discovered by former *Saturday Review* editor Norman Cousins in 1964, who laughed until the laughter healed, organized laughfests in hospitals, and then wrote about humor therapy fifteen years later in *The Anatomy of an Illness* (1979). Many evangelicals believed in the healing properties of laughter from an early date, based on biblical proverbs: "A cheerful heart is a good medicine, but a crushed spirit dries up the bones" (Proverbs 17:22); "Pleasant words are like a honeycomb, sweetness to the soul and health to the body" (Proverbs 16:24). On such foundations Sylvester Graham based his famous declaration that "occasional hilarity and a hearty laugh, healthfully exhilarate and exercise the whole system."[32]

Early into his popular study of the connections between laughter and healing, evangelical Donald E. Demaray cites Mark Twain's *Adventures of Tom Sawyer* (1876), where the story is told about Huckleberry Finn and the old Welshman who "laughed loud and joyously, shook up the details of his anatomy from head to foot, and ended by saying that such a laugh was 'money in a man's pocket, because it cut down the doctor's bill like everything.'"[33] Citing humor as "a wind break for weathering the storm" (Sherwood Eliot Wirt), evangelicals have a long tradition of seeing positive therapeutic links between laughter and the body's physiological functioning. Recent research showing laughter stimulating heart and blood circulation, promoting enhanced respiration, and accelerating the immune system comes as confirmation to a tradition that has lauded the funny bone as connected to the cerebrum, and the cerebrum as connected to the cardiovascular system, and so forth.

Evangelicals are notorious for appropriating laughter's therapeutic value, especially in worship, where they historically have mocked "straight-jacket, tight-laced, cut-and-dried" sermons, as Texas Baptist pioneer preacher Z. N. Morrell put it.[34] They even employed laughter as part of their grief therapy, which in earlier days was called a wake. And increasingly evangelicals can be found appropriating laughter in recovery therapy, a position outlined by the thirteenth-century professor of surgery Henry de Mandeville, who insisted that physicians had an ethical responsibility to patients recovering from surgery to see that family and friends were cheerful and cheering even to the point of sitting down and telling jokes to the patient.

Just as Martin Luther wondered why the devil should get all the good tunes, so Plymouth Church pastor Henry Ward Beecher used to ask why the devil should get all the good jokes.[35] In the African-American evangelical tradition laughter was used by storytelling, sing-songing preachers to give slaves hope and inspiration. Even into the twentieth century, African-American preachers like Georgia's Marshall Keeble used humor and wit to counteract prejudice and even to get whites to laugh at their own racial stereotypes. The use of humor to provoke serious thought is illustrated in one of Keeble's famous openings at a 1964 Texas tent revival: "I'm preaching the gospel in this meeting...so that if a man wants to go to hell, he'll go there with his eyes wide open. Man going to hell, ought to *see* his way down there."[36]

The frontier camp meeting generated many humorous stories and irreverent jokes. "The big revival meeting at the brush arbor tabernacle was a success," one newspaper account read. "We had one conversion, three weddings and seven fights. We were left with more roosters in our flock than last year." Evangelicals received no end of pleasure in telling one another camp-meeting stories about "Uncle Hod, who got religion but lost it on the way home when his buggy broke down" or about "the cripple who, when called on to testify what the Lord had done for him, said, 'He darn near ruint me.'"[37] Early camp meetings themselves were sometimes conducted above the din of "holy laughter," a constant hum of laughing and chuckling that was known to grip worshippers caught up in the beatific joy of the revival.[38]

Theologian Douglas G. Adams has demonstrated conclusively the error of stereotyping eighteenth- and nineteenth-century evangelical preachers as humorless. In fact, one nineteenth-century historian called American Methodist preachers "the greatest wits of the last century in the new world."[39] A diverse array of purposeful humor, most of which was edited out of the public record, was used by evangelical preachers to exercise crowd control, to communicate threatening ideas, and to defend controversial issues — as when itinerant Peter Cartwright, known for his hair-trigger laugh, came to the issue of Methodism's highly trained but poorly educated preachers in this classic exchange: "A prominent divine of another denomination, meaning to be slightly sarcastic, once said to my old friend Mr. Cartwright: 'How is it that you have no doctors of divinity in your denomination?' 'Our divinity is not sick and don't need doctoring,' said the sturdy backwoodsman."[40] But humor in nineteenth-century evangelical pulpits was as natural as it was purposeful — extempore, homey, and matter-of-fact, as matter-of-fact as the circuit rider who used his bowie knife and derringer as paperweights to keep his Bible open on the text while preaching in a windstorm.[41] Beecher himself used humorous illustrations that he believed were good for both community and character building. The two most famous evangelists of the late nineteenth century, Dwight L. Moody in America and Charles H. Spurgeon in England, were both noted for their anecdotal antics. After Moody, humor became a standard feature of the repertoire of evangelical preachers, and the preaching pattern of "a joke, three points, and a deathbed tale" became almost normative. Jokes were now told intentionally to provoke congregational responsiveness, ridicule worldly pretensions, and prod evangelicals toward greater heights of faith.[42] The story of the lazy believer who nailed the Lord's Prayer on the wall at the foot of his bed and who, after falling into bed, was accustomed to say, "Lord, them's my sentiments," was but one example of how humor was used as a behavior modification device.

In fact, the extent of "the increase of levity and fun-making" in late-nineteenth-century evangelical pulpits began to make some leaders nervous about proprieties of public worship being compromised by the church having "caught the funny spirit of the time." W. P. Harrison, the editor of a Southern evangelical periodical, bemoaned the way "preachers are introducing the fopperies of the amusement hall and the oddities of jest-books and comic almanacs into our pulpits" while at the same time disregarding doctrinal preaching and theological instruction. "The house of God is not the place for laughter," he charged, condemning Henry Ward Beecher's Plymouth Church (Brooklyn) in particular and the popularity among evangelicals of "pulpit pleasantry" in general.[43]

The more evangelicals learned the role of laughter as a catalytic agent of personal and social change, the more they began using Jesus himself as an example of someone with a healthy laugh life.[44] The ability to laugh at oneself, an index of a hale and hearty spirituality, evangelicals find evidenced by Jesus in his attitude toward crowds. Everyone loves a big crowd, especially politicians and preachers who are tempted to measure their effectiveness by the number of occupied seats. The big crowds Jesus drew impressed his disciples. But not Jesus. "Wherever there is a carcass, [Jesus said] there the vultures will gather" (Matthew 24:28). There is more than one reason why a crowd assembles, and large numbers may mean something good, or they may not. Evangelicals believe that only the forgiven can truly laugh at themselves, for only with forgiveness can one learn to love oneself. Forgiveness is the tie that binds love and laughter together, allowing Christians to laugh in love.

When I turned five, my parents enrolled me in Bible Memory Association (BMA), a fundamentalist Baptist organization devoted to encouraging Bible memorization among evangelical children and teenagers. If I could recite perfectly twelve verses a week for twelve weeks straight, I was rewarded with a free week at a BMA summer camp. When I returned home after my first trip to "Miracle Camp," I could not stop singing and humming a song the camp director taught us the first day we were there. It is where I first discovered how faith brings back the giggle and gives adults the freedom to embrace and express the inner child through laughter, play, and touching, all of which promote wellness and wholeness. It is also where I began perceiving the smile as really the laugh's whisper.

> You can smile, when you can't say a word
> You can smile, when you cannot be heard
> You can smile, when it's cloudy or fair
> You can smile, anytime, anywhere.

Evangelicals like to smile and laugh a lot, because they have a great deal to smile and laugh about: Jesus, the "joy of our desiring"; resurrection, the punch line of our faith. As Jesus put it himself in these words from the Gospel of John, chapter 16: "In this world you will have trouble. But take heart [that is, *laugh*]! I have overcome the world." Laughter, in the words of one evangelical, is "the rainbow that arches the tears of humanity."[45]

# ·4·

# Sleeping and Dreaming: "Nearer, My God, to Thee"

In a dream, in a vision of the night, when deep sleep falleth upon men, in slumbering upon the bed; then he openeth the ears of men, and sealeth their instruction.

—Job 33:15

Sleep faster. We need the pillows.

—Yiddish proverb

An unexamined dream is like an unopened letter.

—the Talmud

Sleep is such a dull, stupid state of existence, that, even among mere animals, we despise them most which are most drowsy.

—William Law

While I do rest my soul advance:
Make my sleep an holy trance.

—Philip Toynbee

Since we spend something close to a third of our lives in sleep, one would expect that we have extensive knowledge about this mindbody activity. But our ignorance about the natural purposes of sleep is so great that, in spite of burgeoning sleep clinics, sleep laboratories, and more and more bizarre sleep disorders, one of the few things medical specialists in somnology (the scientific study of sleep physiology) can agree on is that we sleep to overcome the sleepiness induced by inadequate sleep.

Throughout much of the evangelical tradition, sleep has been viewed as a regrettable accomplice to waking health. Resentment of sleep now appears as one of the dried fruits in the fashionable contemporary cornucopia of evangelical offerings. But in many evangelical circles this residual tendency to regard sleep with something less than unqualified approbation can still be found. Brandishing its Puritan connection, evangelicalism followed in a long but narrow line of Christian tradition that viewed sleep as wasted time at best, at worst the source of "countless evils," in the words of John Milton: "It dulls and blunts the active mind and is the greatest hindrance to good memory; and what can be more shameful than to snore late into the day and to devote the greatest part of your life to a sort of death."[1]

Evangelicalism inherited from Puritanism a peculiarly negative attitude toward waste, especially waste of time. *Acedia* or sloth may be number four in extant listings of the seven deadly sins, but in the evangelical tradition sloth and every other deadly sin grow up together. Oriented to keeping people awake, evangelicals have been largely opposed to putting people to sleep chemically. Only reluctantly do evangelicals sidle up to the over sixty prescription drugs sold to induce sleep, the most widely taken drugs for other than nonrecreational purposes.

Evangelicals have seldom plumped for sleep for sleep's sake or touted the blessing of sleep as a spiritual gift. To the contrary, the gospel promises a time when "we will not all sleep, but we will all be changed" (1 Corinthians 15:51 NIV). Totally missing in the evangelical tradition are the celebrations of sleep that one finds throughout Western literature. Petrarch's classic look at the bleaker side of sleep could represent evangelicalism's attitudes for much of its history even if Petrarch's example of going to bed in the evening and getting up at midnight could not.

> Too much sleep is the source of vice and infamy, which driveth many headlong and throweth them into perpetual sleep! For it nourisheth lust, maketh heavy the body, weakeneth the mind, dulleth the wit, extinguisheth the memory, diminisheth knowledge, and breedeth stupidity; so that it is not without cause the wakeful and industrious persons are commended: sleep is death, and wakefulness life; take heed then of life and death which thou dost choose! Those who wake early do live the longer.[2]

## I

Of all the branches of the Christian faith, evangelicals have done the most to realize the motto of the Pinkerton Detective Agency: "We Never Sleep." The Methodists played a signal role in setting and then pampering evangelicalism's pet prejudice against sleep, but they did so by invoking Puritan examples and models. John Wesley's classic sermon "On Redeeming the Time" was dedicated exclusively to redeeming the time from sleep. Admitting the necessity of sleep as a requirement of nature that brings "health and vigor both of the body and mind," Wesley spent the bulk of the sermon itemizing the harm done to one's spiritual state, financial position, and physical health by sleeping one minute longer than nature requires: "By *soaking* (as it is emphatically called) so long between warm sheets, the flesh is, as it were, parboiled, and becomes soft and flabby. The nerves, in the mean time, are quite unstrung, and all the train of melancholy symptoms — faintness, tremors, lowness of spirits, (so called) — come on, till life itself is a burden."[3]

Some more liturgically minded evangelicals found theological significance in the near coincidence of St. Luke's day (18 October) and Edison's invention of the light bulb (19 October 1879). It almost seemed as if the festival of the beloved physician had ushered in the doubling of the human lifespan in one technological innovation. Whatever remained of medieval antipathy to working by candlelight, or after "vespers" (and evening services), was finally dispelled by the turning of night into day by electric light.[4] Electric light made possible new ways of organizing the hours of the day and our activities. Today, one regression analysis reveals, a significant portion of sleep time has become simply a matter of economic discretion.[5]

Evangelicals were the pioneers in "sleep restriction" regimens. They adopted all sorts of devices to limit the number of hours of sleep. Perhaps the most popular were customs of early rising. John Wesley set the pace by rising earlier and earlier every morning until he pushed the alarm clock back to 4 A.M. (retiring at 10 P.M.).[6] Grahamite boarding houses, following the teachings of health reformer Sylvester Graham, rang the bell at 5 A.M. and locked the doors at 10 P.M. Dwight L. Moody usually rose at 5 A.M. and "did not need much sleep."[7] Billy Sunday is said to have averaged no more than five hours' sleep a night.[8] The Shakers arose at 5:30 every morning and did all they could to make a little sleep go a long way. In *The American Woman's Home*, Catharine E. Beecher and Harriet Beecher Stowe argue for early rising as a standard of living and set a maximum limit of eight hours' sleep a night, a bracingly low number considering the fact that the typical person in the eighteenth and nineteenth centuries slept 9½ hours each night. (This average had fallen to just under eight hours by the 1950s, and it continues to decline.) Anything more than eight hours, they admonished, was injurious to health.[9]

"Next to intemperance, a quiet conscience, a cheerful mind and active habits," an evangelical columnist wrote in 1845, "I place early rising as a means of health and happiness."[10] The penalty of staying out late attending theater, balls, and parties was poor health.[11]

The evangelical tradition spawned numerous experiments in millennial living, and many of these communitarian movements actually regulated the hours of sleep members of the community could take. The Ephrata Community strictly enforced a limit of three hours of sleep each night.[12] When Oberlin College opened its doors in 1834, students were required to follow Sylvester Graham's recommendation for limiting sleep to seven hours and "keep their beds from 10 o'clock P.M. to 5 o'clock A.M."[13] Charles Fourier proposed a daily schedule for his "Harmonians, many of whom came from evangelical denominations," where sleep was allowed from 10:30 P.M. to 3 A.M. Sleep fasting was practiced by Wesley's friend and successor John Fletcher, who trained himself to sleep only when he could not keep awake. Twice every week he prayed and meditated all night.[14] Attempts to alter sleep patterns are not as common in the evangelical tradition as disciplined efforts at reduced sleep. The scholar Mircea Eliade, who had so much trouble understanding evangelicals, was more like them than he realized when he made do with less sleep, beginning at age 14, by going to sleep five minutes later each night and setting his alarm clock to wake up five minutes earlier each morning until he diminished his sleep time to only four hours a night.

Why have evangelicals fought sleep? First, the Bible does not have many nice things to say about sleep. The Book of Proverbs warns the young Hebrews: "Allow no sleep to your eyes, no slumber to your eyelids" (6:4 NIV). "Go ahead and be lazy," says another proverb. "Sleep on, but you will go hungry" (19:15, Today's English Version, hereafter TEV). A similar sentiment can be found in Proverbs 20:13: "Spend your time sleeping, and you will be poor. Keep busy, and you will have plenty to eat" (TEV). The sluggard is defined in Proverbs 26:14 by his devotion to sleep: "As a door turns on its hinges [that is, without leaving them], so a sluggard turns on his bed." The biblical portrayal of God as neither slumbering nor sleeping (Psalm 121:4) finds its obverse side in Jesus' use of the image of the sleeping man for the spiritual dolt or spiritually indolent: "Therefore, keep awake....If he comes suddenly, do not let him find you sleeping" (Mark 13:35–36 NIV).

Second, both Jesus and Paul used sleep as a metaphor for death, as when Jesus spoke of Jarius's daughter among "those who have fallen asleep" (Luke 8:52). Sleep stood for a little death, and death stood for "sleeping the Big Sleep" in novelist Raymond Chandler's words. Evangelicals' resentment of sleep was in some fashion therefore an affirmation of the resurrection of the dead — here and now.

Third, just as death was never for the evangelical an escape mechanism, so sleep was warned against as a coping mechanism that served as a substitute for dealing with the problems and complexities of the workaday world. In a 1781 letter Wesley warned his niece Sarah against "intemperance in sleep" and attributed all sorts of "nervous diseases," mental disorders, and bodily malfunctions to long sleeping.[15] Evangelicals felt more confirmed than ever in their opposition to excessive sleep when they heard sentiments like that of the eighteenth-century epigrammist Sébastien Chamfort, "To live is a malady from which sleep vouchsafes us relief every sixteen hours. That is a palliative. The remedy is death" or Nietzsche's "No small art it is to sleep: it is necessary to keep awake all day for that purpose."[16]

Fourth, sleeping behavior became for evangelicals an index to character. There was no clearer mark of idleness and self-indulgence, "an inert and feeble mind, infirm of purpose," than long and late sleeping.[17] Tongue-in-cheek, they even dubbed the sleeping sickness that overtook many people on the first day of the week, immobilizing them in bed but never lasting as long as twenty-four hours, the "Sunday sickness" or "worldly fever."[18] The experience of Hester Anne Rogers (1756–95) reflected the evangelical link between sleep patterns and character. Rogers's popular journal became a model of piety for nineteenth-century evangelicals; in fact, the influential theologian Nathan Bangs praised her as "standing first on the list of Christian women" in modern times and recommended her biography to all who "wish to dive into the depths of perfect love, and to become eminently useful."[19] Rogers testified to having trouble sleeping before her conversion. But after the change in her spiritual condition, and her subsequent marriage to a Methodist itinerant, she slept less than ever before because of her "happiness," her "usefulness," and her "communion with God."[20] It was dullness of the head, coldness of the heart, that induced sleep.

Fifth, "Nature's Laws" taught that an hour's sleep before midnight is worth two after it, and evangelicals agreed with Benjamin Franklin that "Early to bed and early to rise, / Makes a man *healthy,* wealthy, and wise."[21] An 1849 article entitled "Hints on Sleep" from the *Water Cure Journal* was widely reported in evangelical periodicals. It lectured against lingering in bed because "breathing the air continually over and over again, renders it a perfect poison." It warned against feather beds and feather pillows, calling them "among the greatest causes of physical debility, horrible dreams, nightmares, and the most unrefreshing sleep that can be." If evangelicals were not to live in opposition to nature, they must "rise, wash, drink some cold water, and if possible go into the open air" immediately upon awakening.[22]

Sleep, then, has been less a blessing for evangelicals, in and of itself, than a source of blessings and of gifts unavailable any other way. "For [God] grants sleep to those he loves" (Psalm 127:2). What are these gifts that evangelicals see coming to them from sleep? First, evangelicals admitted the need for nightly rebirth and recognized that sleep offers physical renewal, as the body is renewed and damaged tissues repaired. And sleep offers mental renewal, as it divides life up into manageable portions so that we can deal with it better. The mind would break down under unremitting consciousness, evangelicals warned, as do cities (like New York City) that never sleep. Evangelicals believed in the renewing powers of sleep described by Shakespeare:

> Sleep that knits up the ravell'd sleave of care,
> The death of each day's life, sore labour's bath,
> Balm of hurt minds, great nature's second course,
> Chief nourisher in life's feast.[23]

Sleep could also be a time of spiritual growth and rebirth, but only if it could be brought "under subjection." There is perhaps no greater evidence for the extent of evangelicalism's emphasis on self-discipline and self-control than its attempt to bring under control the Christian's double-life, or unconscious self.

Evangelical faith works and thinks in the night, indeed through the night. Wesley asked one of his workers, "Does God bid you even in sleep go on?"[24] Faith could move forward even in sleep through a variety of what evangelicals came to call "night watches," a phrase first introduced in Psalm 63:6 (NIV): "On my bed I remember you; I think of you through the watches of the night." "Night watches" included meditation, prayer, dreams, and visions. Like dolphins who never sleep — even during its "naps," half of the dolphin's brain stays awake — the soul is always stocking its supplies, even in sleep.

## II

It is how Albert Einstein thought of the theory of relativity. It is how Abraham Lincoln learned the details of his death by an assassin's bullet shortly before he was killed. It is how novelist William Makepeace Thackeray got the title for his novel *Vanity Fair*. It is how Samuel Taylor Coleridge wrote large portions of "Kubla Khan" and other poems. It is how Robert Louis Stevenson conceived the plot for *Dr. Jekyll and Mr. Hyde*. It is how violinist Guiseppe Tartini composed his famous "Devil's Sonata." It is how Elias Howe decided where to put the eye of the needle while inventing the sewing machine. It is how Samuel Thomson was recruited to take on the dominant therapeutic system of nineteenth-century medicine, seeking to replace it with his own root and herb medical system. It is how Jack Nicklaus thought of a new way to hold his golf club, getting him out of his famous slump in 1964. It is how Friedrich A. Kekulé von Stradonitz discovered the benzene ring, one of the foundations of modern chemistry. The "it," of course, is dreaming.[25] The domain of dreams is the script of destiny.

My two brothers and I grew up in the Mohawk Valley region of upstate New York. Each summer, usually on our way to camp meeting, my history-buff father would stop at the home and fort of Sir William Johnson (1715–74), proprietor of one of the largest estates in the English colonies. (Indeed, there didn't seem to be any historical marker or site we didn't stop to see and photograph.) The story of how Sir William got this immense tract of land from the Mohawk people never failed to fascinate. The Mohawks placed great importance on dreams. Like the Iroquois of New York, they believed that dreams were among their truest friends. They taught their children to value their dreams, to ask their dreams for help, to learn the language of dream symbolism, and to heed what they had to say. Dreams provided Mohawks and Iroquois with direction and assistance — regulating their feasts, dances, games, and hunts, ritualizing every aspect of their life, and giving rein to their terrors, lust, aggression, and irrationalities in nondestructive channels.

Feigning a similar faith in dreams, Johnson began confirming their dreams. When talk was of dreams about tobacco, Johnson gave tobacco to them. When the chief of the Mohawk tribe dreamed that if only he possessed the military apparel of Johnson, he would be as great a leader as King George, again Johnson obliged. Soon it became Johnson's turn to dream. Johnson dreamed that in kindness the Mohawks gave him a large tract of land. The chief of the Mohawks confirmed his dream by giving him sixty-six thousand acres.[26]

I thought of the Native Americans' faith in dreams when we got to camp meeting. When people there stood up and gave their testimony of hearing God's voice speak to them, when saints danced their "sanctified stomp" of praise for night-watch victories and "holyghost showers," when preachers offered vivid accounts of appearances and awakenings, when sickbed stories circulated about ethereal visions and visitations,[27] somehow I knew that my own religious tribe was translating into waking language its moon and starlight experiences.

Evangelicals' greatest desire is, in the words of the popular Stuart Hamblen and George Beverly Shea song, "Just a Closer Walk with Thee." The Bible opens us up to the possibility that a walk with Jesus, getting closer to God, can begin anywhere — not only through "churchy" things like sermons or a visit from a deacon. It began for Moses when he stood in front of an ordinary bush (Exodus 3:2). It happened to Gideon while he was threshing wheat (Judges 6:11). It happened to the disciples while they were fishing (John 21:4–5). It happened to Jacob while he slept on a stone pillow in the desert (Genesis 28:12); for during that sleep, Jacob met God in a dream. Or as evangelicals like to sing: "Yet in my dreams I'd be / nearer, my God, to thee; nearer to thee!"[28]

It has become quite fashionable today to "believe in dreams." Many people are learning how to break down these "bubbles" of soul thoughts "breaking on the surface from the deep below." A person spends some six years of life engaged in dreaming. Many scholars are studying the imaginative activity of this nocturnal self. W. H. Auden praised Sigmund Freud for teaching us to tend our "subliminal uprushes" and steward our sleepthink:

> But he would have us remember most of all
> To be enthusiastic over the night
>   Not only for the sake of wonder
>   It alone has to offer, but also
> Because it needs our love.[29]

Ever since Freud's classic study *The Interpretation of Dreams* (1899), dream theory has rocked generation after generation of theological hardhats. Evangelicals, however, found Freud guilty of a taxonomic error in describing dreams as abnormal psychic phenomena. Even their cursory reading of Scripture revealed the communications function of dreams and tutored them to look at dreams as God speaking or the mind thinking or the self talking to itself while asleep, an imaginative form of storytelling to ourselves. The evangelical mind has been predisposed to find significant self-revelations in the nightmares that swarm out of sleep. In fact, dream chic is so prevalent today in evangelical circles that one can identify with Francisco Umbral's exasperation in calling dreams nothing more than a "messy pile of rubble...To hell with Freud."[30]

Dreams are intrinsically personal myths where the individual is author, actor, audience, and critic all at once. We have been encouraged to interpret dreams, sometimes through the ancient "symbolic" or "decoding" methods of discovering meaning in dreams, sometimes through the modern depth psychology approaches. We have been warned to stop exorcising dreams as we used to exorcise demons. To the extent we are successful in getting rid of our dreams, either flushing them out of our system or repressing them, we succeed in wiping out a language Erich Fromm would call "God's forgotten language," a lost language through which God speaks in myths, in symbols, in alien accents we ignore at our peril.[31]

Even during periods in our cultural history when Americans had the impression that in our dreams we got nearer to the devil than to God, evangelical communions, especially popular evangelical culture, retained the biblical witness that God uses dreams to provide creative inspiration, to increase awareness of the divine, even to solve problems. Evangelicals cut their theological teeth reading the conversion stories of John Bunyan, John New-ton, James Gardiner, and Alexander Duff, all of which gave prominent place to the role of "converting dreams." Charles G. Finney testified publicly to a number of dreams and visions in his autobiography.[32] Horace Bushnell used dreams as evidence that the supernatural was not put to sleep with the apostolic age.[33] A dream kept evangelical theologian Nathan Bangs in ministry when he wanted to give it up; early in his ministry, Bangs became despondent because of the numerous difficulties he experienced and he resolved to abandon the ministry.

> A significant dream relieved him. He thought he was working with a pickax on the top of a basaltic rock. His muscular arm brought down stroke after stroke for hours; but the rock was hardly indented. He said to himself at last, "It is useless; I will pick no more." Suddenly a stranger of dignified mien stood by his side and spoke to him. "You will pick no more?" "No." "Were you not set to this task?" "Yes." "And why abandon it?" "My work is vain; I make no impression on the rock." Solemnly the stranger replied, "What is that to you? Your duty is to pick, whether the rock yields or not. Your work is in your own hands; the result is not. Work on!" He resumed his task. The first blow was given with almost superhuman force, and the rock flew into a thousand pieces. He awoke, pursued his way back…with fresh zeal and energy, and a great revival followed. From that day he never had even a "temptation" to give up his commission.[34]

The more evangelicals have worked the same fields as Pentecostals and neo-Pentecostals, the more likely they have been to fidget nervously and resist receiving these images from God, and the more likely they have been to view dreams and visions as the products of an overheated imagination.

But even that most quarrelsome friend of evangelical truth, theologian Benjamin B. Warfield, argued for "the fitness of dreams to serve as media of divine communications." Warfield admitted that this position "constitutes more or less of a stumbling block to most readers of the Bible" — all the while being careful to distinguish the biblical view of dreams from the superstitious usage of dreams among ancient and folk cultures.[35] Although dreams and visions, or what were called "internal suggestions," characterized the second or "prophetic" age, all three modes of revelation occur in every age and they "occur side by side, broadly speaking, on the same level," Warfield contended. "There is no age in the history of the religion of the Bible, from that of Moses to that of Christ and His apostles, in which all these modes of revelation do not find place."[36] For many evangelicals, visions, visitations, dreams and daydreams were signatures of the Spirit.

I remember being assigned in Sunday school the task of conducting a dream census of the Bible; I discovered that a great part of the Bible is

God speaking to people through dreams. The Book of Genesis is filled with dream material like Jacob's ladder (28:12) or Joseph's speech at Pharaoh's court (41:25–36). Solomon receives the gift of wisdom in a dream (1 Kings 3:5–15). Jeremiah condemns false dream interpreters (Jeremiah 23:25–28; 27:9; 29:8–9), and Daniel interprets Nebuchadnezzar's dreams (Daniel 2 and 4). The first two chapters of Matthew contain no fewer than five dreams. It was a dream that told Joseph to wed the pregnant Mary (1:20). It was a dream that warned the wise men of Herod's intentions (2:12). It was a dream that alerted Joseph to flee with his family to Egypt (2:13), another dream that told them when it was safe to return (2:19), and yet another that led them to settle in Galilee (2:22). It was a dream that so worried Pilate's wife that she cautioned her husband not to lay a hand on this man Jesus (Matthew 27:19). The Bible closes with the Apocalypse of John, a book which in its entirety is a dream. If the Bible were to be purged of the story of God's breakthrough into the human conscious mind via the unconscious, there would be very little left. As Tertullian, lawyer and Latin scholar, noted long ago in his study of dreams entitled *A Treatise on the Soul,* "Almost the greater part of mankind get their knowledge of God from dreams."[37]

Evangelicals are taught that God wants to speak to us today as God spoke to Abraham, Isaac, and Jacob, to Daniel, Jeremiah, and Isaiah. Our problem is that we have not disciplined ourselves to learn the divine languages. In fact, Dale W. Brown states that "the first special gift of the Spirit in the Bible may have been the endowing of Joseph with the gift of interpreting dreams for the common good."[38] Every healthy person still dreams while sleeping. Four or five times a night we dream, whether or not we remember or interpret the dreams. One of the exciting discoveries of the 1950s took place when an American researcher noticed flickerings of the eyeballs under the lids of a sleeping baby. These rapid eye moments (REMs) reveal the phase of our sleeping when we dream; people awakened during REM sleep will usually be able to tell what they were dreaming.

The only people who do not dream are schizophrenics. Their waking life becomes their nightmare. Dreams are essential for normal, healthy human beings because dreams enable us to go safely insane every night of the week. Similarly, dreams can be spiritual mechanisms for the soul to straighten out its knots and kinks. Evangelist Ruth Carter Stapleton used "guided daydreams" as a key ingredient in her healing of memories therapy. As dreams become more and more important to a visual culture, evangelicals listen more retentively to the likes of David Wilkerson (Teen Challenge) and Demos Shakarian (Full Gospel Business Men's Fellowship), who have long argued for renewed attention to dreams and visions in the spiritual culture of evangelicalism.[39] Dream deprivation is one of the factors to which evangelicals attribute the proliferation of sects and cults in America today.

God made each of us a natural storyteller. One way or another we will translate our experiences into a narrative, a story that we tell to ourselves. Dreams are a method of communicating and communing with both ourselves and "the beyond within," as Dietrich Bonhoeffer would put it. By this beam of light we find our way from the unconscious to the conscious story. Dreams bring to our attention things that elude the bonds of reason, revealing truths about ourselves and those around us. By jarring our waking sensibilities, dreams become a means to greater wisdom, integrity, and growth in grace. That is why one of the most profound pieces of advice evangelicals give anyone is "Sleep on it."

Not for the sleep, but for the dreams.

# ·5·

# Sexuality and Morality: "Blest Be the Tie That Binds"

A person's a person, no matter how small.

— Dr. Seuss, *Horton Hears a Who*

If a man loses reverence for any part of life, he will lose his reverence for all life.

— Albert Schweitzer

My two earliest childhood rhymes were learned from my Pilgrim Holiness mother and Free Methodist father. The first was a lullaby many mothers and fathers still sing to their children. As a child I listened to my mother sing it to my two brothers as she rocked and nursed them. It concerns placing a baby high up in a treetop, from which the baby falls, the tree limb and cradle falling after it. It's called "Rock-a-bye baby." The next rhyme was a children's prayer, articulating a different version of a calamity befalling a child. "Now I lay me down to sleep, / I pray the Lord my soul to keep; / If I should die before I wake, / I pray the Lord my soul to take." Evangelical children, even those growing up in hermetically sealed "holiness" households like mine, are not protected from atmospheric pressures of destructive impulses.

The extent of violence that American culture feels toward children, however, I did not discover until my school days. A child of the fifties, I learned that folk metaphor "to give someone the Willies" by reciting in grade school "Little Willie" quatrains, none of which I was allowed to utter before my staunchly evangelical parents. Some of these date from the 1890s, but none of them achieved widespread circulation until they became a prominent part of 1950s humor:

We had a Little Willy!
Now Willie is no more.
For what he thought was $H_2O$
Was really $H_2SO_4$.

In my high school and college years (the 1960s and 1970s) the dead baby joke cycle became even more popular, expanding in the 1970s into sick Jesus jokes ("Do you know why Jesus can't eat M&Ms? Because they fall through the holes in his hands"). The most common dead baby joke was in two parts: "What's red and sits in a corner? A baby chewing razor blades. What's green and sits in a corner? Same baby two weeks later." In the 1980s collecting garbage pail kids replaced dead baby jokes. Reared on pictures of dead bodies in garbage dumps and aborted fetuses in garbage pails, children sensed society's compost heap of resentment and hatred.

Children play out in their fantasy world the awful realities that they cannot face or find protection from in their real life.[1] The sick humor tradition of childhood graphically reveals the cheapening of human life that evangelicals believe both anticipated and attended the introduction of legalized abortion into modern American life. Children transfer their fear of being killed, their rage at infanticide, into defensive fantasies.

Children pick up the messages of our culture: postmodern culture does not like children. For the first time in history, parents can decide what type of children they will raise and discard those deemed "defective." Fully 11 percent of New England couples would abort a child predisposed to obesity.[2] The addition of abortion clinics to modern society sent out powerful social messages about how much children are wanted and needed. In the words of Alan Dundes, "one way of fighting the fear or gilding the guilt is to tell gross dead baby jokes. It is as if one could dehumanize babies and by so doing allow one to destroy them through modern technology."[3] More than any other health issue, abortion became for evangelicals a symbol of modern American social values, although more than evangelicals deemed those values corrupt.

In Oslo, Norway, the 1979 Nobel Peace Prize winner stepped forward to receive her award. In accepting the Peace Prize, she announced that the greatest destroyer of peace in the world today is legalized abortion. It claims the life of 55 million unborn every year, 1.5 million in America alone, a nation where as many as one out of every four pregnancies ends in abortion, a statistic that, interestingly enough, matches the nineteenth-century situation where one in every four infants died within the first year of life.[4]

As Mother Teresa articulated again at the 1994 President's Prayer Breakfast, abortion is the most far-reaching, divisive, and controversial health and public policy issue of the twentieth century. Mother Teresa also symbolized how Roman Catholic involvement in the antiabortion movement has overshadowed the continuous and effective grass-roots leadership given by America's evangelical communities. For evangelicals and many Roman Catholics, abortion is the key issue in world medicine and national politics, "the single most fevered issue joining public policy and moral judgment in American life" (Richard John Neuhaus). It is a symbolic battleground for competing religious, social, and economic value systems. The abortion issue reflects ominous questions about family structure, economic opportunity, changing attitudes toward women, children, and sex, changing relations between men and women, church and state, and by no means least, "*the place and meaning of motherhood.*"[5]

To say that 22 January 1973 was a landmark day in the history of American evangelicalism is to say very little. After *Roe v. Wade,* religion in the United States looked like a city after an earthquake, with geologic changes in the topography of religious life and new fault lines of division within and between evangelicals and American culture. To be sure, from the mid-1960s to the early 1970s prochoice activists achieved a series of stunning successes: laws legalizing the practice in eighteen states; court decisions invalidating prohibitive statutes in a half-dozen other states. But nothing compared to 22 January 1973. On this day the Supreme Court ruled in *Roe v. Wade* (and its companion case *Doe v. Bolton*) that abortion was now legal in America if a mother's health were at stake. The court went on to define *health* as including medical, psychological, social, and economic factors. Women's absolute right to have an abortion during the first three months of pregnancy was guaranteed, and state intervention in the deliberations through the sixth month was severely limited.

Immediately *Roe v. Wade* became for evangelicals a symbol of the dismantling of traditional values and morals, a manifestation of an "anything goes" ethic and "permissiveness" era, and an expression of the modern mentality where, as one college student recently phrased it, "Nothing matters. And what if it did?" The major evangelical organ in the country, *Christianity Today,* responded to *Roe v. Wade* with an angry, two-page editorial. The Supreme Court of the United States "has clearly decided for paganism, and against Christianity."[6]

By this the editors meant that historically the Christian attitude toward abortion contrasted sharply with the prevailing low value put upon infant and unborn life in the ancient world generally and by Roman patrician ideals in particular. In non-Christian cultures, unwanted children were casually disposed of. The Greek philosopher Aristippus called children analogous to "spittle, lice and such like, things unprofitable, which nevertheless are engendered and bred out of our own selves." Ancient Christianity "revived the insensitive conscience of pagan parents who disposed of unwanted baby girls on public garbage heaps, and compassionately sought to lead the weak and unwanted to meaningful spiritual life in Christ."[7]

Until the 1960s, an antiabortion consensus governed Christian church history, and the United States was one of the most difficult nations in which to get an abortion. Michael J. Gorman's portrayal of *Abortion and the Early Church* (1982) is overpowering in its unanimity of witnesses against abortion. The *Didache's* (ca. 100) commandment "You shall not slay the child by abortion" is reiterated in the *Epistle of Barnabas* (ca. 117–31), the *Apocalypse of Peter* (ca. 150), and in early Christian writers like Minucius Felix (2d century), Athenagoras (2d century), Clement of Alexandria (ca. 150–215), Hippolytus (170–236), Tertullian (160–240), Origen (185–254), Cyprian (210–58), Basil (330–79), Ambrose (339–97), John Chrysostom (347–407), Jerome (340–420), and Augustine (354–430).[8] To modern evangelical theologians, from Charles G. Finney and Charles Hodge to Carl F. H. Henry, and C. S. Lewis, abortion was a violent killing of an innocent being.

Abortion itself became loaded with symbolic and emblematic meaning for more than the termination of human life.[9] Abortion took on the character of a "Trojan horse,"[10] the enemy we have admitted into our culture, a social, political, economic, sexual culture where even the devil seemed to have lost its mind, a culture consisting of (or so it seemed to evangelicals) one vast commercial for abortions. The one thing abortion was not for evangelicals was a narrowly focused moral question. Indeed, the abortion issue forced evangelicals to attempt a coherent Christian framework for understanding sexuality, marriage, and family.

As a symbol, *abortion began to stand for the corruption of sexual love.* The abortion issue coincided with the emergence of new candor and celebration among evangelicals of the beauty of sexual love in marriage. That sex was more than the "thou shalt not's" became evident in Marabel Morgan's *Total Woman* (1973), Tim and Beverly LaHaye's *Act of Marriage* (1976), and the global popularity of Walter and Ingrid Trobisch's writings on sex. Evangelicals in the past twenty years have made tremendous progress in "getting behind sexual behavior to sexual being," as Dwight Hervey Small put it in *Christians Celebrate Your Sexuality* (1974).[11]

Taken together, these books denounced Victorian prudery, criticized the push-button use of Puritanism as a symbol of sexual repressiveness, admitted Jesus had sexual desires, and reveled in the "sexiest book in the Bible" — the Song of Songs love poem. In fact, it was the evangelical community in the 1970s and 1980s that provided its members with biblically informed sex manuals for adults, replete with explicit diagrams and tapes widely used as counseling tools and discussion starters about every aspect of lovemaking (including oral-genital play and anal sex).

Abortion cheapened this newly minted evangelical understanding of sexuality, grounded in a deepening theology of creation, as a gift of God to be celebrated as part of humanity's wondrous response to God. For it is in God that we live and move and have our sexual being too (see Acts 17:28). The real pleasure of sexual intercourse is not the sex but the intercourse — not just skins touching and genital grindings but two souls communing. While the evangelical sexual ethic does not allow for the fullest expressions of sex outside of the intimacy and freedom of marriage, evangelicals baptized sex as the ultimate and "primary form of interpersonal communion."[12]

As a symbol, *abortion began to stand for the corruption of civility.* Language hardened into abortion "on demand," and every woman who had an abortion was branded as "murderer." Instead of splashing dash after dash of cold water on the discussion, which would have reminded everyone that no one is *for* abortion, both sides heated up the rhetoric to a punishing temperature. Both sides tried to bury opponents under scalding streams of oratory. Americans could be seen engaged in crusades against the unborn, treating them as alien and an infringement of *our* rights, as if they were our greatest problem and threat.[13] Even mothers could be heard spouting unnatural and uncivil thoughts about pregnancy as an illness or a disease, which could be cured by abortive surgery. And "fatherhood" began to be a name for something sinister and abusive.

Some evangelicals proved especially adept at using the media, with full-color photographs of bloody fetuses in garbage pails or graphic parallels between abortoriums and Nazi gas-oven crematoriums. The book and film series that helped mobilize evangelicals against abortion, Francis Schaeffer and C. Everett Koop's *Whatever Happened to the Human Race?*, featured photos of dolls, symbolizing aborted babies, strewn over the floor of the Dead Sea.[14] A few evangelicals could be heard giving Jesus' answer to those who go around shouting "murderer" to Christian brothers and sisters:

> You have heard that it was said to the people long ago, "Do not murder, and anyone who murders will be subject to judgment." But I tell you that anyone who is angry with his brother will be subject to judgment. Again anyone who says to his brother, "Raca," is answerable to the Sanhedrin. But anyone who says, "You fool!" will be in danger of the fire of hell. (Matthew 5:21–23)

But the noise of Rachel weeping (Jeremiah 31:15; Matthew 2:18) drowned them out.

As a symbol, *abortion began to stand for the corruption of consistency.*

Justice William O. Douglas extended "rights" to trees and air (1972) but denied the same "rights" to the fetus (1973). Philosopher Peter Singer's *Practical Ethics* embraced a utilitarianism that allows the protection of animal life and the practice of vegetarianism but permits the killing of fetuses and in some cases infants.[15] I shall never forget listening to a United Methodist bishop repudiate the pulpit as a "coward's castle." He encouraged both clergy and lay ministers to get involved politically on moral issues of the day like capital punishment, while in the same speech he challenged the Hyde amendment (a 1977 bill designed to ban the use of tax money for abortion on demand), citing the Constitution's separation of church and state and arguing that no one has the right to force particular religious and moral standards on other citizens.

As a symbol, *abortion began to stand for the corruption of categories.* Doctors, nursed on the "heathen" Hippocratic oath and weaned on the ancient medical proverb *Primum non nocere* ("First of all, do no harm"), found themselves performing what has become a common surgical procedure in America today. Mothers, who speak instinctively in terms yoking personality and potentiality — "A baby is coming!" — found themselves justifying the most unnatural thing a mother can do: interruption of pregnancy and termination of the intimacy engendered by pregnancy's fetal family of mother, child, and God. Women who demanded to be seen as subjects, not as objects, found themselves condoning what is to the evangelical mind violence on women by women. Feminists, who successfully repudiated evangelicalism's nineteenth-century "women's sphere doctrine," began espousing the doctrine themselves in demanding total control of their own bodies and complete deference to women's definitions about sexuality, morality, and so forth. Evangelicals, raised on the notion that women are always right in their sphere, began respecting the rights of women without respecting the idea that women are always right.

Liberals, historically on the side of the voiceless, the weak, the oppressed, the immigrant — "A bruised reed he will not break, and a smoldering wick he will not snuff out" (Isaiah 42:3) — abdicated their activist advocacy on behalf of "the ultimate immigrant" and society's most smoldering wicks. In the words of Richard John Neuhaus, the first religious leader to call attention to the theological scandal of liberal views on abortion, "the liberal banner has been planted on the wrong side of the contest."[16] The confusion of categories allowed right-wing politicians to monopolize issues of traditional and family values and use these issues as a ticket to public control of other questions.

As a symbol, *abortion began to stand for the corruption of family.* Few things are more sacred or divinely ordained to evangelicals than the family, notwithstanding Jesus' contrariness. There is an almost feudal quality to the evangelical imagination and belief in a *gemeinschaftlich* world of family loyalties, home truths, organic communities, and nostalgic sentiments. Evangelicals inherited from the Puritans an exalted valuation of marriage and a theological definition of the family as "the school of souls." Evangelicals went beyond seeing the family as a means of grace or even "medium of divine revelation" and actually defined the essence of their faith as "a family religion."[17] Some even have come perilously close to seeing family as almost an end in itself.

The good Christian home, and family home life, became a sacred symbol and biblical norm in nineteenth-century evangelical culture. Home was "the sweetest and most sacred place on earth"; family was "that which most resembles heaven."[18] Gothic revival architecture, domestic rituals (like family worship,[19] family altars, group recitations, Bible-reading and hymn-singing exercises, devout walks), house bibelots and artifacts, and styles of domestic leadership enshrined evangelical values of piety, order, work, self-control, usefulness, and punctuality. Historian Colleen McDannell has shown the degree to which architects designed homes to inspire evangelical piety, illustrated most powerfully in women's education advocate Catharine Beecher's design of a house that could be quickly converted into a church.[20]

For evangelicals, abortion does more than threaten the divine institution of the family, a threat that calls forth periodic proposals for reinforcing the family.[21] Since the family is the original unit of society as well as the bulwark of the church, abortion's erosion of family life pulls down the pillars of both church and state. Evangelicals' well-developed theology of the family is based on the biblical concept of covenant, the Hebrew model of unconditional commitment between God and God's chosen people Israel.[22] Little critical scrutiny is given, however, to whether "the family" is a sufficient metaphor for describing and understanding domestic realities, in spite of the fact that evangelicals themselves have as wide a variety of biological experiences of "normal" family life as almost anyone else.

This lack of self-scrutiny helps to explain why evangelicals have insisted on talking about the "traditional family," often expressed in romanticized terms, envisioning the idealized families depicted in popular culture like Ozzie and Harriet Nelson or the "Brady bunch." Early nineteenth-century revivalism produced changes in the meaning of marriage that are still essential components of today's marriage system. The "law of marriage," which evangelicals viewed as "the first law ever given to mankind," was refocused around character and volition and not around property and obligation.[23]

The distinction between abiding biblical principles and changing cultural standards also helps explain why evangelicalism's relaxed conscience about divorce, which just yesterday was categorized as a crime against God and humanity, has resisted taking the final step that makes divorce an institutionalized part of the marriage system. In a nation with the highest divorce rate in the world, where two out of three first marriages will end in divorce, evangelical acceptance of divorce has been reluctant, but irrepressible.

Until the 1970s, the predominant evangelical perspective on divorce was Erasmian — an interpretation stemming from Erasmus's exegesis of Matthew 5:32 and 19:9, which argued that Jesus allowed divorce and remarriage only in the case of adultery. By the 1980s, evangelicals moved from permitting divorce only under strict conditions (adultery or desertion) to a position best defined as "redemptive realism"[24] — not wanting to make divorce more acceptable, but not wanting to inflict lifelong penalties on people either. The evangelical doctrine of sin always comes around to making allowances for people who, even though they *know* God's will, are too frail of faith to *do* God's will.

By the 1990s, evangelicals were provided with a variety of biblical perspectives from which to choose (typified in *Divorce and Remarriage: Four Christian Views*).[25] But behind each one of these alternatives was a sense of divorce as the lesser of evils, something that could have been avoided if both partners had only applied biblical principles to their marriage, something to be chosen only as a last resort. As Lewis Smedes has pointed out, to accept divorce is not to say that God approves of divorce; it is only to say that God sometimes disapproves of its alternatives even more than divorce itself. Evangelicals also insist on repentance before remarriage.[26] Evangelicals have successfully resisted seeing marriage as simply a contract that can be dissolved at will or ignored. It is more than an honored institution. Marriage is a divine institution for the constitution of the family.

As a symbol, *abortion began to stand for the corruption of community.* The *Epistle of Barnabas* placed the *Didache's* repudiation of abortion in the context of a love of neighbor: "You shall love your neighbor more than your own life. You shall not slay thy child by abortion." To make absolute a woman's "control over her body" and to reduce a moral issue to simply a medical decision excludes, at least to the evangelical mind, other members of the human family — such as males and grandparents and religious communities — who should have a say in moral issues that concern that larger family. Even some feminists have recently begun to question the logic of a defense of abortion on the grounds of reproduction as a private matter and an independent right while at the same time feminism prides itself on fostering a communitarian ethic and a nurturing and protective sisterhood.[27]

A mother has it within her power to choose what she will do with her body, a fact unforgettably etched in the evangelical mind by Marilyn Monroe's twelve abortions. That is not the issue. The question is whether anyone else should have moral standing in that decision, and whether society has the right to rule on whether she made the right choice or not. *Roe v. Wade* placed the state in the position of determining the essence of "meaningful human life," and the physician/patient in the position of deciding when life becomes "meaningful." "Abortion is no more purely a medical problem just because the physician wields the curette," writes E. Fuller Torrey of Stanford University in his influential work *Ethical Issues in Medicine*, "than chemical warfare is purely a problem for pilots because they press the lever releasing the chemical."[28]

As a symbol, *abortion began to stand for the corruption of spirit.* The poverty of spirit that allows accelerating feticide, that sanctions a lifeboat ethics approach to world hunger, that enables humans even to contemplate much less tolerate large-scale destruction of life, makes industrialized nations with legalized abortion poorer than the world's poorest nations. Evangelicals, especially African-American evangelicals, have called attention to this impoverishment by comparing abortion practices with slavery and Nazi extermination of the Jews, although these analogies have been condemned by Jews and liberal Christians alike.[29]

Evangelicals' worst fears of corrupted spirits seemed to be realized, evoking reductive responses to even "moderate" positions on abortion like those of philosopher L. W. Sumner, when philosophers like Mary Ann Warren, Judith Thompson, Michael Tooley, and Peter Singer defined personhood in such a way that one of the two traditional horror crimes for evangelicals, infanticide (the other is witchcraft), is as morally permissible as abortion. "Some human beings are not people [physical 'defectives'] and there may be people who are not human beings [robots and computers]," writes Warren. Since self-consciousness is a criterion for personhood, argues Tooley, infanticide "must be morally acceptable." Indeed, Tooley contends that the revulsion to infanticide "is like the reaction of previous generations to masturbation or oral sex."[30]

To admit that the fetus is "some form of person," as Roger Rosenblatt has recently done, while at the same time managing to argue that termination of that "person's" life should be left to the moral discretion of the individual conscience strikes evangelicals as the same as endowing individuals with the right to terminate life for personal convenience.[31] Perhaps evangelicals have been especially sensitive about utilitarian ethical reasoning because a kind of consequentialism sometimes sneaks into their own ethics, subverting evangelicalism's deontological claims. This may also explain the weight and wordage whenever someone blatantly takes up with utilitarianism: aborted thoughts and grotesque theories, evangelicals announce, will be the result.

As a symbol, *abortion began to stand for the corruption of mind.* An issue deserving the supreme test of moral reasoning and mature discourse got instead hysteria and emotionalism from every side. Little more than a shouting match of slogans and signs, the bumperstickerification of theology and T-shirtification of spirituality were now complete. Placards with slogans like "Every Child a Wanted Child" or "Keep your laws and your morality off my body" and chants of "Not the Church / Not the State / Women must / Control their fate" were pitted in intellectual battle with slogans like "Wanted for murder: 1.5 million women who had abortions last year" and visual representations of aborted fetuses.

But most of all, as a symbol, *abortion began to stand for the corruption of the faith itself,* dividing evangelicals from other members of the Christian community and from other evangelicals themselves. Evangelicals simply cannot understand how brothers and sisters in the faith could conceive of abortion as a moral option, much less a positive religious good. Evangelicals cannot fathom how a hospital with a cross on its roof and "Methodist" in its title could be the abortion center for one of America's major metropolitan centers. Nor can evangelicals comprehend how one so prominent in churchcraft as the bishop of Winchester could crusade to get a prayer like this into the worship book of the Anglican Church — a prayer for after an abortion: "Heavenly Father, you are the Giver of Life and you share with us the care of the life that is given. In your hands we commit in trust the developing life that we have cut short. Look in kindly judgment on the decision that we have made and assure us in all our uncertainty that your love for us can never change. Amen."[32]

Even though nearly all evangelicals oppose abortion, the issue also divides the evangelical community itself.[33] Indeed, it is difficult to get rank-and-file evangelicals to reflect the same mind on this issue.[34] Contrary to what is portrayed in the media, there are many evangelical positions on abortion. Most evangelicals follow Tertullian and permit abortion to save the life of the mother. Many allow abortion in cases of rape and incest. Some evangelicals turn their heads to the destruction of prenatal human life when extreme deformity makes human life problematic. One of the great secrets of the antiabortion movement is that on the eve of *Roe v. Wade,* the Southern Baptist Convention was calling for liberalized abortion laws.

Others such as theologian John Jefferson Davis can defend abortion when the mother's life is endangered, justifying surgical intervention "as an effort to salvage the life that has some real prospect of survival," but they can support neither abortion for rape (the child has committed no crime and should not be punished for another's deeds) nor predetermined birth defects (a Christian life-style "accepts God's providence"; such defects "can play a part in the sovereign plan of God").[35] The Christian Medical and Dental Society (CMDS) was founded as the Christian Medical Society (CMS) in 1931 to "think biblically" about ethical issues and to "impact the world for Jesus Christ through medicine and dentistry." The society, clearly opposing the practice of abortion, recognizes the rights of patients and physicians to "follow the dictates of individual conscience before God" yet affirms the final authority of "Scripture which teaches the sanctity of human life."[36]

The major issue for evangelicals is not whether abortion should be permitted. Most evangelicals follow Carl F. H. Henry, Harold Lindsell, and others and permit it under rigid circumstances during most of a woman's pregnancy.[37] The major issue for evangelicals is whether the fetus is a human life before birth. Even though evangelicals condemn premarital sex as undesirable or immoral, they oppose legal abortions on the grounds of the humanity of the embryo, not the promiscuity of the mother and father. The Bible says God loved us before we existed. That is why we were created. That is why abortion is wrong. It is as simple as that for evangelicals.

In other words, for all evangelicals, no matter how divided on particulars, the major issues are biblical and theological, not sociological and psychological. Granted, the linkages among religious variables in abortion decisions are complex, and sometimes contradictory.[38] But the influence of religious doctrine in abortion attitudes is significantly more direct among evangelicals than in most other major religious bodies. The primary biblical and theological question, which raises a host of theological questions — including those arising from biblical doctrines of providence, creation, death, and evil — is, When does human life begin? Evangelicals know that the philosophical literature on abortion denies that this is the question to ask. There is even one evangelical theologian who dismisses the question as casuistry.[39] But evangelicals also know that when one ignores this question the argument ends up most often defending infanticide.

The worst offense of *Roe v. Wade*, according to evangelicals, is that this question of when life begins does not concern the court: "We need not resolve the difficult decision of when life begins. When those trained in the respective disciplines of medicine, philosophy, and theology are unable to arrive at any consensus, the judiciary, at this point in the development of man's knowledge, is not in a position to speculate as to the answer."

Evangelicals look to the Bible as the one sure guide through the quicksands of ethical turmoil and confusion. To be sure, it is not only evangelicals who look to the Bible for answers to the question of when human life begins. Also, to be sure, some evangelicals draw upon the Bible merely to brandish the most verses that sanction preconceived prejudices and to make these the law of the land. But for most evangelicals, the Bible provides a clear answer to the fundamental social question of whether humans can arrogate to themselves what belongs to God — decisions of life and death, the taking of human life, and the like. Moral issues that impinge on public life require a public response. The only adequate response, one evangelical concludes, "must be rooted in the individual and societal expression of persons whose consciences are *in*formed by the principle that God alone is Lord of life and Lord of death."[40]

The problem is that "the Bible says nothing directly and almost nothing indirectly on the problems of contraception and abortion," writes C. E. Cerling, Jr.[41] There is only one passage that touches on abortion, and this concerns a spontaneous abortion incidental to a quarrel (Exodus 21:22–23). Other portions of the First Testament that have shaped evangelical views on abortion include Genesis 9:6, where "whoever sheds the blood of man, by man his blood shall be shed; for in the image of God has God made man"; Job 10:8–12, where God cares for us even before we were born; Zechariah 12:1, where God is described as the one "who forms the spirit of a man within him"; and Hosea 9:14, where miscarriage is part of God's curse on Israel for her disobedience. The most important Hebrew text for evangelicals, however, is what has come to be known as "the pregnant woman's psalm." In Psalm 139, especially verses 13–16, God expresses deep love for the human zygote.

> For you created my inmost being;
>     you knit me together in my
>         mother's womb.
> . . . . . . . . . . . . . . . . . . . . . . . .
> My frame was not hidden from you
>     when I was made in the secret
>         place.
> When I was woven together in the
>     depths of the earth,
>         your eyes saw my unformed body.
> All the days ordained for me
>     were written in your book
>         before one of them came to be.

This is the most complete biblical statement pertaining to fetal life, and the clearest biblical statement that the fetus is more than a protoplasmic mass.

In the Second Testament, John the Baptist salutes the unborn Christ by leaping for joy in his mother's womb (Luke 1:41); to evangelicals, this passage is reminiscent of Yahweh's calling of prophets before their birth (Jeremiah 1:5 and Isaiah 49:5). Evangelicals out of the Wesleyan tradition find Luke 1:13–15 especially important because it shows that not only does God know us before our births (Ephesians 1:4–6), but God sanctifies the unborn human being:

"and he will be filled with the Holy Spirit, while yet in his mother's womb."[42] There is also the biblical condemnation of *pharmakeia*, the giving of magical potions and drugs by medicine men, particularly a potion to induce abortion (see Galatians 5:20; compare Revelation 9:21, 21:8, 22:15).

There is no question abortion kills something. The question is, what does it kill? Is the fetus a member of the human community or not? The biblical answer to this question is consistent from an evangelical perspective: Scriptures support the humanity of prenatal life, giving that life civil rights. What is more, evangelicals point to embryological findings of rapid development that further portray the fetus not as a dependent vegetable but as an active creature: regular heartbeat between four and five weeks of age; spontaneous movement by six weeks old; detectable brain waves by six to seven weeks; organs and limbs formed by eight weeks, with gender observable by nine weeks; face features recognizable by ten weeks, with babies who suck thumbs *in utero* turning out to be thumb suckers after birth.

*Abortion* means literally "to stop from rising" or "to cut off from birth." Indeed, theologian John R. W. Stott contends that the lid was closed on the question of when life begins when the genetic code was cracked. The moment the ovum is fertilized, the three constituent features of life are present: creation, continuity, communion.[43] Novelist and physician Walker Percy agrees, arguing from a biological standpoint that the onset of individual life at the moment a single cell is fertilized is not a dogma of the church but a fact of science. Evangelicals have given strong support to traducianism, the doctrine that a fetus is a person from the moment of conception.[44]

Evangelicals have been some of the staunchest detractors of what Albert C. Outler called "magic-moment-theories" of when the defenseless deserve to be defended.[45] A prime reason for the enormous expenditure of evangelical energies opposing these magic-moment theories is not that they perpetuate damaging body-soul dualisms, as Outler reveals so brilliantly, but that evangelicals believe the exact moment of personhood "lies in the freedom of God," as Kenneth Kantzer puts it.[46] They also believe that the burden of proof should be on those who support abortion to show that we are not persons from conception.

For some the magic moment is "viability" — that is, the point in the second trimester of pregnancy when the child can function independently of the mother. But we can never function independently of one another. We can never exist totally on our own. Theologically mature human life always needs another to actuate its potential for authenticity and relatedness. Furthermore, the advance of technology is pushing the point of "viability" further and further back; neonatal wards can now sustain life from as early as twenty weeks.

For others the magic moment is the attainment of rationality or language or some other worthy characteristic. James D. Watson, Nobel Prize winner in genetics, has proposed that children not be declared living until three days after birth to give parents a choice of destroying their "deformed" children, who are defined as devoid of "meaningful humanhood."[47] But are there any such things as "unworthy humans"? Do not all of us exhibit various levels of worthy attainments and deformities? We are all imperfect, marred by sin and faulty design. As God loves us and does not destroy us, imperfect as we are, so God calls us to love and treat our imperfect offspring similarly.

For some the magic moment is being wanted by either the parent or the society in which one lives. Since most abortions today occur for reasons of convenience — with the significant exception of China, countries where the abortion rate is highest are plump with riches, not poverty-stricken — a mother's "interests" are being given priority over an infant's life. For most evangelicals the real stake in abortion is one of selfishness and irresponsibility; a powerless, dependent life is to be sacrificed either on the altar of self-interest and convenience or as a cover-up for corrupt morals (fornication and adultery). Evangelicals distinguish between being wanted (by society, by parents) and having value (to God and others). The notion that the fetus becomes a person before birth the moment the mother "accepts" and "consents to the pregnancy," as one ethicist argues, is beyond comprehension for evangelicals.[48] To not want to bring an "unwanted" child into the world begs the question — unwanted by whom? The child certainly has no chance to want or unwant himself or herself; as for the parents, "Breathes there a parent with soul so dead / who never to himself hath said, / these are my own, the ones I bred — / I must have had holes inside my head." The theological question is whether this life is unwanted by God. A child is God's gift. To reject a child is to reject God. Life is not our own. We are not our own. We are God's, gifted with life as God's loan and blessing.

God's affirmation of life with love requires our affirmation of life with love. The sanctity of human life depends on the value God places on it, not on our personal needs, or wants, or convenience. Malcolm Muggeridge dubbed the path from abortion to active euthanasia "a slippery slope," introducing a very powerful term in the debate. Evangelicals have refused to replace a "sanctity of life" ethic with a "quality of life" ethic, a doctrine of essence with a doctrine of achievement.

> The choice, then, between the 'sanctity of life' ethic based on the idea of the image of God, and the 'quality of life' ethic based on brain function, is a choice between an ethic that protects all human beings in principle, and an ethic with a sliding scale of human worth based on estimates of intelligence and mental function.[49]

For the Supreme Court the magic moment is "the capability of meaningful life" (*Roe v. Wade*, x). But "the biblical standard is not 'meaninglessness' but *innocence*."[50] Besides, once the state acts like Pilate, washing its hands of protecting anyone who lacks "the capability of meaningful life," the state then arrogates to itself the right to definitions that belong only to God. Even more slippery are the lengths one takes in defining *meaningless*. Once the psychological barriers against taking human life are down, every excuse conceivable floods in.

For a number of Christians the magic moment is "ensoulment" or "hominization," the moment a body becomes a being. First propounded by Augustine, then picked up by Jerome and Aquinas, and recently revived, this theory depicts the development of the soul through stages, from vegetative to animal to rational to divine. The fetus becomes a person when God gives it a soul. Besides the fact that this theory carts into the present some embarrassingly antiquated distinctions (Augustine gave an ensoulment period of forty days for males and eighty days for females), the "creationist" approach is both tautological and beside the point. Tautological in that the problem has shifted from when life begins to when the soul begins, but the problem is still the same. Beside the point in that, in the words of Dietrich Bonhoeffer, "To raise the question whether we are here concerned already with a human being or not is merely to confuse the issue. The simple fact is that God certainly intended to create a human being and that this nascent human being has been deliberately deprived of his life."[51] Or in words centuries older, from Tertullian: "He is a man while yet a man still to be even as every fruit is already present in seed."[52]

If abortion is immoral, is every act of abortion equally immoral? For evangelicals this is not the same question as whether every act of killing is equally immoral. Abortion may be a "crime," an evil act, and still be permissible to do, as society allows certain "crimes" and "killings" to take place. "Killing" is not morally wrong under all circumstances. Evangelicals insist that the distinction be maintained between what is morally good versus what is legally permissible, what is *my* right legally to do versus what is morally right to do. *Roe v. Wade* raised with a vengeance this issue of what happens when law and life come into conflict, distinguishing the embryo's legal status from its moral status, and deciding that the legal status would be determined by the woman's physician.

Evangelicals believe that opposition to abortion is not a religious rule peculiar to a certain faith tradition but a universal moral prohibition like that against rape and robbery. For this reason few evangelicals are both prochoice and antiabortion.[53] The failure of the entire Christian tradition to demand the fetus be granted legal standing as a person, thereby providing fetal life with legal protection, is a prime example to evangelicals of the acculturation of the church and its selling out to the surrounding culture.

To those who argue that some women will have an abortion whether it is legal or not and that illegal abortions drive women to back-alley butchers, evangelicals counter with studies showing that abortions became safe long before they became legal and that before *Roe v. Wade* illegal abortions were approaching 10 percent (135,000 per year) of what they are today (1.6 million).[54] In fact, in every country where abortion on demand has become a legal right, illegal abortions have increased rather than decreased.

At some time we all find ourselves, or place ourselves, in tragic situations where choosing the lesser evil is the only recourse. This position has been most fully explored in the evangelical community by John Warwick Montgomery.[55] But even in cases where life conflicts with life — in these "hard" cases of rape, incest, or possible loss of the mother's life — evangelicals insist that abortion is still an evil and must always be confessed as an evil.[56] For mothers whose own health, physical or sometimes even mental, is seriously endangered, there is a high tolerance for abortion. Evangelicals throughout their history have accorded the mother both a higher legal and moral standing than the infant. Indeed, Christians adopted the Jewish position, where the rabbis assumed the existence of a human being before birth but held that this human being does not have equal status to the mother until birth.[57] Evangelicals have generally not taken the Roman Catholic position that abortion is never justifiable, regardless of maternal danger or circumstances of impregnation.

The National Association of Evangelicals, which comprises over forty evangelical denominations representing fifty thousand churches, "recognizes the necessity for therapeutic abortions to safeguard the health or the life of the mother" or in cases of rape.[58] The second largest African-American denomination, the African Methodist Episcopal Church, opposes abortion except in cases of rape and incest or to save the mother's life.[59] The Lutheran Church–Missouri Synod, "independent" Christian Churches and Churches of Christ, and Baptist Bible Fellowships all are on record prohibiting abortion — except to save the mother's life. Only the Southern Baptists, comprising almost a quarter of the evangelical community, have hardened their opposition against abortion, opposing it as of 1988 even in cases of rape and incest. Normative evangelical practice in extreme cases is to judge abortion the lesser of two evils as long as "the doctor has not introduced death into the case," in the words of Oliver O'Donovan.[60] Death is already present when birth poses a threat to the mother's sanity or survival.

But the "hard" cases of rape, incest, life-incompatible birth defects, or threatened maternal life are a rarity, involving only 2 to 3 percent of all abortions. The vast majority of abortions are for "soft" reasons — "birth control of last resort," feminist theologian Beverly Wildung Harrison calls them as she attacks the "moral schizophrenia" of those that distinguish between abortion and birth control.[61] For evangelicals the distinction is theologically critical, and the conflation of the two morally abhorrent. To sacrifice "life," not for the health of others but for their happiness (not wanting more children, not wanting to marry, not able to afford more children), is to tolerate thoughts that can drag a culture swiftly to the bottom. Life must not be destroyed in order to solve personal, political, and economic problems (like food and shelter for existing populations or population control).

The evangelical tradition, in fact, pioneered in family planning and birth control. Two scholars of historical fertility have discovered a significant causal connection between family limitation and evangelical religion in nineteenth-century America. The difference in fertility patterns between evangelical and nonevangelical women were "dramatic" in the nineteenth century, when infant death "was the central reality of maternal experience."[62]

Conscious family planning and birth spacing strategies allowed evangelical women greater time for revival and reform activities outside the home as well as more time to spend on "fewer children of greater spiritual quality."[63] Large numbers of evangelical women turned to hydropathy, at least in part because hydropathists offered women help in controlling childbearing, help denied them by orthodox medicine's refusal to give women any right to birth control and contraceptive information.[64]

Nonreligious factors play a much larger role in evangelical views on contraception than on abortion. In fact, outside influences have shaped evangelical approaches to human sexuality more than evangelicals like to admit — from the "sexzak" of Marabel Morgan, the evangelical equivalent of Masters and Johnson (the two most responsible along with Kinsey for introducing to the modern world "a new pleasure: the pleasure of talking about sex"),[65] to erotic literature lurking on Christian bookshelves in the sheep's clothing of a Song of Solomon picture book and guidebook.

Opposition to contraception in twentieth-century evangelicalism has come from two secular influences. First, the fundamentalist wing opposed contraception until the 1930s, not primarily because of religious directives but because of fear of depopulation, "race suicide," and views on the place of women.[66] The best storks used to be the busiest birds.

Second, evangelicals support rulings that require government-financed clinics to notify parents when minors are given prescription contraceptives, not because of opposition to birth control, as popularly presented, but because "the facts of life" as presented by health-care providers are too likely to be all technology, no morality. Evangelicals believe in teaching children words increasingly missing from common speech — words like *promiscuity* and *fornication* and *self-discipline*. They insist on parental involvement in children's sexual life.

Contrary to popular perception, evangelicals have produced some of the best literature on sexual education for children and teenagers, educating kids on everything from masturbation to sexual abuse to date rape[67] and leading the Christian church in the development of sophisticated models and methods of combating "ignorance and evil by the judicious impartation of sex knowledge." The book from which this last quotation was taken, *Where Do They Come From?* (1917), was one such pioneering attempt at providing parents with a resource they might use with their children. Good evangelical parents, this book argued, did not "try to keep from their children the knowledge of sex." For evangelicals the real question was never whether to educate children about sex but rather who was to be their teacher. Children will learn — if not from parents or Sunday school teachers, then from "older children or degraded adults."[68]

Similarly, the contemporary debate is not over sex education in the schools, but whether sex education will be taught within a context of values and morality.[69] The morality of contraception for the unmarried, writes one evangelical scholar, "is like the question of whether a bank robber should use a Ford or a Plymouth as his getaway car."[70] To focus on "protection" is to forget the more important question of whether one should sin — rob a bank or engage in premarital sex — in the first place.

Evangelicalism's role in constructing sexual expression for evangelical singles extends over a broad range. Clearly the prescriptive literature on "Sex and the Single Person" would make contraception a nonissue for singles since premarital intercourse is forbidden. Masturbation is no longer the stigma it once was when Adam Clarke, in his commentary on Genesis 38 (1810), called masturbation "one of the most destructive evils ever practiced by fallen man."[71] Indeed, one contemporary evangelical author calls masturbation "God's greatest invention," subject of course to all the abuses that attend any gift of creation.[72] Still nervous over the role of fantasy, evangelicals are generally accepting of masturbation as an immature but nonharmful sexual expression that can be useful as a preventative measure. Because the Bible says nothing directly about masturbation, evangelicals contend that it could be right or wrong, depending on what the believer discerns God wills for him or her.

But studies have shown a fair amount of deviation from traditional precepts of evangelical morality both in the basic sexual attitudes of evangelical singles (on such matters as premarital sex, oral-genital sex, and mutual masturbation) and their behavior patterns, especially if those polled were currently in a relationship. The strongest disapproval ranking went to homosexuality.[73]

Homosexuality would rank high on the evangelical list of problems facing this nation. More inclined to perceive homosexuals as "inverts" rather than "perverts," evangelicals almost uniformly denounce the bad exchange that has taken place in homosexual inversion and consider homosexuality as unnatural as idolatry. Evangelicals are divided about homosexuality. Is this a "sexual identity disorder," often induced by unhealthy and unstable home environments, which can be treated — as insisted by James Dobson of Focus on the Family, Bob Davies, the "ex-gay" director of the umbrella organization Exodus International, and Robert P. Dugan, executive of the National Association of Evangelicals? Or is sexual orientation an inborn trait (like left-handedness), so that no psychotherapy or "ex-gay" movement could alter these genetic, congenital homoerotic impulses — as maintained by Ralph Blair, a New York City psychologist and founder of Evangelicals Concerned, by Mark Olson, editor and publisher of *The Other Side*, and by evangelical feminist theologians Letha Dawson Scanzoni, Nancy A. Hardesty, and Virginia Mollenkott.[74]

Whereas both sides of this nature/nurture dispute agree that the Bible is the source of authority on issues of morality and sexuality, those who believe homosexuality is a learned behavior think that we are taught more about homosexuality by biblical condemnations of such behavior (they cite Leviticus 18:22, 20:13; Genesis 19; 1 Corinthians 6:9; Romans 1:26–27). Those who believe that homosexuality is an innate or genetic characteristic hold that we are taught more about homosexuality through the biblical themes of grace, redemption, creation, and covenant. The former group has founded "transforming congregations" that hold out the hope of healing for homosexuals. The latter group has established "reconciling congregations" where gays and lesbians can worship in love and acceptance.

The majority of evangelicals advocate compassion and love for the homosexual, while at the same time they insist on repentance for "deviant" acts. Long before the AIDS pandemic, one evangelical theologian reminded the community that "the homosexual is not a special class of sinner that is the particular object of a special divine wrath."[75] Indeed, in an interview on the PTL Club broadcast historian-theologian Richard Lovelace said that "most of the repenting that needs to be done on this issue of homosexuality needs to be done by straight people, including straight Christians. By far the greater sin in our church is the sin of neglect, fear, hatred, just wanting to brush these people under the rug."[76] Healing, rather than punishment, is the preferred public evangelical response to homosexual behavior,[77] but self-control and abstinence are the only alternatives for "unhealed" evangelical homosexuals.[78] It is not the business of the state to find and punish consenting adult homosexuals, most evangelicals warn. But it is not the business of the state either to promote or normalize the homosexual life-style through legislation or social policy.

"Alex Davidson" is the pen name of the evangelical who wrote letters to a friend that comprise *The Returns of Love,* testimonies from personal experience that even though God may not heal the homosexual of his condition, the Spirit can be present to control his conduct and help him to live with the denial of sexual fulfillment.[79] Letha Dawson Scanzoni, Virginia Mollenkott, and Ralph Blair, who find nothing in the Bible to prohibit or condemn the formation of loving, lasting, same-sex relationships, are lonely voices in the evangelical community.[80]

Similar moralizing attends evangelical opposition to widespread distribution, especially in the public schools, of contraceptive information, services, and devices. There is also, however, the admission that "the approaches of abstinence, pill, and abortion are seriously flawed as widespread social answers."[81] Evangelicals are likely to oppose the reasoning behind making contraceptives available to teenagers (without parental support) because such reasoning is likely to be based on a view of sex that has shed the moral-ethical values of traditional Christianity. The assumption that the sexual behavior patterns of teenagers cannot be changed is the bone of contention evangelicals have with Planned Parenthood, who deem it an ethical duty to tell women with unwanted pregnancies about all their options, including abortion.

Evangelicals have held out for the principle that the use of contraceptives would not be right in all circumstances. For example, evangelicals do not accept contraceptive use to escape the consequences of fornication, to permit torrid, transient sexual encounters, or to avoid permanently the responsibility of children. But increasingly it is difficult to find evangelical theologians who do not line up behind the belief that God calls married couples to responsible family planning. John J. Davis, for example, writes:

> Man's calling is not simply to let "nature take its course," but to consciously redirect nature toward the fulfillment of the divine plan. Just as God himself created the human race and recreated a fallen humanity according to a conscious plan, so it would follow that man, as God's vice regent on earth, should imitate God by exercising his procreative gifts according to a conscious plan.[82]

For most married evangelicals, contraception is an accepted practice, seen largely not as a religious issue but as a medical and scientific one. This was affirmed in 1969 by a group of evangelicals who put together "A Protestant

Affirmation of the Control of Human Reproduction," which stated that the prevention of conception is not sinful as long as the "reasons for it are in harmony with the total revelation of God for married life."[83] More recent evangelical studies go further in uncoupling sexual intimacy from reproduction. "The first word dealing with marriage and sex in the Bible, Genesis 2:24," writes David Fraser in the *Reformed Journal*, "strongly implies the completeness of erotic love without children. It ends with the phrase '…they shall be one flesh,' without any mention of children."[84] Reflecting John Milton's claim in *Paradise Lost* (1665) that the joys of sex are shared by the angels, Fraser asserts that "erotic love is complete apart from children. The woman is not simply a womb, a garden in which to sow seed to increase the tribe or produce the Savior. What binds the couple is love itself, love apart from its sociological or religious functions."[85]

The evangelical resistance is strong, however, to this final break in the diminishing ties between sexual fulfillment and reproduction, an incremental divorce which began in the nineteenth century and became a pressing moral and ideological issue in the West with the work of Thomas Robert Malthus. This is especially true for the few evangelicals working on a biblical, ethical response to homosexuality. Here the inextricability of the relational and procreational purposes of sexual intercourse grounds their opposition to homosexuality in a doctrine of creation.[86] While virtually no one insists on a simple one-to-one connection any more between coitus and conception, the moral dimension of teleology is still a prime consideration in evangelical discussions of contraception. Marriage is more than an organism for orgasm. In the words of an old mountain proverb, "There goes more to marrying than four legs in bed."

It is precisely here that evangelicals are most vulnerable to criticism. In the forefront of right-to-life legislation, evangelicals are often in the rearguard of reaction against compulsory sex education, contraceptive information, or reproductive advice. Evangelical Christians are somewhat less favorable to sex education in the public schools than the general population, and one study in the early 1980s of evangelical colleges revealed that few of them offered a well-integrated course on human sexuality.[87]

Not all evangelicals have been as prescient as Billy Sunday who, early in the twentieth century, predicted sex education would soon be a part of high school curriculums and confessed, "I would rather have my children taught sex hygiene than Greek and Latin."[88] Evangelicals appear more ready to criticize present-day public school attempts at sex education than to support them.[89] They are also not eager to face up to realities in which the "practice of pediatric medicine now includes gynecology, birth control advice, and the treatment of venereal disease."[90]

Evangelicals have become all too content to leave to the courts issues of artificial insemination, genetic engineering, in vitro fertilization, and other reproductive technologies.[91] There are now eleven different means of human reproduction with which the courts are struggling without much help from the church. Ethicist Gilbert Meilaender has called attention to the separation of genetic, gestational, and social parentage in striking fashion: "The day is at hand when a child can be born with five 'parents,' the man who donated the sperm, the woman who donated the egg, the woman who received the embryo after sperm and egg were united in the laboratory and carried the fetus to term, and the (probably infertile) couple who commissioned the process and will undertake to raise the child."[92] The moral concern of children denied secure self-identity, as that has been traditionally defined in terms of genetic continuity and parental origins, renders reproductive technologies involving third-party donors extremely suspect. Evangelicals have not shown the same introspective sensitivity, however, to the commercialization of reproduction as it manifests itself in the variety of "free market–contract" models of surrogacy that are now available. The moral ambiguity here lies more in the threat of heterologous artificial fertilization (gametes from a third party) to the sacred mother-child bond and the exclusive domain of marriage in procreation and parenthood. German Lutheran theologian Helmut Thielicke's dated diatribe on the evils of nonprocreative sex, still of widespread influence in evangelical circles thirty years after *The Ethics of Sex* was published, advocates that couples suffer in silence the pain of infertility rather than divorce "love-making" from "life-giving."[93]

Evangelicals perceive venereal disease and varieties of sexual contacts as not unrelated to the current epidemic of infertility. The sperm count of American males has fallen by 30 percent in the last century. One in six married couples in childbearing years is having fertility problems that necessitate medical intervention. Generally, artificial insemination by the husband (AIH) presents nowhere near the difficulty that artificial insemination by a donor (AID) does. Some evangelical theologians like Norman Geisler make a case for both AIH and AID technologies. Others, like Helmut Thielicke, draw the line at AID.[94]

Surrogate motherhood is seen by evangelicals as the "mirror image" of donor insemination, with similar controversial line-ups. Evangelicals have proven to be extremely cautious over both sex selection for "ideal" babies and in vitro fertilization (IVF), primarily because of moral ambiguities concerning the risk of birth defects to the fetus and what happens to the "extra embryos" (in the blastocyst stage) left over from the superovulating procedures.

The latter consideration has played a major role in evangelical reactions to the French abortifacient RU-486, also known as the "morning-after abortion pill."[95] Whereas contraceptives prevent the union of a sperm with an egg, RU-486 prevents a fertilized egg from implanting in the uterine wall. In combination with prostaglandin, it strips the uterus, induces labor, and expels the fertilized egg. Hailed by the drug's inventor, Etienne-Emile Baulieu, as the most important invention of the twentieth century, RU-486 is widely celebrated for its promise of privatizing abortion.

Some evangelicals have been quick to point out, however, that the full RU-486 treatment takes three weeks and includes several clinical visits. Its success rate is only 10 percent that of surgical suction procedures, and its safety is still being debated.[96] The real question for evangelicals is not safety or privacy or effectiveness. "The question is whether it is right to destroy innocent human lives.... Efficiency in killing, after all, is no virtue."[97]

On the nascent topic of gene therapy and genetic engineering, evangelicals have not yet contributed more to the discussion than raising the sobering question first posed by Karl Mannheim: "Who plans the planners?" A few astute evangelicals have connected the striving for genetic reconstruction of disease-free, unblemished human beings with America's obsessive healthism. But if past discussions are any predictors, one can count on evangelicals to do two things: both to celebrate the beginning of an age wherein humans have more power to cure diseases and make of themselves and their lives what they will through natural processes, and yet to warn that history is more than a matter of choice, that life has limits, that no one should have genes changed without his or her informed consent, and that individuals should not be allowed to retrofit themselves when such alterations are likely to cause harm to others.

Ethical leadership in issues of medical technology often comes more from the evangelical front lines than from ivory towers. For example, the use of fetal tissue in research and transplantation, which promises great benefits for patients with Alzheimer's, Parkinson's, and diabetes, would loom no larger for evangelicals than organ donor transplants if it were not for abortion's raising the awful specter of infanticide, as portrayed graphically in "King On, Jorund's Son," a Nordic legend familiar to Lutheran evangelicals. On was a king of the Swedes who sacrificed his sons to Odin so that he might live sixty years longer. One son killed every tenth year gave King On another ten years of life, although he lived in a progressively weakened condition, until he could only drink out of a horn "like a weaned infant."

> In Upsal's town the cruel king
> Slaughtered his sons at Odin's shrine —
> To get from Odin length of life.
> He lived until he had to turn
> His toothless mouth to the deer's horn;

And he who shed his children's blood
Sucked through the ox's horn his food.
At length till Death has tracked him down,
Slowly, but sure, in Upsal's town.[98]

The transplantation of fetal brain cells in Alzheimer's patients, one of the few treatments with potential for reversing the forgotten life of Alzheimer's disease, raises the possibility of the harvest of fetal crops for medical purposes, as some medical researchers are claiming is the current situation in Europe. Ironically, there are more sustained discussions on bioethics in the scientific community than in the religious community, evangelicals not excepted. It has been left to the Christian Medical and Dental Society (CMDS) to exert moral leadership on this issue of fetal tissue research.

In 1989 CMDS distributed widely to educational institutions and denominational agencies standards that opposed "the use of electively aborted fetuses for research or transplantation" but endorsed the use of "the tissue of spontaneously aborted, non-viable fetuses, with parental consent, for research or transplantation."[99] Evangelical senator Mark Hatfield and Southern Baptist minister Guy Walden, whose son's enzyme deficiency was treated in 1990 by a transplant of fetal cells obtained from an ectopic pregnancy, both argue that fetal tissue treatments are consistent with a prolife posture.[100] Other prolife political activists within the evangelical community vigorously disagree (as does the National Right to Life Committee [NRLC]).

Evangelicals have also proved themselves to be the least prepared to vote or pay taxes for programs designed to provide better alternatives to abortion or to support the needs of children through quality adoption programs, foster care programs, or guaranteed health and educational opportunities. "Perhaps the most important insight clarified in the abortion debate," writes antiabortionist Sidney Callahan, "is the shocking lack of support available to American women in childbearing and child rearing."[101] Some evangelical scholars, like John Jefferson Davis, do challenge the Christian community with the responsibility to back up its antiabortion stands "with tangible spiritual, emotional, and financial help for women who are facing difficult pregnancies."[102]

The problem is that evangelicals who are antiabortion are not necessarily prolife. Indeed, for too many life begins at conception and ends at birth — that is, the concern about the unborn child's well-being does not extend to the child's life after birth. But "a true prolife perspective must include a concern for justice in all its forms," says a black evangelical who subsumes the abortion battle within a broader crusade against injustice.[103] Antiabortion too often means nothing more than probirth. And prochoice too often equals proself.

Blame for the belief that life begins at conception and ends at birth has not been overgenerously apportioned to evangelicals. Evangelicals are indefensible latecomers to movements dedicated to getting rid of the conditions that make abortion seem so necessary for some.[104] Evangelicals have yet to demonstrate enough interest or support in getting this country to care for children who are not wanted or cared for.

Jerry Falwell founded Moral Majority in 1979, adopting the "right to life" movement as a key plank in its platform. Falwell tells of an encounter with a reporter that transformed his thinking about what the "human life" argument entails.

> "You say you are against abortion?" she began.
> "Yes," I smiled and nodded....
> "But what practical alternative to abortion do pregnant girls have when they are facing an unwanted pregnancy?" she asked.
> "They can have the baby," I answered quickly, too quickly to suit the bright young woman who was questioning me....
> I decided that the reporter was right. It wasn't enough to be against abortion. Millions of babies were being killed, and I would go on fighting to save their lives, but what about the other victims of abortion, the mothers of those babies who desperately need help to save their babies?

Falwell's book *If I Should Die before I Wake* (1986) represents his awakening, and it may signal evangelicalism's awakening, to the fact that Christians must "work just as hard for the health and happiness of the girls and women who are facing unwanted pregnancies and for the future of their babies after they are born."[105] Likewise a Focus on the Family editor states bluntly that adoption will not replace abortion until Christians appropriate some of their "eagerness to adopt the easily adopted" into a "willingness to sacrifice for the hard-to-adopt."[106]

Yet antiabortionists still often fight for the very things that make abortion seem to some such a necessity. Too often "prolife" and "anti–family planning" go together. The prolife movement is hardly on the front lines for social services, whether for poverty-stricken adults or disadvantaged children. From within the evangelical community, Southern Baptist historian and theologian William J. Leonard lambasts "those whose rhetoric exalts the rights of the unborn, but whose social and legislative actions systematically undermine the rights of the 'born,'" those who clamor for rights of the unborn but are "relatively silent about the rights of the born."[107]

There are those in the evangelical community who are presenting a consistent prolife umbrella. A special issue of *Sojourners* entitled "What Does It Mean to Be Pro-Life?" set forth "the seamless garment" agenda on abortion (also known as "the consistent ethic of life" argument) and on the three moral disputes that lie on either side of it — contraception, infanticide, and euthanasia; this publication has been widely reprinted and circulated.[108] But in the main, evangelicals have been a retrograde force in disconnecting abortion from the modern conurbations that provide abortion with such strong life-support systems.

Ever since 1975, when C. Everett Koop and theologian Harold O. J. Brown met at Billy Graham's Minneapolis residence to found the Christian Action Council, the first Protestant action group against abortion, there has been an efflorescence of evangelical activity against abortion. In spite of *Roe v. Wade*'s widespread endorsement by the intellectual and cultural community, the prolife movement has shown dramatic resilience, endurance, and even growth in the past twenty years.[109]

The pivotal year appears to have been 1986, when the momentum started to shift toward the prolife side.[110] Old-line Protestants began the slow process of reassessment and realignment on this moral issue. A broadening base of support for the evangelical position was evident as prominent atheists and humanists came forward to argue for the recriminalization of abortion — not on religious or moral grounds so much as on the basis of civil rights for unborn humans. Gordon C. Zahn, a liberal sociologist, developed the case against abortion from a humanist value system, and he insisted that the connection between abortion and Auschwitz is more than an analogy.[111] Two of America's leading abortionists, Joseph Randall and Bernard N. Nathanson, the latter in charge of the world's busiest abortion clinic, changed their minds and adopted antiabortion as their noblest passion.[112]

Feminists began to see that evangelicals were more right than they knew. In supporting abortion women were not as liberal, or liberated, as they thought. The increasing numbers of "wrong-sex" abortions, as family planning was distorted into gender planning, pointed out the scurvy connections between feticide and femicide. Feminists for Life (FFL), a group of women who support both the equal rights and human rights amendment to the Constitution, was founded on the grounds that abortion is nothing more than the violent "remedy of a male-dominated society that expects women to conform to the needs of men." Abortion does nothing for women except "unpregnant" them so they can be more readily accepted and integrated into a man's world, hostile to the needs of women. To promote the rights of women by denying rights to the unborn is to imitate male attitudes and aggressiveness in dismissing undeveloped life. These feminist antiabortionists, some evangelical, some not, are the heirs of nineteenth-century feminists, some evangelical, some not, who spearheaded opposition to abortion and, in the case of Elizabeth Cady Stanton, lobbied for tougher laws against abortion to put an end to male irresponsibility.[113]

Jewish theologians and leaders have begun to come out against abortion, although they have not denounced it as murder.[114] With increasing rates of survival for premature infants and with surgeons able to operate successfully on the unborn, medical advances have made the proabortion position more and more problematic from the standpoint of biology and medical ethics for groups like Prolifers for Survival and the National Youth Pro-Life Coalition.[115] As child abuse has climbed by nearly 400 percent since 1973, evangelicalism has effectively focused attention on abortion as the ultimate form of child abuse.

Antiabortion values have been conveyed with great impact by evangelicals who have seen themselves as spiritual descendants of the antislavery movement. The comparison of the antiabortion struggle with the civil rights struggle, *Roe v. Wade* with *Dred Scott v. Sanford*, the antiabortionist mindset with the abolitionist mindset, is not merely a rhetorical one.[116] Judge John T. Noonan, Jr., argues that abortionism is "driven by a deep logic" toward its own destruction in an exact parallel to the slavery movement of the nineteenth century.[117] In what *Sojourners* calls "the biggest and most controversial new development on the abortion front," evangelicals have begun mimicking the tactics of the civil rights and antiwar movements as well as resurrecting "higher law" doctrines of the abolitionist evangelical crusades.[118] For an increasing number of evangelicals, civil disobedience represents a last-resort, last-ditch exercise of personal conscience against governmental policy.

Operation Rescue organizes direct "nonviolent" action against abortion clinics, shutting down clinics and targeting "abortionist" physicians. Every January an annual March for Life draws thousands to Washington, D.C., to protest the Supreme Court's 1973 decision. Increased political activity has given evangelicals marked success in blocking the election of prochoice candidates on a county, regional, and national basis. While in the larger culture *Roe v. Wade* may mean little more than two ways to cross a river, the struggle on the legal front to overturn the decision is stronger than ever before.[119] The Supreme Court has reversed itself one hundred times in two hundred years; evangelicals believe it will do so again.

Although evangelicals oppose vigilantism as unbiblical, an increasing incidence of bombing or arson against abortion clinics, which began in 1984 by a militant group called "Army of God" and culminated in the 1993 murder of a physician, testifies to the growing despair and frustration among evangelicals who hold their desperate dream of hope amid a spiritual slumberland. The borrowing of tactics from the fight against slavery also extends to the borrowing of rhetoric; evangelicals cite William Lloyd Garrison's response to the notion that he was too impassioned about his cause:

> On this subject I do not wish to think, or speak, or write with moderation. No! No! Tell a man whose house is on fire to give a moderate alarm; tell him moderately to rescue his wife from the hands of a ravisher; tell the mother to gradually extricate her babe from the fire into which he has fallen; but urge me not to rise moderately in a cause like the present.[120]

Evangelicals have found, like their abolitionist forebears, that it is hard to be unemotional about a subject that has such deep and persisting emotional resonance.

For all their faults, says literary critic J. D. Enright, antiabortionists "...let live. We would not like to see the opposing principle achieve general acceptance."[121] Evangelicals have respected and reflected one of humanity's most fundamental moral intuitions — it is wrong to take life.[122] For this reason evangelicals believe they are bound to win this issue in the long run. No one wins by insisting on a right to destroy. In Francis A. Schaeffer's parting words to the world, evangelicals must not take a "lowered view of life."[123] Evangelicalism should take a high view. It must be life-affirming.

# ·6·

# Eating, Drinking, and Bathing: "Cleanliness Is Next to Godliness"

Affect in things about thee cleanlinesse,
   That all may gladly board thee, as a flowre.
Slovens take up their stock of noisomnesse
   Beforehand, and anticipate their last houre.
Let thy minde's sweetnesse have his operation
Upon thy body, clothes, and habitation.

— George Herbert, "The Church Porch"

The average American digs his grave with his teeth.

— Billy Sunday

Well do I remember Holy Communion on one hot summer's day, and the cool silver cup containing delicious grape juice that passed along the congregation — and Mother's restraining hand when I drank too much of it.

— Charlie Chaplin

The early nineteenth century in industrial America was an unwashed age. Disease and dirt were rampant. Filth was "the premier public health problem in the nineteenth century."[1] Bathtubs had not yet become a household fixture; there were only 401 baths in the whole city of Philadelphia in 1826. By 1906, only 20 percent of Pittsburgh's homes contained a bathtub.

The city air itself was filled with odors that literally made people sick. Few could escape inhaling noxious and noisome *materiae morbae* (matters of disease). Philosopher Immanuel Kant, who gave moderns the intellectual scaffolding on which we built today's privatized, deodorant society bent on eliminating odors, was responding to a situation

115

barely conceivable to us modern men and women. The streets stank of manure, the courtyards of urine, the stairwells stank of moldering wood and rat droppings,...the unaired parlours stank of stale dust, the bedrooms of greasy sheets....People stank of sweat and unwashed clothes; from their mouths came the stench of rotting teeth...and from their bodies came the stench of rancid cheese and sour milk and tumorous disease.[2]

Little wonder that Kant banished the sense of smell from his aesthetics and helped fashion the modern concept of the "private individual," which, when coupled with the "olfactive revolution" of the eighteenth and nineteenth centuries, led individuals to become self-conscious about body odors. Homes unventilated during the long winter months produced what physicians dubbed the "prayer meeting smell" — a blended perfume of barn, dairy, and dwelling house "accented by perspiring piety."[3]

As if breathing were not difficult enough in this environment, tortuosities called corsets, stays, and garters twisted women's midriffs into hourglass shapes. Their viselike grips often caused fainting and damage to internal organs. Hoop skirts and petticoats, which led the fashion parade in the 1850s, often weighed fifteen pounds or more, dragging the ground and sweeping into their folds every filth imaginable. Bustles brought into church so much "wadding and padding" that maximum seating capacity in evangelical Protestant churches was reduced by one-sixth, and getting out of church took much longer as aisles could only accommodate two abreast whereas before the bustle three abreast could move conveniently.[4]

Eating habits were thuggish. Conduct disorders like blowing of the nose on tablecloths were not uncommon. Fruits and vegetables were rare. The American diet was famous for its richness in "the beef, the birds, and the multitudinous bibbles" summarized in a mid-century issue of *Harper's Weekly*. Gargantuan amounts of meat (mostly high-fat "hog's flesh") were consumed, with five or six (or at holidays as many as thirty) kinds of animal food and fish served at one setting.[5] Taverns featured such "delicacies" as pancakes fried in bear grease (also good for "aches and cold swellings"). "Where I behold a table set out in all its magnificence, I fancy I see gouts and dropsies, fever and lethargies, with other innumerable distempers, lying in ambuscade among the dishes," said one nineteenth-century witness.[6] In addition to this rich diet, Americans took into their bodies other harmful products. In the antebellum era, per capita consumption of tobacco in America ranked eight times higher than in France, three times higher than in England.[7] Americans' per capita consumption of alcohol reached an all-time high in 1830. Crudity and frivolity reigned in the American dietary regimen. "A hog stuffed with tobacco in an alcohol gravy" was a favorite oblation to the devil offered by evangelist Peter Akers.[8]

# I

One of the favorite pulpit stories from the later nineteenth century concerns the preacher's son who was called in from play by his mother. As he ran in the kitchen door and headed for the evening meal at the dining room table, his mother stopped him and said: "Go wash your hands." The boy protested, "Why do I always have to wash my hands?" "To get rid of the germs," his mother replied. The boy then said in disgust: "All I ever hear around this house is germs and Jesus, and I've never seen either one."

Evangelicals pioneered in clamoring for hygienic measures aimed at preserving health and improving "life-style." William and Catherine Booth started the Salvation Army with the slogan "Soap, Soup, and Salvation." Their calls for environmental hygiene were not merely expressions of disgust at the horrendous lack of personal and public hygiene. Their reaction was a positive expression of a moral and religious understanding of cleanliness.[9] Until evangelicals rediscovered it, "Cleanliness is next to godliness" was but an idle, ancient proverb first attributed to the second-century haggadist, the saintly scholar Phinehas ben Jair. In fact, medieval Christians looked on the wearing of hairshirts (with their attendant vermin) and not taking baths as signs of holiness.

Evangelicals like John Wesley disturbed the dust on this centuries-old epigram, pointing out the theological dangers of dirt and making cleanliness a shelf-mate to morality and medicine, not simply cosmetics.[10] By the nineteenth century inner and outer cleanliness were organic conditions of the same cup. Indeed, cleanliness symbolized for evangelicals a state of being morally whole, physically well, and mentally happy. Benjamin Rush, a Philadelphia physician and Wesley admirer, described how cleanliness was becoming "a physical means of promoting virtue," a phenomenon carried to embarrassing extremes almost a century later when Henry Ward Beecher appeared in Pear's Soap ads, claiming that "if Cleanliness is next to Godliness Soap must be considered as a Means of Grace and a Clergyman who recommends moral things should be willing to recommend Soap."[11]

There was also a promise of spiritual sanctification through reformed hygienic practices. "Christian physiology," as it came to be called, was one cornerstone in the millennial endeavor of building the kingdom of God. One historian has phrased the evangelical moral-social crusade calling for personal and public hygiene "a redirecting of biological science toward the social goals of contemporary revivalism."[12] In evangelical circles, cleanliness was a theological category of great moral strength and social importance.

Public health as we know it today developed from the sanitary reform movement spearheaded by American and British evangelicals in the mid-nineteenth century. Evangelicals were among the first to call for decent housing, tenement reforms, clean drinking water, adequate city sewerage, and other improvements in the disposal of human and animal ordure. Evangelicals agitated on behalf of environmental concerns and declaimed against the human cost of industrialization, calling for improved living conditions.

Beginning in the 1840s, evangelicals led the crusade in America's cities for sanitary reforms; they staffed boards of health and founded numerous sanitary societies. Evangelical reformers lobbied for quarantine regulations and for embargoed funerals of the infected dead. They fought for slaughterhouse regulations. The modern concept of "social services" is a direct outgrowth of evangelicalism's campaign against filth, disease, and destitution, aided in the late nineteenth century, as we shall see, by dramatic advances in the health sciences, especially microbiology and immunology.

Except for significant silence in tobacco-growing regions, evangelicals attacked the uncivilized use of tobacco, both for its filth on the floor and its fouling the air. One nineteenth-century evangelical merchant in southern Ohio described "vile tobacco spit" in a poem as "Filth of the mouth, fog of the mind, / Filthiest of filthy kind."[13] Evangelicals visited the poor, preaching the moral deterrence of detergents. They sought to free women from the dreadful imprisonment of bodices and corsets. They espoused good food and moderation in eating and drinking. Revivalist Billy Sunday, who always left the table hungry, constantly quoted his friends the Mayo brothers to the effect that "half of what you eat is half more than you need."[14]

Charles E. Rosenberg and Carroll Smith-Rosenberg have demonstrated the degree to which America's first generation of public health leaders — people like Edwin Snow of Providence, H. G. Clark of Boston, and Robert M. Hartley, John H. Griscom, and Samuel B. Halliday of New York City — were shaped by evangelical beliefs in the spiritual indissolubility of morality, health, and environment.[15] As Griscom put it in his 1842 classic statement on sanitary conditions, "The coincidence, or parallelism, of moral degradation and physical disease, is plainly apparent to any experienced observer."[16] To these pioneer public health reformers belongs the distinction of raising America's consciousness about nightmarish sanitary conditions in burgeoning urban centers.

It was the evangelicals' involvement in their own network of voluntary societies that alerted them to the miserable health conditions of the nation's slums. One of the missionary strategies introduced by these voluntary societies was systematic house-to-house visitation. Middle-class evangelicals like

Samuel Halliday, who worked for voluntary societies in inner-city missions, and Robert Hartley, who labored as a tract distributor for the New York City Tract Society, encountered firsthand the slum conditions of both large and small cities.

Methodist itinerant W. Lee Spottswood tells of accompanying a volunteer missionary on his rounds one day in Clearfield, Pennsylvania. At an early stop they found themselves "in a filthy basement, dimly lighted and destitute of every comfort." In a corner on a bed of rags lay a sick man. "Why, John," asked the missionary, "what's the matter with you?" The man replied: "Oh, not much — I've just got the smallpox." The itinerant admitted, "I got out of that place in a hurry." He confessed, further, "I paid no more pastoral calls with the city missionary."[17] But from these trying experiences evangelicals returned with increased clarity and charity to lead public health movements and to create some of America's first "protosocial welfare agencies" like the New York Association for Improving the Condition of the Poor.[18]

It was most commonly the temperance issue, however, that triggered evangelicals' entry into the public health arena. Nothing could stab awake the evangelical conscience so sharply or drive evangelical women and men into the streets, slums, back alleys, and doorways of the neighborhood so quickly as the sobering mission of temperance. The moral strategies of temperance benevolence societies — cash, clothing, compassion, and conversion — required intimate personal contact with the destitute and disadvantaged. Temperance became for nineteenth-century evangelicals a rallying cry for reform because of this firsthand exposure to alcoholism's debilitating effects on individual well-being and family life.[19] In the twentieth century, evangelical responses to the problems of alcoholism and the bowery, in this case Episcopalian Sam Shoemaker's opening in 1926 of Calvary Mission on the lower east side of New York's Gas House district, inspired Bill Wilson to write the famous Twelve Steps and cofound Alcoholics Anonymous, establishing it on evangelical principles picked up from the Student Volunteer Movement, John R. Mott, the Oxford Group, and the Young Men's Christian Association.[20]

Evangelical blurring of differences between sanitation and salvation were acted out on a large scale in millennial crusades like temperance, the most pervasive social reform movement in American evangelical history, and, microcosmically, in the liturgy of the Lord's Supper, where evangelicals raised sanitary issues relating both to the cup's contents and container. Indeed, even more than temperance psychology, it was microbiology and germ theory that caused American churches to substitute grape juice and individual communion cups for wine and the common chalice.

## II

The temperance movement began early in the nineteenth century when evangelicals began speaking out on the issue of "spirituous liquors," as the famous New England Tract Society temperance *Tract No. 3* called them in 1814, and when evangelicals started lobbying for temperance laws. By the 1830s, a sizable number of evangelicals had succeeded in making total abstinence the official handshake of the temperance movement. For many evangelicals, in James C. Whorton's words, "moderation was just excess in embryo. The same distrust of human nature redirected the campaign against alcohol abuse, corrupting genuine temperance into teetotalism."[21]

The question was how "total" was total. In the first half of the nineteenth century, most evangelicals exempted communion wine and "medical liquor" from their definition of total abstinence. The moderate position on medicinal alcohol is typified in these words from physician John Redman Coxe in 1831: "Vinous spirits, in small doses, and properly diluted, may be applied to useful purposes in the cure of diseases; whilst in larger ones they produce the most deleterious effects."[22] But as long as alcohol was justified medicinally, its manufacture and traffic could always be excused, evangelicals came to believe, and its extermination was impossible. Similarly, as long as wine was justified at communion, religion legitimated alcohol's wider social usage. Long before Billy Sunday sang his battle hymn "De Brewer's Big Hosses" and delivered his most famous "booze" sermon, the masses of evangelicals came to a consensus about those "dirty, low-down, whisky-soaked, beer-guzzling,...peanut-brained, weasel-eyed, hog-jowled, beetle-browed, bull-necked, foul-mouthed" monsters that owned the saloons and liquor factories.

The first church body to take the pledge of total abstinence — and I am here treading heavily in the footnotes of Betty A. O'Brien's article on Lord's Supper practices — was the 1835 Pennsylvania Conference of the Evangelical Association. It concluded its resolution against "King Alcohol" with these words: "Resolved, That we consider the use of fermented-wine in the Sacrament of the Lord's Supper contrary to the total-abstinence principles of our church."[23] Similarly, in 1841 the Freewill Baptists resolved to use "none but unfermented wine at the Lord's Supper."[24]

The theological rendering of this relationship between temperance principles and sacramental practices was not an easy one. But it would have been much more factious and factitious if mid-nineteenth-century evangelicals had esteemed and observed the ordinance of communion as enthusiastically as they did other religious exercises. Evangelicalism was blessed with an abundance — sacramental services, love feasts, prayer meetings, camp meetings, watch-nights and revival services — that worked to feed, speed, and lead spiritual cubs into lionhood.[25]

The founder of American biblical literature, Congregationalist Moses Stuart, leaned the weight of his immense learning and eloquence against the use of "wine and strong drink" through the development of the "two wine theory."[26] Whenever the Bible refers to wine as something good, according to this theory, it could only mean wine that was not fermented, supposedly a common drink in the ancient world. Conversely, whenever the Bible denounces drunkenness, revelry, and the like, it could only mean fermented, intoxicating wine.[27] Another respected evangelical scholar, Eliphalet Nott, president of Union College, promulgated Stuart's two-wine theory in his writings.

At the same time, Stuart argued that wine was an expedient symbol, albeit a nonessential one, in the celebration of the Lord's Supper. Yet it was not worth making a fuss about, Stuart concluded. Besides, Jesus so "mingled" the wine with water, predictably three parts water to one part wine, figured one Baptist biblical scholar, that it was too weak and watery a solution to offend anyone.[28] Another Congregationalist minister, Calvin Chapin, took an even more radical approach, arguing not only that the liquid need not be wine, but that "it need not be any liquid having the *name* of wine."[29] Interestingly enough, missionaries were often the loudest defenders of communion wine and the stoutest objectors to any change in the ritual.[30]

Evangelical leaders were not of one mind on this issue. Methodist theologian Nathan Bangs was so adamant in support of wine that he believed "we might dispense with *water* at *baptism* with as much propriety as we could *wine* in the *sacrament* of the Lord's Supper."[31] Most antebellum evangelical clergy agreed with Bangs. They did not see any moral hypocrisy between wine at the Lord's table and temperance or even total abstinence everywhere else.[32] When the temperance literature itself began to raise the question of the moral witness of the American churches' use of fermented wine at communion, clergy became so outraged at this "meddling" in their affairs that they threatened the temperance movement with mass withdrawal.

Congregationalist pastor and general agent of the American Temperance Society, Nathaniel Hewit, warned that "if temperance societies insist on the condemnation of unadulterated wine, and its exclusion from the church... they must make up their minds to witness the succession of the church of Christ from all further fellowship with them."[33] The *American Temperance Intelligencer* found out just how serious such threats could be. In 1835 this periodical became the first to publish articles proposing grape juice or water as fitting substitutes for wine at communion. The journal and its editor Edward Delavan incurred such wrath from clergy that the journal was forced to cease publication the following year.[34]

While temperance groups and presses kept the pressure on America's churches for the sacramental use of nonalcoholic wine, even printing recipes for home preparation of unfermented grape juice,[35] most religious periodicals covered denominational indecision and inertia with various alibis and ad libs. By 1880, only the Methodist Episcopal Church's *Book of Discipline* carried the stipulation "Let none but the pure juice of the grape be used in administering the Lord's Supper, whenever practicable" (the loophole in the last phrase was not dropped until 1916).[36]

Sustained debate on the nature of the wine used by Jesus at the Last Supper did not alter the dominant pattern. As late as the early 1890s, the use of fermented wine or grape juice was still one of the most prominent but unsettled questions of the day. Fermented wine continued to be used in the sacrament by all Protestant Episcopal and Roman Catholic churches, by almost all Presbyterian, Congregational, and Lutheran churches, by most Baptist churches, and surprisingly, given the official proscriptions (which stopped short, however, of prohibitions), by a "considerable" number of Methodist Episcopal churches.[37] Some evangelical churches experimented in the administration of the Lord's Supper with nongrape substitutes, including water and, with a sense of the ludicrous, cider, tamarind water, molasses and water, and buttermilk. But they tampered thus to universal disparagement.[38] Presbyterian theologian Archibald Alexander Hodge spoke for the more liturgical segment of evangelicalism when he uttered an emphatic "No!" to any attempts to modify the blessed sacrament, even in the elevated interests of temperance.[39]

Evangelical tolerance of differing table standards for home and church disappeared into the scientific gloaming — the growing haze of awareness that threw a chill instead of a charm over alcoholic consumption. The health issues raised by science's nervous assessments of wine's "purity" and "drugged" additives surfaced repeatedly in the resolutions and literature of America's evangelical denominations in the 1860s, 1870s, and 1880s. Churches should at least use homemade wines to avoid the marketplace's "foul mixtures" and "adulterated" concoctions made of the "vilest compounds" imaginable. One 1886 article in the quarterly review of the Evangelical Lutheran Church even printed side-by-side a comparative table on the composition on grape juice and wine. Wine contained

1. Alcohol

2. OEnanthic Acid

3. OEnanthic Ether

4. Essential, or volatile oils

5. Acetic Acid

6. Sulphate of Potash

7. Bouquet, or Aroma

8. Chlorides of Potassium and Sodium

9. Tannin and coloring matter

10. Undecomposed Sugar, Gum, etc.[40]

Methodist annual conferences, which were the first to enforce total abstinence principles at the Lord's table, made it clear in their resolutions and speeches that "personal safety" and "suspicious ingredients" made the substitution of "healthful, innocent, unintoxicating wine" imperative.[41]

The Women's Christian Temperance Union (WCTU), founded in 1874, was the largest nondenominational mass women's organization. At the second WCTU convention the most hotly debated topic centered on the banishment of wine at communion. The ensuing WCTU boycott of communion services until churches used grape juice instead of wine was justified on the basis of the duty of a pure example and concern for the "weaker" brother (that is, the reformed drunkard, also known as the "repentant dipsomaniac," and the "yet unfallen hereditary legatee of alcohol").[42] Clearly, American evangelicals "want a Christ that needs no apology, for whose acts we must not blush with shame, but whose example is worthy of our imitation."[43] Temperance advocates questioned how something as pure as the blood of Jesus could be symbolized by an "adulterated liquid" — a "disagreeable, fermented composition of who knows just what."[44]

It is within the context of this health-conscious debate that the labors of a certain evangelical physician must be interpreted. The novel "pasteurizing" experiments with locally grown grapes of Thomas Bramwell Welch (1825–1903) — a Vineland, New Jersey, dentist, Methodist communion steward, and erstwhile Wesleyan Methodist preacher — were as important to the replacement of the contents of the chalice as another physician's labors, as we shall see, would be to the replacement of the chalice itself. In his will, Welch's son Charles, also a dentist and his father's business partner, states that "unfermented grape juice was born in 1869 out of a passion to serve God by helping His Church to give its communion 'the fruit of the vine,' instead of the 'cup of devils.'"[45] But within four years the pasteurizing business floundered, forced to close because of lack of interest.

Revived two years later, it became incorporated in 1887 as the Welch Grape Juice Company. With greater attention to home uses and to health concerns, Welch's sales slowly increased, supplemented by advertisements in denominational publications, free samples to churches willing to try grape juice at communion, and a pamphlet distributed by the company entitled "What Wine Shall We Use at the Lord's Supper?"[46] It was not until American Protestants became convinced that "boughten" wine was, as we shall see in the next section, filled with "poisons" that grape juice became their drink of choice at communion. In the words of a Swedenborgian physician, "No vegetable juice on earth so strictly resembles the blood, as does the pure unfermented juice of grapes, for it contains albuminous matter to nourish the brain, muscles and nerves, acid and alkaline salts for the tendons and bones, and sweet to warm the body and make glad the heart of man."[47]

## III

Evangelicals eventually succeeded in flushing wine from the church's tables into the drains of urban America's newly constructed water-flushed sewers. What gave the grape juice movement its unifying and staying power were the same impulses that prompted another major liturgical innovation: the change in the mode as well as means of administering communion. With unprecedented resourcefulness of liturgical improvisation evangelicals experimented with an exotic array of alternatives to the common cup — with varying degrees of enthusiasm. Common spoons had sometimes been used in church history, but like the common chalice they were customarily passed from lip to lip. This time "communion spoons" were introduced, with everyone receiving his or her own spoon. What people also received, and resented, however, was the noise — clanging spoons, slurping sounds, and dripping lips.

"Fistulas" or long pipes (that is, straws) also have an ancient pedigree among communion utensils, used on and off (mostly off) since the ninth century in the Western church to prevent effusion.[48] This time evangelicals called them communion syphons, and produced them in two elegant styles: jointed silver or glass. But the problems were the same as those that prevented their earlier adoption. No matter how graceful one tried to be, picking straws out of a pocket and sucking wine through a slender tube stuck in a cup could not be made into good table manners. And some wine still returned to the cup after touching the lips.

Two of the more radical departures from tradition were the scalloped chalice and the gelatine capsules.

The California Communion Cup, as it came to be known, was invented by an Oakland, California, Episcopal clergyman and physician at the request of women from some of San Francisco's wealthiest Episcopal churches. Scalloped in such a way that the celebrant "never touches any wine excepting that which he actually consumes," one chalice could contain as many as fifteen scallops.[49] Variant versions of the scalloped chalice, such as the Double Trinity Cup with six large scallops in the rim or the Boston Cup with revolving silver scoops, never were given widespread consideration because it was not clear whether the wine could flow back from the lips into the cup.

Although the proposal of putting wine in gelatine capsules "in the ordinary or soft grape form" was not infrequent, there is no evidence that wine pills were actually passed out at any communion service.[50] Gelatine capsules brought their own problems — for example, how to prevent people who can't swallow capsules from choking, and how to get the pills down without reintroducing liquid and thus multiplying the problem. One might as well simply give everyone a grape or perhaps, as one minister suggested, a "wine laden wafer." Only clergy seemed to take seriously the proposal to add some form of antiseptic to the wine. This measure, physicians were quick to point out, would change the taste of the wine, would hardly destroy all the bacteria, and most definitely would do nothing to purify the outside of the cup.[51]

How does one explain the relatively abrupt adoption of what one English paper called the most revolutionary liturgical departure in the history of the post-Reformation church[52] — a change in the common mode of administering the sacrament of the Lord's Supper? The most apparent factor is popularization of germ theory that attended the emerging science of microbiology. In the 1870s and 1880s Louis Pasteur of France, Robert Koch of Germany, and Joseph Lister of England demonstrated the ironclad connection between illness and bacteria. Evangelicals greeted news of the existence of pathogenic organisms as scientific confirmation of their long-standing religious convictions correlating physical and moral cleanliness. Dirt and disease had long been moral metaphors for sin, the sickness of the soul. It now appeared as if the evangelical proverb "Cleanliness is next to godliness" had become a scientific maxim.

The new bacteriological creed defined disease as what happened after human and germ had met. At least twenty-two infectious diseases were supposedly communicated by the meeting of mouths, including such specters as diphtheria, typhus, tuberculosis, and syphilis. Just as medieval Christians had taken protective measures against evil spirits that taunted their souls, Americans set about to protect their bodies against invasion from disease-causing germs.[53] *Pollution* and *impurity* were words much used in the pulpit, as hygienic laws and phobias replaced the *Malleus Maleficarum* (the standard handbook on witchcraft used as a defense against satanism by Catholics and Protestants alike from the fifteenth to the mid-nineteenth century). Witnesses were excused from kissing the Bible. Bank tellers were instructed to moisten their fingers with damp sponges instead of their lips. Teachers began supervising the distribution of lead pencils among public school children. Some school boards required that books be covered with fresh paper monthly. The common drinking cup was banned at soda fountains, stores, schools, railroad stations, and other public places. "The public drinking fountain," one report read, "is beyond doubt the chief medium for the spread of contagious diseases in civilized communities."[54] There was even the introduction of individual drinking cups in public water troughs for horses, a cement monstrosity first introduced in Philadelphia by the Pennsylvania Society for Prevention of Cruelty to Animals. It is not surprising, then, that almost all observers have viewed sanitation as the primary cause of the switch from the shared communion cup to individual cups.[55]

But the popularization of scientific concepts about germ theory linked to public health concerns revealed something about the evangelical tradition that had largely been obscured in the public debate over evolution: the degree to which scientific authority had already taken precedence over the authority of church and doctrine. In the words of Charles Forbes, Presbyterian physician and inventor of the individual communion cup, "While so striking an instance of the practical interference of science with religion is unparalleled in the history of Christianity, it is evident that intelligent American Christians need only to be convinced that a religious custom is possibly attended with danger to lead them to so amend it that it will not be objectionable to any reasonably minded person."[56]

It was evangelical laymen in general, but Christian physicians in particular, who launched the movement and led the campaign to replace the common chalice with individual cups. Clergy characteristically misjudged the distance between pulpit and pew on this issue. For example, clergy reacted to the first recorded suggestion that individual cups be substituted for the chalice with paradigmatic resistance. In 1882 A. Van Derwerken of Brooklyn, New York, proposed switching to individual communion cups, but his pastor so opposed the idea that Van Derwerken delayed for six years an article for the *Annals of Hygiene* elaborating his position.

The slowness of clergy to retire their silver goblets and pick up terraced trays was evident when Presbyterian clergy met in New York City in 1894 to discuss the issue. Once again, the proposal to change conventional practice "received little support."[57] But no one, clergy especially, could ignore the newspaper reports of doubled church attendance and "packed houses" that allegedly occurred where individual cups were used. A standard rule of thumb had been that 40 percent of a church's membership would show up on a communion Sunday. With the adoption of the individual cups, that figure supposedly increased to 80 percent. Even those among the faithful 40 percent who were not boycotting communion began stepping forward and admitting that they had "only *pretended* to drink from the same cup."[58]

Baptist and Presbyterian laity confessed the loudest, although the Congregationalists were actually the first to adopt individual cups on the basis of hygienic principles (at the First Congregational Church of Saco, Maine, in November 1893). More than one church had experiences similar to that of the Presbyterian Church of Rome, New York, which was pressured into the change, partly by the spectacle of members of the congregation competing with one another to donate the new communion outfits.[59] Even when brouhahas ensued over the proposed change, as at Old South Congregational Church in Boston, for most members the furor had less to do with the theology of the change than with the fact that the new communion vessels permanently shelved "precious old heirlooms" that had been in use for many generations.[60]

On 13 May 1894, the collaboration between the physician Charles Forbes (Rochester Pathological Society) and the Reverend Henry H. Stebbens, a longtime advocate of sanitary reform, resulted in individual communion cups being used for the first time in the Central Presbyterian Church, Rochester, New York. Within one month after their simultaneous introduction in the city's flagship Presbyterian and Baptist churches, twenty other Rochester churches either were already using them or had sent purchase orders to Forbes's Sanitary Communion Outfit Company.

Much as Rochester, the flash point for "the burned-over district," had pointed the way earlier in the century for the identity and direction of evangelicalism, the city again became a catalyst for other cities, moving and encouraging evangelicalism in new directions. By 1905 "practically all denominations and sects [were] using the individual cups" stated one report.[61] By 1930 one estimate was that over 140,000 churches had adopted the individual cups as normative liturgical practice.[62]

The Methodists proved the most resistant to change, due largely to the crusade led by the influential James M. Buckley, for thirty-two years editor of the New York edition of the *Christian Advocate* and one of the most authoritative voices in the largest evangelical denomination. He insisted on calling this "the saloon method" of distributing the bread and wine, and he castigated the individual cups as "one of the most inconsistent and repugnant innovations ever foisted upon any part of the Christian Church."[63] Neither Buckley's crusade nor a resolution of discouragement passed in 1898 by the Board of Bishops ever resulted in any general conference action or disciplinary provision prohibiting the use of individual cups. In fact, by 1912 the Methodists' own Church Supply Company in Chicago was advertising cups in their catalogue. Likewise, the General Assembly of the Presbyterian church refused to direct churches to use either the common cup or the individual cup; they left this decision to individual church sessions, which almost always chose the latter.[64]

It was medical authority, however, that supplied the clinical support to sustain the momentum until the individual communion cup achieved general acceptance. In the *Chautauquan*, physician Felix L. Oswald warned Americans in 1893 that "our national health" was imperiled by the "thousands of uncontrollable gates of immigration" through which would pass willynilly devastating epidemics such as the "impending plague" of the "Asiatic cholera," a virulent epidemic "postponed" for a year by the intervention of an unusually severe winter.[65] Earlier, in 1887, Utica surgeon Marshall Orlando Terry presented to the Oneida County Homeopathic Medical Society an address entitled "The Poisoned Chalice," in which he argued that one of the most sacred symbols of the faith was actually a deathtrap. The Last Supper lured innocent old ladies, "pure in mind and body," into sipping from cups contaminated by the lips of the most degenerate and "physically impure" persons imaginable.[66] An anonymous physician published a pamphlet in 1895 entitled *Medical Testimony for the Individual Communion Cup* and mailed it to the clergy of several annual conferences in the Methodist Episcopal Church.[67]

Prominent evangelical physicians like William S. Ely, Martland L. Mallory, and Charles Forbes led thirty-five of their colleagues in the Rochester Pathological Society to adopt unanimously in December 1893 a resolution recommending "that the communion ordinance of churches be so modified as to lessen the liability to the transmission of contagious diseases which we believe attaches to the prevalent method of observance of the ordinance."[68] Medical societies around the country were quickly inundated with papers calling for the adoption of the individual communion cup.[69] In 1897 the American Public Health Association commended churches that had put aside the common cup and slapped the unsanitary hands of those that had not. Not to be left out, dentists lent their weight to the reform, replete with graphic descriptions of "neglected teeth, vitiated oral secretions, diseased gums."[70]

A few evangelical physicians, like the Philadelphia Presbyterian William H. Walling, complained that the germ theory had become too much of a fad and noted that people are continually surrounded with microbes in their carpets and pets, on door handles and coins, throughout their water and air. Sipping from the common chalice was about as dangerous to one's health as stepping foot inside church. Physicians outside the evangelical tradition were more likely to look on the individual cup movement as momentary modishness. Indeed, some argued, science's search for bacilli in saliva was being used for purposes outside the best interests of science.[71] But at a time when respected bodies such as the Maryland State Board of Health were making headlines by putting grape juice under a microscope and finding salicylic acid, judicious perspectives like those of Walling were largely ignored.[72]

Medicine permitted no back talk, once bacteriological tests of the wine at the bottom of the communion cup allegedly revealed that microbes did not have spiritual scruples and could conceivably contaminate anyone, even the saints. Those who ventured to contradict the "dispassionate medical and hygienic view-point" were themselves "open to ridicule and the suspicion of ignorance, indifference, narrowness, or wanton and stubborn animadversion."[73] This would be one of the first of many lessons for American religion in the authoritative voice of the new priesthood, now wearing white coats instead of black robes. Religion could declaim against sexual promiscuity all it wanted, marshaling every sort of ethical reason against ad hoc hopping in bed, but it was not until science warned against the dangers of promiscuity — the risk of herpes, and then AIDS — that Americans took notice and began to alter their sexual habits and promiscuous patterns.

Nonmedical factors, especially commercial and class interests, deserve the greatest share of historical attention in explaining the genesis of the communion cup movement. To be sure, medical and scientific elements were present from the first. But evangelicals were too shrill in their denials of any concerns other than sanitation; here is a too-often-expressed defensiveness, this one from the *Evangelist:* "It is not at all a matter of the rich and poor, nor merely of the cleanly and uncleanly, but emphatically of the diseased and the well — the unavoidable transfer of disease germs from lip to lip."[74] The fact that it was, more than evangelicals liked to admit, a matter of rich and poor, clean and unclean, can be seen from various standpoints.

First, no one ever proved the theory of the communication of infectious diseases at worship. The *Christian Advocate* laid down the challenge on 21 February 1895, calling upon the eighteen hundred physicians who were subscribers to the periodical, or anyone else, to identify any case of disease presumptively caught from the common cup. No one came forward with a single case of actual infection resulting from the common cup.[75] There was as much danger in the common cup, its editor concluded, as there was in going to church.

Second, the easiest and most obvious solution to the problem, as one lay person "not presuming to instruct the clergy" noted, would be to return to the ancient practice of dipping the bread in the cup. But the venerable tradition of intinction, first mentioned by a Latin author in the fifth century and by the tenth a fairly common European manner of administering the sacrament, never was even an option, much less a serious contender, as a way out of evangelical Protestantism's dilemma.[76]

Third, evangelicals shared in the cultural and corporate valuation of efficiency and expediency. As they watched the clock at work, evangelicals began watching the clock at worship, even expecting a "time-clock" service of one hour. In one sense, convenience had already caused evangelical Protestants to make the break with the common cup. Traditional communion services were about twice as long as regular Sunday services. The need to save time had dictated that larger churches use from two to thirty cups. Furthermore, many preachers had long held a cup in each hand, presenting one to the women and the other to the men.[77] Moustache cups were also in use for male communicants, many of whom had long, tobacco-stained moustaches that might otherwise drag the dregs in the cup.[78] The individual communion cup "shortens the service," one ad promised. "Long waits are avoided," and as many as eighteen hundred congregants can be served in eleven minutes. The big news coming out of Bishop John Heyl Vincent's presiding at the 84th Ohio Annual Conference on 25 September 1895 was not that for the first time in Christian history a bishop officiated at the Lord's table using individual communion cups. It was rather that "only about half the usual time was occupied."[79]

Fourth, the entrepreneurial spirit of competition and economic incentive spilled over into the church from the culture of the Gilded Age. Cities vied with cities; denominations with denominations; clergy with clergy; and firm with firm for the orders of America's churches. Presbyterians tended to use "the Rochester Plan," started by Charles Forbes, who founded the Sanitary Communion Outfit Company. (A national mecca for sanitary reform, Rochester was also the proud home of the Hyde Fountain Company, which made the only drinking fountain on the market in the late 1890s that shot up a jet of water.) Methodists tended to use the "Ryan Individual Communion Cup," patented by their own clergyman and physician E. W. Ryan. Ryan's method featured the option of two styles of seating: the "simultaneous method" for large churches and the "distributive method" for small churches.

Rejecting the claim of Rochester, New York, as the first to have used individual communion cups was the Thomas Communion Service Company of Lima, Ohio. It was founded by the Reverend John Gethin Thomas, pastor of the Congregational Church of Vaughnsville, Ohio (seven miles north of Lima). Inspired by Leonardo da Vinci's portrayal of each disciple with his own goblet in *The Last Supper,* Thomas designed an individual communion set used by Market Street Presbyterian Church in the spring of 1894. Thomas's company boasted that by 1907 its trays had been purchased by over three thousand churches. Rochester's Sanitary Communion Outfit Company countered in their ads that by 1907 they had sold over four thousand sets.

Other manufacturers also conducted ad campaigns in denominational periodicals, hawked their communion wares at church conventions, hired retired clergy as sales agents, and offered pastors commissions to introduce their products. The Dietz Communion Service in Chicago sold "noiseless" cushioned trays that competed with the "self-collecting cushioned trays" of the Thomas Communion Service in Ohio. Other competitors included the Globe Furniture Company of Northville, Michigan; the Individual Communion Service Company of Philadelphia, which offered church clients a complete "dignified and beautiful service manufactured by the company"; and the Le Pace Individual Communion Cup Company of Toronto, Canada, whose ads pictured a unique "Unbreakable Pointed Top Style" individual cup, which "Requires No Tipping Back of the Head." By 1895 the respected silversmiths of Reed and Barton were selling "silver plated communion sets having individual cups" out of their offices in Chicago, Philadelphia, New York City, and Taunton, Massachusetts. The competition was so severe and rampant, in fact, that some suspected "trade enterprise" at the bottom of the discussion. "It is a new way of making money, and the church is the proposed victim."[80]

The "victim" played its part well. It proved itself almost incapable of resisting rosewood chalice holders with nickel-plated trimmings, polished mahogany trays, or "silver, bell-shaped wine cups with gold lining" passed among the pews in "holders of oak, silver-tipped." Evangelical churches were ready for ostentatious displays of respectability and affluence on their altars. Indeed, the pastor who started the movement, Henry Stebbens of Rochester's Central Presbyterian Church, summed up nicely the psychological appeal of the new cups by making them symbols of the image evangelicals wanted to convey in American culture: "beautiful, chaste, rich, refined, and decidedly cleanly."[81]

Finally and most importantly, the whole exchange over the issue of individual cups centered in the connotations associated with that word *individual.* The evangelical equipoise between the community and the individual was now broken. "The world is convinced and converted in units and by units," a columnist in the *Christian Observer* wrote under the heading "Individual Christianity." "Christianity is not dispensed in the bulk."[82] While at the same time complaining about a notion of freedom that is identified with individual personal liberty, a writer in the *Reformed Quarterly Review* under the title "Individual Freedom" admitted that "the tendency of this age, especially in our country, is toward the extreme of individualism."[83] Evangelicalism tilted so far in the direction of the individual that the twofold meaning of *communion* existed only in antiquarian detail and broken-backed defense. Holy Communion meant "Communion with Christ" completely, "communion with each other" scarcely at all.[84]

Evangelicals stated this with surprising ease and pride. "The effort to prove that 'communion' or fellowship is an essential part of this sacrament, and therefore the necessity of a common cup, is not satisfactory" one minister argued. "All that can be said concerning the fellowship feature is secondary or inferential."[85] Irish-born Methodist Episcopal minister and soon-to-be district superintendent Joseph Pullman contended from the perspective of his parish in Patchogue, New York, that the issue was theological, not scientific. The Lord's Supper was a ritual of union, not communion. "The ordinance is memorial of Christ, and exclusively of Christ, and the communicant has lost his way if in the ordinance he has for a moment gotten away from Jesus Christ to consideration about the unity of believers." Biblically speaking, the eucharistic celebration contains "not a hint of fellowship of believers one with another, or of their union in one body." Indeed, the symbol of the individual cup is more in keeping with the fundamental purpose of the supper, namely, "the fellowship of the individual disciple with his divine Lord and Master[.] He takes that little cup in his hand, filled from the common wine, and, forgetful of all but the sacrifice of the cross, he enters into undisturbed fellowship with Jesus."[86] In eating the Lord's Supper, everyone was eating his or her own supper. In drinking the cup of salvation and purifying the soul, each person was performing an individual cleansing ritual that matched perfectly in time and theology the "cleanliness rituals" evangelicals were learning at home in their newly acquired bathtubs. (The more affluent even had newly installed separate rooms with complex plumbing systems where cleansing rituals could take place.)[87] The privatization of evangelical religion was now complete.

The real reason for the individual cup movement, the Reverend S. S. Rahn observed, was not fear of fatal microbes lurking in the communion cup or dread of contagious colds or disorderly worship. It was rather "the horror of sipping after one whose mouth is, perchance, not clean and whose breath is not sweet."[88] The common cup hindered the cultivation of religious devotion by permitting "sickening thoughts" to invade one's worship space of prayer and meditation: thoughts of having to drink wine that had become little more than mouthwash, or the troubling awareness that "others are waiting for you."[89] "All joy of the divine communion is lost in the thought of the brother who preceded."[90] The individual cup, on the other hand, promoted greater solemnity and increased meditation by allowing each person to hold the communion cup for more than a moment.

Besides, others argued, the "usages of polite society" require individual cups. As a "matter of taste" if not of science, the church must accommodate those who find it "indelicate" and "offensive" to take from a cup passed to them from people they do not know. No longer the friend of the downtrodden and rejected even among defenders of the common cup, Jesus was now "the world's model *gentleman* for all time and under all circumstances." He would not want his disciples to set a higher standard of fastidiousness for family tables than those that apply to the Lord's table. Jesus would not want his meal to "cause the gorge to rise in persons of cleanly habits."[91] Evangelicalism's appeals to gentility and agreeable message to the "more refined" and the "intelligent portion of our people" necessitated a change from the awkward and inconvenient custom of passing a chalice that ladies' gloved hands had difficulty grasping, which caused mundane worries about the possibility of spilling the cup's contents on a neighbor's dress.[92] "The Church of Jesus Christ stands for progress, and its example should always be on the side of the highest, most refined civilization."[93] Indeed, if the church wants "the rich and the poor, the refined and the unrefined, to mingle together in the same communion, we must give up the common cup."[94]

Evangelical congregations, in the words of one observer, were becoming too "'awful nice, you know,' to drink from the cup with brother Christians."[95] James M. Buckley called them "caste churches" and warned about the long-term effects on the church's psyche of diminished moral horizons. The internal damage of "ostracizing" persons who are "physically disagreeable," whose "countenance is repulsive, whose manners are disagreeable, or whose motives may be adjudged evil" was already showing up. Religious societies were being reduced to "clubs in which any member would be permitted to blackball unsatisfactory applicants."[96]

But those like Buckley who attacked the individual cup for its "isolating tendency" missed the point. For the fact that "there is *no fellowship of communion* in its use" was the knockdown argument in its favor. For too long evangelicals felt, but had not expressed, the exhaustion of acts of love in a society of strangers. As one put it, Christians have been "held under suppression from motives of kindly forbearance, as if under an unavoidable stress of duty to be fraternal."[97] The report of a special committee formed by Boston's Old South Church to investigate individual communion cups states this explicitly. "Formerly the church was in many respects a large family" where everyone knew one another and was part of an organic communal life. "We now know but little regarding the actual life of those around us." Even the best-dressed, best-looking Christian communicant in the congregation may be a carrier of a most horrid, unspeakable disease. Besides, "the increase of a mixed population in large communities" made the question of whether to use the same drinking vessel "of very serious importance, both from a sanitary as well as from an aesthetic point of view."[98] Blacks and the sick frequently stayed away on Communion Sunday for fear of arousing public prejudice. But immigrants, strangers, and the poor did not.

One dissenter on the eleven-member special committee from Old South Church braved a minority report. The loving cup is so named and so special, Henry D. Hyde entreated, because of its "common use as it passes from hand to hand among close friends, but not closer friends than Christian communicants should be." The loss of the "loving cup" would diminish not only the horizontal identity Christians have with each other but the historic continuity that links past, present, and future in an apostolic chain. "How many lips have pressed these cups in their first communion! How many saints have held them at their last communion! How much more will they be prized by those who shall come after us!" Instead of the spirit of class and smug self-righteousness, Hyde pleaded, the church must manifest the spirit of Christ, which draws together rather than divides the community. "The Church, to be efficient, must be robust, hearty, sympathetic, reaching out to all classes, including the rich, the common people, the needy and the outcast, and avoiding an exclusive perfumed dilettantism."[99] This was the original vision of sanitation and salvation with which evangelicals began the nineteenth century. It was perhaps best expressed in the words of Josiah Conder's communion hymn:

> All who bear the Saviour's name,
>   Here their common faith proclaim;
> Though diverse in tongue or rite,
>   Here, one body, we unite;
> Breaking thus one mystic bread,
>   Members of one common Head.[100]

By the end of the century, when street vendors and sidewalk hawkers in immigrant-packed cities like Philadelphia included the hominy man, the pepper-pot woman, the crab man, the catfish woman, and the peanut merchant, evangelicals were singing a different hymn: "I come to the Garden alone." The new eye-catching tiered trays sitting on the table every Communion Sunday gave eloquent testimony to the changes whereby evangelicalism developed its own tiered consciousness.

# ·7·

# Praying and Healing: "Standing on the Promises"

It is the love of the physician that heals the patient.

—Sándor Ferenczi

I dressed his wounds, God healed him.

—Carving over the portals to the
French Academy of Medical Science

My system's founded on this truth,
Man's Air and Water, Fire and Earth;
And death is cold, and life is heat
These temper'd well, your health's complete.

—Samuel Thomson

O what peace we often forfeit,
O what needless pain we bear,
All because we do not carry
Everything to God in prayer.

—Joseph M. Scriven

Thomas Franklin Day was a professor at San Francisco Theological Seminary. He recalled with great tenderness his family's Presbyterian Sabbath customs in Ohio in the 1850s. There was church, of course, every Sunday morning. But after church, when dinner was over, "Father would take from their wrappers *The Evangelist* and *The Herald and Presbyter*, which we took turns at reading." Intermingled with reading these religious weeklies went memorization and recitation of the Catechism. "It was a proud day

135

when any of us could repeat the answers to all the questions from the first to the one hundred and seventh."[1]

What was it about these religious periodicals that so captivated even their youngest readers like Thomas Franklin Day? Each one was a nosebag of new ideas and information designed to keep evangelicals spiritually invigorated and headed in the right direction.

Always stuffed in that nosebag were feature columns (the earliest ones were called "Medical Intelligence," the later ones most often "Health and Disease" or "Health and Healing") that kept evangelical readers abreast of developments in the health and medicine arena. A sampling of evangelical denominational weeklies reveals regular departments in all of them designed to make accessible to the widest possible audience the most recent scientific developments in medical matters.[2]

A list of some of the topics treated in one year (1882) suggests the scope of this unique partnership between evangelical religion and medicine: "Milk-Poisoning"; "Milk as a Remedy"; "Throat Diseases"; "What Causes Consumption"; "The Tubercle Parasite"; "The Soap Cure" (for boils and other inflammations); "Headaches in Children"; "Insomnia" and "Asthma" (allegedly treated by "compound oxygen" for which there appeared numerous ads); "Proper Clothing"; "Effects of Gymnastics" (the jogging craze of the late nineteenth century); "A Sure and Effectual Remedy" (for smallpox and scarlet fever); "How to Remove Insects from the Ear"; "Thefto-Therapy"; "Water as a Beverage"; "Well-Water and Typhoid Fever"; "Water in Disease"; "The Operation for Removing Cancers of the Stomach"; "The Practice of Medicine and Riches"; "Poultice Making"; "On the Hygiene of Bedrooms"; "Influence of Soil on Health."

Sometimes the medical column received front-page treatment, as when one evangelical weekly made a lead article of what to do "When Doctors Disagree."[3] Other times evangelical periodicals would print lengthy (eight to ten pages) review articles of major books germane to their readers' health and medicine interests.[4] These weeklies and periodicals also kept their evangelical readers informed about the dangers of quack remedies, including "Mrs. Winslow's Soothing Syrup," a cough syrup with enough morphine ("morphia") in it to kill children under one year of age, and "St. Jacob's Oil," a red-colored liniment having as its major ingredient turpentine. At the same time that these periodicals accepted health ads for "Ball's Health Preserving Corset," "Perry Davis' Vegetable Pain Killer," "Benson's Plaster for the Kidneys," "Smith's Patent Perforated Buckskin Undergarments — TO PRESERVE HEALTH," "Dr. Kline's Great Nerve Restorer" for brain and nerve disorders (trial bottles sent free to "Fit patients"), "Dr. John Bull's Smith Tonic Syrup" (if after three or four doses the patient needs a cathartic, "a single dose of 'Dr. Bull's Vegetable Family Pills' will be sufficient"), "Dr. Bigger's Huckleberry Cordial" (for diarrhea, dysentery, and "children teething"), and miscellaneous ads for cancer cures, acid phosphate, cocoa, cod liver oil, and cashmere bouquet soap, they also could expose quack medical advertisements, many of which appeared in *Popular Science Monthly*, including "Voltaic Belts," "Graeffenberg's Vegetable Pills," "Parker's Ginger Tonic," "Mrs. Pinkham's Vegetable Compound," "Kidney-wort," and so forth. Evangelical editors took strong positions against those who attacked health movements and measures fashionable at the time.

## I

The portrait of "Medicus" and "Clericus," physicians and clergy, as partners in healing is a common one throughout the evangelical tradition. It was symbolized for them in two biblical figures, the missionaries Luke and Paul, the one a beloved physician whose care was for the body, the other a spiritual leader whose care was for the soul. The two together provided evangelicals with a holistic model of Jesus' ministry of "teaching, preaching, and healing" as described by Matthew. In his famous sermon on "The Beloved Physician," Phillips Brooks put it memorably, as always:

> As [Luke] and Paul are seen travelling on together over land and sea, those two figures taken together represent in a broad way the total care of man for man....As we watch their figures, climbing side by side over mountains, sleeping side by side on the decks of little Mediterranean boats, standing side by side in the midst of little groups of hard-won disciples, — may we not say of them that they may be considered as recognizing and representing between them the double nature and the double need of man? Body and soul as man is, the ministry that would redeem him and relieve him must have a word to speak to, and a hand to lay upon, both soul and body.[5]

As we have seen throughout this study, health meant for evangelicals a right relationship to God that expressed itself in a state of holistic balance among body, mind, and spirit. Healing was that which restores right relationship and perfect balance. Baptist-affiliated E. G. Robinson, president of Brown University, lectured to Yale students in 1882 on the "economy of Christianity" and the various professional partners in a balanced economy: a social organism needs educators and lawyers; a physical organism needs physicians; a moral organism needs religious leaders; a healthy organism needs all of the above.[6] Evangelical ministers still teach their people to send for a minister when they become ill almost as quickly as they send for or see a physician. In the words of one evangelical "Doctor's Confession," both physician and cleric are necessary for the treatment and restoration of a whole being, "though from opposite sides — one the physician of the body, the other the physician of the soul."[7]

The healing gospel of evangelicalism proclaims all healing as God's activity. In fact, God always heals: "Bless the Lord, O my soul, and forget not all his benefits: who forgives all your iniquities, who heals all your diseases" (Psalm 103:2 NKJV; compare Revelation 21:3–4). But God works through a variety of what evangelicals learned from their Puritan forebears to call means, including death (the final healing act). John Gunn, author of the popular antebellum health guide *Domestic Medicine* (first edition, 1830; 100th edition, 1870), spoke of how "the great Father of the Universe, has clothed our soul with means, and those means powerful ones, of curing our diseases."[8] God is not going to do for us what God has made us to do for ourselves.

Prominent among these means are the hands of both physicians and ministers. "The medical and theological professions have a natural bond of union," another evangelical stated in 1865. "They once were united; they should always be friendly and cooperate with each other....Neither should be ignorant of the other. Either studied alone leads inevitably to erroneous theory and to dangerous practice."[9] God helps the sick through medicine and surgery as surely as through faith and prayer.

Evangelicalism furnishes some of the best specimens of physician and clergy cooperation in healing the sick. John Wesley pioneered this model and personally set the example, as E. Brooks Holifield has pointed out so deftly in an earlier volume in this series.[10] Wesley's *Primitive Physick* (1747), which was reprinted at least eleven times in the colonies between 1764 and 1795, often was bound with other works like John Theobald's *Every Man His Own Physician* (1770), which emphasized a spirit of cooperation between all the healing parties. If we are all healers, then to paraphrase Wesley, the world is our hospital.

## II

It was not until the latter part of the nineteenth century that evangelicals built hospitals, or what they liked to call "healing homes." Although evangelical denominations got around to establishing healing agencies largely after they supplied themselves earlier in the century with colleges, academies, seminaries, and missionary agencies, the development of the hospital system in America owed a great deal to the social initiatives of antebellum evangelicals' voluntarism.

Antebellum evangelicalism had its greatest achievements on the health front in medical missions. Famous for placing physicians and hospitals on the mission field, evangelicals were no slouches at home either. In fact, medical trainees getting educated for their mission work often did their field training with the poor and immigrants in the slums of the United States. Variously called "social work," "slum work," "rescue work," "gospel welfare work," behind every designation was a personalized caring for the sick and injured. Medical aid, provided through both physicians and nurses, was combined with welfare work and spiritual renewal by evangelicals.[11] Evangelicals deployed orders of Christian nurses, called deaconesses, to minister to America's urban sick in places where no one else would go.

The second phase of evangelical hospital development, which occurred after the Civil War, was shaped by the establishment of specialized hospitals for certain diseases or categories of persons. Evangelical denominations did not get earnest about founding hospitals until the last third of the nineteenth century, and did so then often in response to Catholic hospitals or in competition with other evangelical denominations.[12] But when they did get involved, they did so with verve and tenacity.

Evangelicals played an important role in the phenomenal increase in the reported number of hospitals from 1872 (178) to 1910 (4,000 plus). Some evangelical groups, such as the Salvation Army, achieved recognition in the wider culture for "adopting the newer and sounder methods of hospital and home care."[13] The first American medical mission opened in 1879 by the Alliance; it gave medical treatment to 40,000 Philadelphians in nine years. By 1910, at least one-fourth of all hospitals in Chicago were related to evangelical denominations or movements.[14] This does not even include clinics, dispensaries, convalescent homes, and homes for the aged, orphans, or unwed mothers (the Salvation Army established thirty-four homes for "wayward girls" or "fallen women" — many with the most modern maternity facilities attached).

Evangelicals and their churches continue to raise enormous sums of money for the support of health-care and social service agencies. There are currently over five hundred hospitals affiliated with the American Protestant Hospital Association, most of them started by evangelicals.

## III

As in the ancient church and in the lineage of some Puritan priest-physicians (Cotton Mather, Thomas Harwood, Manasseh Cutler), early evangelical leaders were looked up to as health experts. Some, like Church of the Brethren ministers Christopher Sower and Elder John Kline, were well-known and loved (Elder Kline was frequently referred to as "Dr. Kline, the Beloved Physician").[15] Evangelical ministers assumed an important health-care role, especially in frontier areas where there was little access to professional medical help.

Pastoral care meant medical care. In remote areas, responsibility for ministering to the sick resided largely with the minister of the congregation. This tradition of physician-priests was facilitated by the fact that "from the 1820s through the end of the antebellum period, a medical practitioner in America could lack an M.D. degree, be unlicensed, belong to no professional society, and not read (much less write for) a medical journal, yet still undeniably be a regular physician" and be recognized as such by lay people and by other medical men.[16] There was a hazy boundary between lay and professional in the early evangelical era.

Itinerants who did not do double duty as physicians were still often the only educated people seen in rural areas and hence were looked upon as medical experts. William G. Rothstein calls them "root and herb doctors."[17] They and sectarian practitioners were almost the exclusive alternatives to self-medication, which was, in early nineteenth-century America, a practical necessity more than a democratic philosophy that all of us are healers — *Every Man His Own Physician*, to quote the title of the 1836 book by Samuel B. Emmons.[18] The domestic management of illness meant that natural therapies and folk remedies were stressed, nonprofessional health-care options were preferred, and the physician not called until the last recourse. Given these conditions it was inevitable that clergy be consulted on the whole range of health issues, from sick babies to burst appendixes. They were expected to be somewhere between snake oil salesmen and orthodox medicine men.

Some enterprising evangelicals even patented medicinal remedies, which they sold in conjunction with their revival meetings. For example, itinerant preacher Lorenzo Dow often sold bottles of "Lorenzo Dow's Family Medicine" after his preaching meetings.[19] Dow's contemporary, Baptist preacher Peter Smith, traveled the Ohio Valley and hawked his book of treatments *The Indian Doctor's Dispensatory* (1813). Clergy did not see themselves as replacing physicians, only supplementing them and serving as their plenipotentiaries. Although this phenomenon of physician-ministers is today largely forgotten, every now and then residual reminders appear. The theologian on whom evangelicals have always kept a watch, Dietrich Bonhoeffer, reportedly carried bottles of sleeping pills and tranquilizers to give people in time of stress.[20]

Not only did pastoral care include medical care, but medical care entailed pastoral care. Evangelical physicians in the nineteenth century believed that their "mental management" of patients was as important as their medicinal and therapeutic treatments.[21] The solidarity of the mind with the body is such, one 1880s health column admonished evangelicals, that the human will "has the power of itself to relieve pain and in some cases to heal disease." Evangelical physicians were known to mix their prescriptions with prayer, and "without in any way depreciating the value of drugs as remedies" to recognize that "the will is in certain cases the more powerful, if not the only, agent in securing recovery."[22]

Again, much of this tradition is lost today except in residual and reflective form. Or it is preserved in stories from the mission field. Aylward Shorter tells the story of a Chinese doctor practicing in a Tanzanian hospital. A patient to whom he had just given some medicine said in appreciation, " 'God bless you, doctor.' To which the Chinese Communist replied: 'I don't believe in God.' 'Then,' said the African patient, 'I don't want your medicine!' "[23]

In the nineteenth century, the authority and identity of both the physician and clergy were based on the same foundation: morality. Evangelicals believed one should honor a physician for the same reason one honored a cleric. Both were the community's missionaries of morality.[24] As historian John H. Warner puts it in *Therapeutic Perspective*, the physician of the nineteenth century was "to act as a moral agent in a religious sense." He was expected to assume significant responsibility for "directing the flight" of souls into eternity, and for functioning as what evangelicals called a "missionary to the bedside" of dying patients: "Being a moral man was deemed crucial not merely to the physician's standing in the community, but also to his effectiveness as a healer....'Moral influence' was both a source and an expression of the physician's healing power and was regarded as an active force that daily made a difference in the sickroom."[25]

Modern science and the professionalization of modern life labored to separate Medicus and Clericus until evangelicalism's high model of partnership became a subdominant part of its tradition. Euphoric over the fact that they could really heal, physicians for much of the twentieth century decided to go it alone in the healing enterprise. Except for some individuals, and a very few institutions (like the Park Ridge Center, sponsor of this series), modern medicine has displayed little interest in the social, environmental, and moral aspects of healing.

Until recently the church has obliged medicine's wish to go it alone, itself euphoric over modern medicine's "miracles" and unsure about its own offerings to the healing enterprise. Once science brought medicine "almost to the border of the miraculous," in the words of one evangelical,[26] the pastoral function of the church upheld a safe, respectful distance from medical and healing matters. Religion joined the rest of culture in cheering on medical technology as it, in Ivan Illich's words, began "to reclaim the right to perform miracles."[27] Hence the clerical and medical professions became separate but unequal colleagues in a joint task to which each side makes a different contribution.

The "extra" that the church and clergy bring to healing came to be seen too often as precisely that: a contribution that is above and beyond that which is necessary for healing to take place. When medicine has done all it can do, which is everything humanly possible, religion is supposed to take over. But it is time for the evangelical tradition to collect its thoughts, and its traditions.

The healing forces of faith, hope, and love are not incidental to health and medicine. Like an antibiotic, faith, hope, and love enter the system quickly and do their work slowly. But the body gets well. Curing, or the removal of the disease, may take place with medical means alone. But healing, or the triumphal reentry into one's total environment, only takes place in partnership with faith. Medical healing is the knowledge of God manifested through science. Spiritual healing is the knowledge of God manifested through faith. It is the same knowledge. It is the same God.

# IV

James Erwin was sick, sick enough to seek treatment by a regular physician. Given large dosages of calomel and jalap, he was sent home to rest. Instead Erwin turned his horse in another direction and tried to keep his appointment to preach. On the way he collapsed off his horse in the midst of a rainstorm, lay in the mud for hours in his wet clothes, and prayed. The "covenant-keeping God" answered his prayer, "covered [him] with his feathers," and became for him "as a shadow of a great rock in a weary land."[28]

In two areas of their life together, the nineteenth-century union of Clericus and Medicus resembled a stormy marriage that bends and twists but never quite breaks. The first fight was over proper sickroom protocols and the moral management of dying patients. Surprisingly, these clerical protocols for the sickroom boast a past but not a history.

Evangelical ministers bore the burden of knowing that they would be speaking the last words to the dying, seconds prior to that person's standing before the throne. Clergy prayers for the sick and dying were sometimes less for one's health and recovery than for repentance and forgiveness before one's hellish future.[29] Some physicians looked askance at clergy stirring up "religious excitements." They especially condemned the "disastrous effects" of sickroom shedding of tears for sins.

Some physicians tried to keep clergy out of the sickroom for precisely this reason. Itinerant Elnathan Corrington Gavitt related from personal experience how physicians could forbid anyone but nurses from entering the sickroom, expressly prohibiting "anything like religious excitement" until it was apparent the patient would not last the night. Then the minister was sent for, with more than one patient outliving through prayer the physician's verdict of imminent death.[30]

Evangelical clergy advocated the principle of equal access to the sickroom by both physician and clergy, "for often his [the clergy's] visit will be as beneficial, sometimes more so," argued another itinerant, James Erwin. "Indeed, we ought to be as ready to *send* for the minister to pray, as for the physician to prescribe....Many owe their lives to answered prayer, offered in the sick room."[31] It is interesting to track in these sickroom protocols the increasing deference of clergy toward physicians as the pace of professionalized medicine picked up in American life.[32]

The second fight between Clericus and Medicus revolved around evangelicals having to make theological judgments about two basic kinds of healing coming out of the medical community: allopathic medicine and homeopathic medicine. Allopathic medicine is "regular," orthodox medicine, the "heroic" intervention through palliatives and placebos. Homeopathic medicine is "sectarian medicine," the gentle therapy of natural healing based on the biomedical belief in the delicate integration of mental, physical, and spiritual health. In allopathy, opposites heal; in homeopathy, like heals like. In allopathy the physician is in charge and intrusiveness is not uncommon. In homeopathy a close cooperation between patient and doctor is required, and nature is granted large healing powers and a central role to play. In allopathy the natural world is often out of kilter and needs jerking and twisting to be put right, so nature is never allowed to take its course. In homeopathy there is a mysterious harmony in the natural world, which when discovered brings healing. Allopathy is physicians' medicine and often quite costly. Homeopathy became known as people's medicine and was often quite cheap. In allopathy, "my power is made perfect in weakness" (2 Corinthians 12:9). In homeopathy, "by his wounds you have been healed" (1 Peter 2:24).

Homeopathy sidles up to depth psychology, which says that for healing to take place, one needs to bring suffering and pain to the surface. Accordingly, the healing power of Mathias Grünewald's *St. Anthony's Fire* (the Isenheim Altarpiece painted to bring comfort to those afflicted with St. Anthony's fire) is precisely in the images of tortured victims wracked with pain, watched by sufferers of the disease. In India this kind of medicine attempts to heal the aged and dying by burying them momentarily in a womb-shaped grave. Allopathy, in contrast, sidles up to humanist psychology, which compensates with the opposite. If you're downcast, the remedy is to have an "upper" or an upbeat individual pick up your spirits.

These two nonreligious forms of healing were, are, and ever shall be in some sort of conflict. By the 1920s the allopathic or "old school" physicians would win, aided by revolutionary developments in biological medicine (beginning with germ theory in the 1870s, the isolation of the tubercle bacillus in 1882, and immunization) and chemical medicine (beginning with aspirin, now consumed at the rate of over 21,000 tons a year, or 250 tablets per person per year). Homeopaths were much slower coming to terms with scientific modernity. But Mary Lamar Riley has shown in her study of nineteenth-century household health guides, how-to-live books, schoolbooks, popular periodicals, and lectures that the homeopathic agenda was subsumed into the regular therapeutics of allopathic medicine — a phenomenon Marshall Scott Legan shows was duplicated in the case of hydropathy.[33] The blending of homeopathy and hydrotherapy into the topography of American medicine is symbolized in the introduction of nutrition and dietetic departments into hospital staffs in the 1920s and 1930s and the incorporation of water therapies, such as whirlpool baths and "moist heat" services, into hospital rehabilitation centers by the 1940s and 1950s.

But the antipathy between the two was especially acute in the nineteenth century.[34] For one thing, homeopathy became more than an approach and mind-set. It also became a specific movement inspired by Samuel Christian Friedrich Hahnemann, whose theories included two fundamental principles: what caused symptoms in a well person will cure similar symptoms in a sick person ("the law of similars"), and medicines are more effective the smaller the dose ("the law of infinitesimals"). Homeopathic therapy became an inexpensive, natural, democratic, holistic, nonmechanistic approach to sickness and health that grew into a major medical sect.

What galled "orthodox" allopathic doctors the most was that homeopaths had the annoying habit of almost always being right. It worked. "Until the latter part of the century," Judith Walzer Leavitt and Ronald L. Numbers have written, "doctors possessed few specified remedies besides quinine for malaria, digitalis for dropsy, and lime juice for scurvy."[35] Boundary issues raised by the historical processes of professionalization assumed greater and greater importance in the light of the challenge of this homeopathic movement, and actually led to the founding of the American Medical Association in 1846.

Often as not nineteenth-century evangelicals were eager to try, then came to decry, the clinical power of allopathic medicine. Too many of the orthodox therapies simply were invalid, and they sometimes made things worse, Charles G. Finney was overheard saying in a lecture to Oberlin College students. Evangelicals also were temperamentally less suited to orthodox medicine's almost "high church" treatment of patients: regular physicians expected their patients to be acquiescent and play a relatively passive role in the healing process. Orthodox medicine was a "priestly function," Walker

Rumble observes; "guidance and cooperation typified the doctor-patient relationship, not mutual participation."[36] Accustomed to playing an active role
in the salvation process, evangelicals were drawn to those who offered them
an active role in the healing process.

This helps explain why so many evangelicals were attracted to alternative
methods of healing, which Norman Gevitz calls "unorthodox medical movements." Popular homeopathic crusaders, self-help treatments, folk and faith
healing, psychological, diet, and fitness programs — all had as their mission
the infusion of science with a spiritual dimension and holistic consciousness.
It would be too much to call these early-nineteenth-century versions of holistic healing the medicine of American evangelicalism. It is not too much to
say that evangelical religion was the path, and portal, through which many
Americans entered health reform and healthism.

"Medicine did not make an effective contribution to human welfare until
the middle of the twentieth century," contends Jonathan Miller in *The Body
in Question*.[37] Another historian of medicine argues that 1912 was probably
the first year when a visit to a doctor was likely to be beneficial to the patient.[38] One publication calling itself "a weekly magazine of contemporary
literature and thought" reported in 1903 "On the Progress of Medicine since
1803." In looking back the author admitted that "faith healing and homeopathy" had been "safer weapons than the mercury and bloodletting" treatments
fashionable in allopathic medicine.[39]

Of course, much of twentieth-century establishment medicine leaves little
scope for its practitioners' self-righteousness. Medical resistance to the discovery of vitamins — a discovery made not by scientists of medicine but by
chemists working at agricultural outposts — delayed for decades recognition
of the nutritional importance of vitamins, according to historians of nutrition
science.[40] Medicine's Vitamin-C complex still makes Linus Pauling a cast-off,
even a crackpot figure. In many ways a Gregor Mendel figure herself, Barbara McClintock was awarded the Nobel Prize in medicine in 1983 for a
discovery made forty years earlier but whose significance was denied and
denounced by colleagues.[41]

Two advanced medical technologies of my childhood — the tonsillectomy
(an operation then performed with far greater frequency than today) and
the hemicorporectomy (in which the surgeon literally cut the cancer patient
in two, leaving nothing below the waist) — testify to the halting advance of
science in every generation. The Upjohn Company debated whether to list
murder and attempted murder as complicating side effects of the use of the
sleeping drug Halcion.

If every discipline needs the corrective voice of a heckler, evangelicals
provided medicine with its share. Although they were early supporters of

blood transfusions, some evangelicals questioned the therapeutic use of vene-section, or bloodletting and/or blistering, from the very beginnings of their history.[42] Regular physicians admitted it had been abused, but they clung to both its therapeutic and symbolic importance until the mid-1850s and early 1860s. In fact, "therapeutics" like venesection, calomel, and tartar emetic le-gitimated and defined professional identity in allopathic medicine, according to John Harley Warner:

> Venesection was an insignia of the regular physician, a function evinced by the names of medical journals such as the *Western Lancet.* External attacks on the principle redoubled its symbolic significance, for faith in blood-letting was a clearly recognizable badge of professional regularity. It was therefore important to regular physicians that bloodletting not be rejected in principle, whatever might be its status in actual practice.[43]

Because evangelicals dismissed the quietist notion of passive resignation to sickness and believed instead that people had some control over their own destinies through individual and communal effort, and because they held the ideal of a partnership with physicians, evangelicals like James Erwin turned again and again to professional physicians for help. Unfortunately, too many of the physicians Erwin saw valued the "heroic" therapeutics of "bleeding and blistering" as the panacea for all of life's ills; or, in the words of one nineteenth-century physician when asked to give his general plan of attack in combating disease: "First I pukes 'em, then I sweats 'em, / Then if they wants to die, I lets 'em!" Antimony-laden tartar emetics and mineral poisons, especially calomel, a poisonous salt of mercury, were less and less prescribed by the orthodox medical profession from the 1820s to 1870s even though they were, at the same time, more and more defended by the same group. But they were prescribed frequently enough, both with and without bleeding, to cause Erwin to become "as helpless as an infant." After repeated treatments, he says, "I made up my mind that I would not be bled again; that such frequent drainage would exhaust the source of life, and I preferred to die a natural death, rather than be guilty of suicide by consenting to a course of treatment that insured certain dissolution."[44]

Another evangelical minister who had difficulty with his liver and lungs sought treatment of a physician, who bled him "a quart at a time, and blis-tered all across my breast." He tried preaching with a ten-by-eight-inch blister-plaster on his chest. But it filled up with blood and broke under the exertions of preaching, spewing blood all over the preaching desk.[45] Expe-riences of this kind gave rise to a strong evangelical tradition of skepticism about practices of "modern medicine," as this 1809 poem phrased it:

The lancet's us'd to take the blood,
The poisonous mercury for our good;
They nitre give to kill the heat,
They tell the patient not to eat.

They opium give to ease the pain,
This kills in part, then lives again,
To take the life which doth remain,
They then the lancet use again.

The blister's us'd to help distress,
And break the patient of his rest;
With setons they will tear the skin,
With physic clear what is within.

. . . . . . . . . . . . . . . . . . . . . .

MERCURY — ARS'NIC — OPIUM too —
PHYSIC — BLISTERS — LANCE — *adieu!*
And all who use them we deny,
Excepting when we wish to die.[46]

Laudanum and its sister medicine, Dover's Powder, were highly prescribed in antebellum America. Both contained tinctures of opium. As with
mercurial purgatives and bleeding plasters, both were in declining usage
by the 1860s. But the shift was not away from opium use but toward
more powerful opium compounds and higher dosages of it when prescribed.
Almost half (48.2 percent) of the prescriptions at Massachusetts General Hospital in the 1840s and over half (59 percent) in the 1850s had some form of
opium or opiate in them.[47]

An unexplored chapter in evangelical history is the surprising number
of evangelical leaders like Elizabeth Atkinson Finney, the second wife of
Charles G. Finney, who labored under severe addictions to opium caused by
laudanum prescriptions.[48] The problem is further evidenced by the presence
of ads for opium cures on the pages of evangelical newspapers.[49]

Little wonder, therefore, that revivalists and other evangelical leaders
joined forces with evangelical physicians like Russell T. Trall, Joel Shew,
James Caleb Jackson, William A. Alcott, Thomas Blackwood, John Romig,
Isaac Jennings, John Bell, Josiah Burlingame, A. G. Goodlett, Larkin B.
Coles, Arthur Grimshaw, Richard Carter, and Charles Cullis, to name but
a few, to found healing movements that experimented with nonaggressive,
nondepletive therapies. Many began frequenting osteopaths, orthopaths, chi-
ropractors, physiobotanics, eclectics, and hydropaths. Many also wound up
converting to the botanic system known as Thomsonianism, which purged
the body through heat-restoring botanicals (for example, cayenne pepper and

the emetic lobelia) rather than through leeches, calomel, alcohol, coffee, tea, and tobacco.

By 1840 herbalist Samuel Thomson estimated that three million persons had adopted his self-help system of rigorous therapy in natural foods. Historians have put the figures somewhat smaller, since by the 1850s the Thomsonian system disappeared as a unique medical sect except in frontier settlements. This was partly due to Thomson's own greed and gruff; it was also partly due to the success of his ideas at infiltrating other movements. Thomsonian doctors, for example, were influential in shaping Joseph Smith's views on health and healing.

But everyone is agreed that sectarian medical men comprised roughly 10 percent of the total number of physicians between 1835 and 1860, and almost 20 percent during the last decades of the nineteenth century.[50] By the dawning of the twentieth century, homeopathic physicians constituted over 12 percent of the total number of physicians in America.[51]

The weakening of orthodox authority and the therapeutic changes taking place in mid-nineteenth-century America can also be seen in the estimated 50 percent of the population of Ohio that allegedly acted as their own physicians, bent on curing themselves with only the nonviolent therapies associated with Thomsonians. Sectarian healing practitioners like hydropaths — who specialized in bathing, steam, massage, wet compresses, and cold water — also provided evangelicals with what Katherine Kish Sklar nicely calls "socially approved sensual experiences." A few sectarians went further and actually treated sexual disorders. At least 213 water-cure establishments opened during the last half of the nineteenth century. The lasting impact of evangelicalism's health reform movement can be seen in the establishment of the American Temperance Society (1826), the American Physiological Society (1837), and the American Vegetarian Society (1850).

Some evangelicals pointed to the basic problem with both allopathic and homeopathic medicine: all treatments and medications were based on bodily symptoms. Little attention was given to the mind and spirit. Among these evangelicals, for whom "healthful living was not just an opportunity, it was a religious duty,"[52] were some of the first to advocate what we today know as holistic medicine, if by that is meant the healing harmonization and interrelatedness of mind, body, and spirit. The alternatives they came up with were variations of religious healing Catherine Albanese calls "physical religion," which she defines as "healing religion" in which "acts of caring and curing constituted the central ritual enterprise for believers."[53] The evangelical critique of allopathic and homeopathic medicine also sowed the seeds for reform movements like Swedenborgianism, mesmerism, mind-cure, and Christian Science. Thanks to this coalition of health reformers around natural law, by the eve of the Civil War evangelical theology had been translated into scientific language and marketed for popular consumption.[54] Until 24 November 1859, when all 1,250 copies of Charles Darwin's *Origin of Species* sold out on the first day of its publication, evangelicals were at the forefront of popularizing scientific explanations and educating Americans in the compatibility and reciprocity of scientific arguments and religious faith.

Thanks to James Whorton, Stephen Nissenbaum, and Ronald Numbers, the "Christian Physiology" movement is perhaps the best studied of these health reform alternatives, which equated physiology with evangelical morality and stressed individual self-reliance and nature's curative powers. Two diverse figures loom large in this movement that secularized evangelicalism's perfectionist and pietist temper.

Sylvester Graham was a third-generation Presbyterian minister who was made at the time into a bran-bread fanatic by the learned medical tradition. They mocked his vegetarian diet featuring fruits, pure water, and unbolted wheat bran bread. A mob of butchers and bakers actually attacked him in Boston. Until recently historians saw Graham as a crackpot figure whose biggest gifts to history were the graham cracker, cold shower, hard mattress, masturbation anxieties, and once-a-month sex in marriage.

It is true, as Warner says, that "Grahamism was the antithesis of the *Playboy* philosophy: if it feels good, don't do it."[55] Graham didn't like flesh on the body any more than he liked flesh in the diet. But Graham educated evangelicals to see the laws of health as binding as the laws of holiness. His stress on individual self-reliance and nature's curative powers became part of the family traits of evangelicalism, even if individual evangelical leaders and institutions like Charles G. Finney and Oberlin College couldn't follow him all the way into his "hygienic millennium."[56] Some evangelicals, however, did: James Caleb Jackson and Ellen Gould White integrated Grahamite regimens of bathing, eating, and exercise into their millennial movements.

William Andrus Alcott, cousin of Bronson Alcott, was a Pestalozzian educator and Yale-trained physician who educated evangelicals to see illness as an unnatural, avoidable state of affairs. In the course of his prolific writings — thirty-one volumes on health, forty-four volumes for the Sabbath-school library, nineteen volumes on education, and fourteen volumes on the home and school — Alcott persisted in lifting up health as the natural condition of the human being. Illness was caused by human transgressions. In perhaps his most powerful and memorable image (and he was a master of metaphor), Alcott argued that one could "manufacture" health or disease. It was all a matter of human choice. Both were the "product of manufacture, just as truly and certainly, as cloth, paper, or pins."[57]

A valetudinarian way of life was not part of God's plan for human beings.

A diseased body was caused by diseased living, which these evangelicals defined as defiance of the physical laws of nature. God authored two books and expects us to master the laws of both: Scripture and nature. In fact, better to be strict about obeying the physical laws of nature than the moral laws of Scripture, Alcott argued, since Jesus atoned for the latter but "there is no known atonement for our transgressions of physical law."[58] Like good Arminians, Albanese notes, "revivalists and health reformers alike preached a 'can-do' religion, in which grace became the divine blessing on human effort."[59]

V

Few journeys have led evangelicals through as many bramble patches, which are almost impossible to get through without getting all scratched up, than the one that goes through miracles and faith healing. Let us begin with miracles.

The Enlightenment colors of evangelicalism are shown by its standard definition of miracles as a violation of nature by a volition of God. Or, in C. S. Lewis's widely touted definition of miracles, "we do not mean that they are contradictions or outrages; we mean that, left to [nature's] own resources [nature] could never produce them."[60]

Surely the first-century church knew nothing of this in its understanding of the miraculous. The notion that this is a law-abiding universe is an Enlightenment notion. Early Christians did not think in terms of hard and fast laws of nature being abrogated by God's action. Rather, the miraculous was God's lifting creatures and creation into higher and higher plateaus, not where laws of nature no longer hold but where people can see better, reach higher, and serve stronger than ever before. A miracle was when one could say he had "never seen anything like this" before (Mark 2:12).

Both professionalism and dispensationalism have been employed to finesse the problem of miracles. Toward the end of his life, magician Harry Houdini wrote an exposé entitled *Miracle Mongers and Their Methods* (1920) in which he dismissed all miracles and discredited the supernatural as nothing more than attributing to God what is technical and professional legerdemain. "Wonder workers," he said, are simply masters of stage illusions, expert tricks, and professional stunts.[61]

In evangelical history, miracles received the biggest dressing down by one of their own. Benjamin B. Warfield's classic *Counterfeit Miracles* took up where Luther and Calvin and Wesley left off. All three argued in one form or another that miracles were, in Calvin's words, a "temporary gift," although Wesley pushed God's withdrawal of miracles well into the third century and then only because of the church's decay of faith.[62] All three reformers contended that God allowed the spoken Word to preempt the healing gifts.

Warfield tightened up the arguments to contain supernatural gifts with a narrow divine dispensation. Miracles belong "exclusively to the Apostolic age."[63] To launch the faith and manifest Christ's deity,[64] God supplied believers with supernatural proof after supernatural proof. But the apostolic dispensation's use of *apodeixis* (a technical Greek term for proof observable through signs and wonders rather than reason or logic; compare 1 Corinthians 2:4–5) authenticated the gospel and accomplished God's plan for miracles. After the apostolic age, however, there is no more miraculous healing. Jesus' promise in John 14:12 that "greater works than these will you do" refers only to spiritual works. The prodigies promised in 1 Corinthians 12 are applicable and available only to the apostolic age. "The days of miracles have passed away," a mid-nineteenth-century Methodist bishop asserted somewhat wistfully.[65]

Ironically, this dispensational idea was fought back in the nineteenth century by none other than Horace Bushnell, an evangelical theologian influential in the formation of a liberal wing to evangelicalism. The difference between Warfield and Bushnell, the two theologians that evangelicals have most quoted to set forth their respective positions, is not whether God answers prayer for healing. Warfield said that many times. The dispute concerns whether God answers prayer within the limits of medicine and loving care. Or, to use Bushnell's formulation, which sets forth his understanding of the difference, "the problem was, how to use natural causes with a faith in supernatural helps."[66]

Chiding fellow evangelicals for the way in which "we believe so little, and deny so much," Bushnell deemed it of little wonder that "we have difficulty in sustaining the historic facts of Christianity, when the most Christian, most evangelical teachers, assume, so readily, the utter incredibility of any such gifts and wonders as the gospels report, and as they themselves have it for a righteousness to believe."[67]

Bushnell professed himself to have no difficulty in believing that "supernatural facts, such as healings, tongues, and other gifts may as well be manifested now as at any former time," and that "there has never been a formal discontinuance." Bushnell wrote *Nature and the Supernatural* to fight against a naturalistic, deistic conception of the world where the spiritual world and natural world are split into separate systems. The spiritual world, he argued, is not governed by cause and effect. It knows its own laws. It is even of a higher order than the natural. It is only faith's openness to the supernatural, Bushnell argued, that can "lift the church out of the abysses of a mere second-hand religion, keeping it alive and open to the realities of God's immediate visitation."[68] Bushnell's position was never stamped out completely, but went underground and surfaced in the holiness and Pentecostal movement's insistence on the accessibility and availability of the full range of the Spirit's gifts to the church today.

The contemporary evangelical community is split over this issue. The dispute is more than a friendly theological pillow fight. At stake are basic fears about worldly bedfellows like rationalism, naturalism, monism (for example, primitivism, pantheism), and extreme dualism. Fuller Theological Seminary ethicist Lewis B. Smedes and Fuller theologian Colin Brown do not feel that "we can appropriately celebrate the miraculous healings of sick people in a world of chronic and unhealed pain." Smedes calls this "a new triumphalist narcissism" where divine acts become arbitrary, "whimsical signals."[69]

Evangelicals like Smedes do not deny that healings ever take place but argue that they are not to be lifted up as an everyday occurrence and celebrated before the community. Fundamentally, miracles make them nervous. The "independent miracles" of Jesus' time, miracles that were independent of medical treatment, are no longer possible. Healings can still take place, they admit, though rarely.

Another segment of the evangelical community contends for miracles and claims that Christians should expect to do those things depicted in the Gospels. "Power encounters" are necessary steps in the process of soul making. Healing is a normative life process. It is not abnormal and intrusive, but a reflection of a healing God who is constantly healing. Theologian George I. Mavrodes counters Smedes with the argument that precisely those things that Smedes doesn't like in modern miracles — "that they are not the final answer to suffering, that they are occasional and particular, that some of them happen to bourgeois and middle-class people rather than to the desperately poor, that some are healed and many are not, that they do not confront the demonic powers in 'the big battleground'" of "systems that determine the lives of millions of people at a crack" — all of these objections can be leveled at Jesus' ministry as well.[70]

Some evangelicals, however, interpret a miracle less as a violation of natural law than as an expression of divine sovereignty. Henry Stob fails to see the big deal about miracles. There are those who are open to the presence of the supernatural all around, in both the miraculous and the mundane.

> Everything is for them a "sign" of God, one of His "mighty deeds." Each is marvelous in their eyes, a "wonder," fit to evoke astonishment and praise.
>     What we call miracles are in the New Testament called "signs" (*semeia*), "mighty works" (*dunameis*), and "wonders" (*terata*). But what we call nonmiraculous or natural events are in the Bible also viewed as signs and mighty works and wonders. In the biblical view, God is behind *everything,*

the usual and the unusual, the common and the strange; and He is behind them equally.[71]

The difficulty of this position Stob recognizes: "If miracles are everywhere, they have lost all meaning." When the distinction between creator and creation is lost, as it is in pantheistic monism, "all talk of miracles becomes meaningless."[72]

Some evangelicals, especially those from the Presbyterian and Church of Christ traditions,[73] have been most vigorous in embracing scientific approaches to healing and denying miraculous ones. But most evangelicals have sought to keep faith with the biblical testimony of miracles and the modern tradition of science at the same time. "Miracles are possible only in a determinate universe, the kind of universe that makes science possible. Conversely, science is possible only in a universe that is under the control of an intelligent Creator, the kind of universe in which miracle is possible."[74]

## VI

Only recently has there been in the evangelical mind a separation of sacred and profane healing. The healing power of medicine is itself part of God's healing action in creation. "I am the Lord, your healer," reads Exodus 15:26. Doctors treat. God heals. Medical and spiritual means cooperate in the economy of healing. Calvin taught his followers to use medical means for healing but also to pray and take the sacraments. Wesley taught his followers the same. Use physicians, but pray for the sick, he told his followers, and he added the new admonition of administering their own remedies and taking their cures into their own hands.

Evangelicals have not found it easy to steer the difficult course between the belief in a God who answers prayer and the espousal of an abracadabra faith. In a religion of miraculism, "signs and wonders" and "power shows" attune the believers' attention to the channel for the healing gifts and not to the source of the healing itself. Evangelicals do not claim any magic wand to ward off illness and disease. But they have braved ridicule to suggest that just as mind and spirit play a significant role in the onset of disease, the mental and spiritual also play an important role in the cure of disease.[75] But mind and spirit are not to replace science and technology in healing. In the words of Baptist theologian Augustus Hopkins Strong, whose systematic theology is still a favorite among evangelicals today, "Medicines and physicians are the rope thrown to us by God; we cannot expect miraculous help while we neglect the help God has already given us."[76]

In recent years evangelicals have been particularly sensitive to their image as being hostile to scientific advancement and indifferent to medical ethics, an image gained somewhat deservedly by their forebears' response to Darwin. This may be one reason why so many evangelical leaders believe in miracles and healings but play down their experiences of them.

Harold Lindsell tells the marvelous story of missionary Rowland V. Bingham's healing as an "illustration of answered prayer" at the same time he enounces the "principle that God usually does not do miraculously what can be done through normal processes. Therefore, the *normal* means of answering prayer is through secondary agencies."[77] In 1975 an interdisciplinary, international meeting of evangelical scholars took place at Wheaton College to look at "Human Engineering and the Future of Man."[78] The delegates were very conscious of evangelicalism's nay-saying, nagging reputation in its response to new technological developments. These evangelicals also admitted their past guilt for "undue fear and suspicion towards researchers and scientists in general," especially toward nonevangelical researchers and scientists in the fields of applied genetics and biomedical technology.[79]

## VII

But while evangelicals have tried to reshape their image of hostility to science, they have not abandoned the key plank in their theology that medicine is only a part, and at times only a small part, of the healing process. Spiritual "instrumentalities," healing arts, and holy curatives are vitally important as well.

Evangelicals have advocated basically six spiritual therapeutics in their healing regimen: communion, fasting, anointings, laying on of hands, readings from sacred texts, and prayer. Communion has not been as popular a spiritual therapeutic as one might imagine, but many evangelicals have shared St. Ignatius of Antioch's estimation of the eucharist as "the medicine of immortality." After visiting a dying smallpox victim and exposing himself to the dread disease, one frontier circuit rider announced that he "would sooner risk [his] own life than that a member should die without the sacrament, when they express a desire to communicate in the dying hour."[80] In the 1840s Presbyterians began taking communion to the sickroom, but Southern Presbyterians did not provide for sickbed communion until 1863.

Fasting has been a favorite evangelical curative, partly because of the biblical injunction that some healing "does not go out except by prayer and fasting" (Matthew 17:21 NKJV). Very few evangelicals were like Jacob Albright, the founder of the Evangelical Association, who declared "Darum fastete ich Unfangs ganze Wochen lang" (I fasted for weeks at a time).[81] The common standard, observed increasingly in the breach as the nineteenth century progressed[82] and only recently making a comeback, was fasting once a week, with cooking and eating time replaced with the preparation and consumption of "angel's food" — the manna of confession, contrition, and intercession that feeds the soul. Fasting for evangelicals meant not changing or cutting back on foods, but total abstinence from food and drink. In eighteenth-century evangelicalism fasting became almost an identifying badge and boundary marker from the world, a world which could satirize evangelicals' fasting, like Samuel Johnson in his humorous epigram: "Serviat ut menti corpus, jejunia serva; / Ut mens utatur corpore, sume cibos" (If you want the body to be useful to the mind, fast; if you want the mind to be useful to the body, eat).[83]

Evangelicals from the Wesleyan tradition practiced fasting as a religious duty. It was part of their "general rules," and fasts were required on the Friday preceding every quarterly meeting. Wesley was an ardent devotee of frequent fasts; he believed they should be kept as strictly as the Sabbath. He contended fasting gave the believer unique access to the mercy seat. Consequently, in the early days of Methodism there was fasting twice a week, and throughout the century they even fasted and prayed for rain in times of drought. All evangelicals observed special and solemn fasts such as national days of fasting and prayer for health and healing of the nation.[84] This was picked up by the new American nation, which in times of crisis throughout its history appointed national days of fasting and prayer.

Fasting meant more than abstaining from food and drink. It also meant "refraining from all sinful pleasures, and from all temporal business, except works of necessity and works of charity." This social dimension of fasting evangelicals took seriously: "The fast which God has chosen for us requires also works of charity, dealing bread to the hungry (at least as much as is saved by fasting), sheltering the homeless and friendless, and covering the naked with garments."[85] Good Samaritan fasting also helped evangelicals escape one of the spiritual dangers of fasting, a quid pro quo barter described this way by one evangelical: so much discomfort equals so much grace...and God is the banker handling transactions in human pain.

The spiritual therapeutic of anointings is more popular today than it ever has been in evangelical history. Prior to the charismatic movement, which softened long-standing antagonisms to anointings, evangelicals looked with jaundiced eyes on those who anointed the sick and dying with oil. They learned this in part from their beloved Johann Albrecht Bengel, who argued in his *Gnomon oder Zeiger des Neuen Testaments* (1742) that the oil mentioned in James 5 is only a sign.[86] In fact, the 1882 issue of the *Christian Advocate* featured two attacks on anointing rituals. Reports of miraculous healings from a faith-cure camp meeting conducted by Dr. Charles Cullis at

Old Orchard Beach, where a total of six hundred "invalids" went up to be prayed over and anointed, received the skeptical query: "If it is the prayer of faith that is to heal the sick, why not all of them, as well as five out of a hundred?" The editors also rebuked the report of a city missionary who anointed with oil someone dying of cancer, and then three months later telegraphed the country's daily papers that the tumor was shrinking: "We claim to have faith, but there is still incredulity enough about us to lead us to ask what other agencies have been at work during these three months?"[87] Evangelical reluctance to approve religious therapies using physical objects that have been such a popular and prominent feature of mass piety throughout Christian history, whether it be worry beads, rosary beads, cruciforms, or crystals, may have played an as yet unexplored role in giving rise to Pentecostal, neo-Pentecostal, and New Age movements.

The laying on of hands has been a prominent feature of the evangelical Presbyterian community of discipline, work, and worship called Iona Community, since 1938 situated in the ancient abbey on the Isle of Iona in Scotland. But like anointings, its healing and liturgical possibilities are more apparent to contemporary evangelicals than they had been to the vast majority of their forebears, some of the earliest of whom associated the laying on of hands with Shaker rituals for healing the sick.

Reading to the sick from sacred texts is a therapeutic and healing ritual for evangelicals. It once was believed that reading a certain verse of Scripture could stop bleeding (Ezekiel 16:6). Other scriptures, when coupled with secret sayings and prayers (some of which could be passed only to the opposite sex) had special curative powers.[88] Sortilege, or what evangelicals today dub the "lucky-dip" method of Bible reading, is a lingering feature of these folk uses of Bible readings.

Of all the spiritual therapeutics, however, the one most cherished by evangelicals is prayer. Few things evangelicals do are filled with as much spiritual physic as prayer; frequent prayer is the lifeblood of evangelicalism. It is often the first thing evangelicals do when they rise, of a morning, and the last thing they do before retiring. Prayer was second only to preaching as the most prominent feature of evangelical worship for much of its history, and prayers were often so lengthy (Charles G. Finney would pray twenty to thirty minutes) that warnings went out about wearying prayers. The Methodist *Discipline* admonished its ministers not to pray "above eight to ten minutes (at most) without an intermission," and the Baptists surveyed the fifty-five recorded prayers in the Bible and found that thirty-nine of them could be uttered in from one minute to two seconds.[89] Francis Asbury counseled his preachers, while on the road, to spend ten minutes of every hour in prayer. Prayer was often the only payment required by frontier families for a night's lodging. One "Methodist tavern" had as an admission requirement for clergy a parlor prayer that had to pass muster before the preacher was granted a free night's room and board for himself and his horse.[90]

One of the most powerful visual memories of my childhood is of preachers going directly from their knees into the pulpit. Similarly, one of my most powerful childhood auditory memories is of the thunder — the sound of an entire church getting on its knees and then erupting in individual, audible, thunderous prayer as soon as the preacher said, "Let us pray." In rebuke of and reaction to "formalism," most evangelicals proudly pray extempore, which means there are few published prayers for the ill and dying in evangelical literature. For example, I know of no evangelical denomination that used liturgical prayers for the sick in their worship from 1800 through 1850. Princeton's Samuel Miller, who put together *Thoughts on Public Prayer* (1848), included in it no prayers for the sick and dying at all. R. Milton Winter concludes that among the evangelicals most likely to have such things, there was "little formal provision of prayers for the sick in services of worship or of forms of prayer and administration of the sacraments for sickroom use."[91]

The connection between prayer and healing was assumed in evangelicalism. The memoirs and journals of ministers are filled with prayer-healing stories of preachers who "took hold of God's strength" and gave effectual and prevailing prayers that issued in instantaneous healings, simultaneous recoveries, announcements of accomplished healing that later proved true, and so forth. But these accounts are almost formulaic. When physicians walk out and throw up their hands, prayer steps in. Religious healing becomes, then, little more than a supplement to failed practical medicine.

Within the holiness wing of the evangelical tradition, however, there emerged certain impulses and ideas that helped encourage the development of healing doctrines. The "prayer of faith" was one of them. Its first recorded use was by Methodists like Hester Anne Rogers, who used the prayer of faith to expect the blessing of healing, and she obtained it.[92] It was Charles G. Finney, however, who popularized the prayer of faith among the broader evangelical community; in his words, "faith *always obtains the blessing.*"[93]

There have been more than a few who have argued that prayer is nothing more than a psychic placebo. One scientist in the 1880s challenged religious faith to a duel. Ten patients would be found who were suffering from the same disease. They would then be divided up into two groups — five placed in care of the church and treated exclusively with religious healing, five placed in care of physicians and treated exclusively with scientific treatment.[94] Evangelicals no more took up this challenge than they cheered the findings of a 1982–83 study carried out at San Francisco General Medical Center's coronary care unit, which suggested that hospitalized heart patients had fewer medical complications when prayed for than when not.[95] Contemporary evangelicals shrugged off this study (published in the *Southern Medical Journal*) just as their counterparts had ignored the scientist's challenge one hundred years earlier, for the exact same reason. The only proof of prayer's efficacy for the sick is not in physical healing or betterment in well-being. Millions of American evangelicals prayed hard, long, and in unison for President Garfield's recovery. He died. God's mysterious purposes preempt simple considerations of life and health. As Adoniram Judson Gordon put it, "We must remember both Melita and Miletum. In one place Paul healed the father of Publius by his prayers [Acts 28:8]; in the other he left Trophimus sick [2 Timothy 4:20]."[96] Healing has relative, secondary value. Bodily well-being is not the essence of religion.

## VIII

This is the essence of the dispute between the mainstream evangelical tradition and its faith-healing tributaries such as "prayer-cure" and "faith-cure" and "mind-cure." With the turn of the century came an explosive interest in healing. Guardians and guilds of spiritual healing began to multiply. Some of these became new denominations, like Christian Science. Others were isolated outcroppings of the "psychic principle" — the power of the mind to heal — like Boston's Immanuel Movement and Immanuel Church, known as "the first Protestant church that has ever declared openly in favour of mental or psychic healing as a department of its work."[97]

But within the broader evangelical world there emerged what historian Donald Dayton calls a "healing ethos," which was not expunged from evangelicalism until the Pentecostal movement appeared on the scene. In Dayton's words, "the early decades of the twentieth century saw a real scramble to avoid identification with Pentecostalism."[98] Even before then, certain evangelicals distanced themselves from the "faith-cure" craze, retreating into the posture that "Christianity's mission is to the soul, and not to the body. The spiritual-supernatural and not the physical-supernatural is what is required."[99]

It has only been in recent years, a product of the "charismatic revival" of the 1960s and 1970s, that evangelicals have realized that their lost heart in healing was a loss of something near the heart of the Christian faith. Jeff Kirby describes how "no one, at least in my suburban evangelical environment, believed or expected such things" as the prayer of faith or healing.[100]

Popular evangelicalism's interest in healing is demonstrated in Ruth Carter Stapleton's *Gift of Inner Healing* and *The Healing of Memories* and

Catherine Marshall's *Something More.* Some evangelical scholars even detect the unfolding of what Rodney Clapp calls "a centrist view of healing," which removes itself from the extremes at both ends of all supernatural noes and all yeses but is open to God's surprises and interventions.[101] These evangelicals who believe in healing, however, are less inclined than charismatics simply to people the present with first-century "demons" and "possessions" and more likely to try to understand and explore the experiences that created that language and then attempt a new language. By the second decade of the twentieth century, evangelicals found themselves having to fend off a bewildering array of mental healers, or as they were known popularly at the time, "psychotherapists" and "faith healers" — Mary Baker Eddy, Ida Mingle, F. F. Bosworth, and Aimee Semple McPherson. Fights with earlier generations of faith-cure figures — people like Charles Cullis, W. E. Boardman, Carrie Judd Montgomery, A. B. Simpson, Adoniram Judson Gordon — had seemed like family squabbles. Now the fights became more like blood feuds. What exactly were the points of dispute?

For one thing, healing is for evangelicals a hard-won faith, not to be claimed glibly or without struggle as some push-button healers were wont to do. Some faith healers even went so far as to denounce the combination of "means" and "faith" as ridiculous as "harnessing a tortoise with a locomotive."

To the contrary, evangelicals insisted, God does not work through the supernatural when medical and natural means can effect the cure. Indeed, "the positive refusal of medical and surgical aid is nothing less than a sin, inasmuch as it is a rejection of two of the most useful agencies" God has given us.[102] Evangelicals took offense at attacks on science and especially resented the designation "Christian Science," both words of which were deemed an affront to their respective constituencies. This is not to mention the fact that, regardless of what is claimed, faith healers use "means," whether they admit to it or not. Indeed, one physician defined faith cure as "a spiritual delusion mistaking faith in prayer for faith in God."[103]

The second thing evangelicals did not appreciate about faith-healing movements was their claim for a scriptural foundation. "Anybody who can be relieved of actual distress by a series of syllogisms ought to be allowed to do so," one evangelical periodical editor argued toward the end of the nineteenth century. Just don't say it's scriptural.[104]

Evangelicals took special umbrage at the cardinal tenet of the faith-cure movement, which found healing in atonement — "Christ bore our sickness on the cross" — and rewrote Scripture to accommodate their find: "God be merciful to me, *a sick one!*"[105] Faith-cure physician, mathematician, musician, and sheep rancher Captain R. Kelso Carter, who wrote the gospel song

"Standing on the Promises" to celebrate the healing promises of the gospel, also authored a popular defense of the doctrine of *The Atonement for Sin and Sickness; A Full Salvation for Soul and Body* (1884). Evangelist F. F. Bosworth argued that there is exactly the same basis for physical healing as there is for the healing of the soul.[106]

Such doctrines of a double gospel, where the sacraments came to symbolize remission of sin for the soul (wine) and the remission of disease for the body (bread), were viewed as double-dealing attempts to seduce the biblically untutored. Faith healers fused evangelicalism's concepts of salvation and health — parallel modes of divine activity — into one divine work. And evangelicals resented it.

The use of scriptural scaffolding to make an unscriptural attack on medicine as "satanic" particularly offended evangelicals. In fact, evangelicals could be quite vituperative against those like the "Faith Tabernacle" who led the charge.[107] Most Pentecostal groups that practice faith healing — like the Assemblies of God and the Pentecostal Fellowship of North America — embrace standard medical therapies. (One of the things that has made Oral Roberts acceptable to evangelicals is his support for medicine, as symbolized by his ill-fated, $150-million City of Faith Medical and Research Center, which opened in 1978 and closed in 1989.)

Third, evangelicals resented the movement's cruel identification of sickness with sin, or healing with holiness.[108] It is destructive to make disease into a direct function of faith. It stigmatizes the sufferer, demonizes the sickbed, and lionizes those who impeach Scriptures. It condemns a person for tuberculosis (the great killer of nineteenth-century Americans) as much as for theft. The "evil effects" of this notion were not hard for evangelicals to find. The deaths in the early 1980s of over fifty members of the "Faith Assembly" (near Fort Wayne, Indiana) who rejected medical treatment are but one example of thousands.[109]

Fourth, evangelicals question why faith healers, if they are really interested in healing, do not seem to be interested in health.

Finally, healing has always been reserved for and revered as the business of the divine. Evangelicals could not aspire to the pride involved in hurling oneself at the ultimate unknown, as if one could make special deals with supernatural powers.

For evangelicals, there are at least three certain conditions and criteria for healing. "If these things be in you, and abound, they make you that ye shall neither be barren nor unfruitful" (2 Peter 1:8 KJV). All three of "these things" are present in Jesus' healings, which comprise an amazing proportion of gospel verses given his short ministry. First, "Do you want to be well again?" as Jesus asked the man at Bethesda who had been sick for thirty-eight years (John 5:7). There are many people who simply do not want to be healed of their disease.

Second, "Your faith has saved you" (Luke 17:19), Jesus said more than once. There is the triggering, releasing power of faith. Faith releases healing, just as unbelief limits healing. Physicians can no sooner heal those who refuse medical treatment than the Great Physician can heal those who refuse spiritual treatment. Physical wholeness requires spiritual responsiveness. Faith begets faith: faith in Christ and the faith of Christ. This faith requirement can be seen in the centurion's plea for his servant; in the Syro-Phoenician woman's begging of deliverance for her daughter; in the father and his lunatic son; in Martha and Mary weeping over Lazarus; in the Bethesda blind man's submission; and so forth. This is also why some segments of the healing community are known as the faith movement.[110]

Third, Jesus heals with "bleeding hands," as T. S. Eliot reminds us. This is the chief qualification for becoming a healer oneself, stretching out one's hands and making them vulnerable to those in need. It is in the very nature of Jesus' healing love to require "hands-on" contact.

# ·8·

# Aging and Saging:
# "This Ol' House"

Let us cherish and love old age, for it is full of pleasure if one knows how to use it.

— Seneca

The best time for a man to sow his wild oats is between the ages of eighty-five and ninety.

— Billy Sunday

When you meet a dragon that has eaten a swan, do you guess by the few feathers left around the mouth?

— Ray Bradbury

I'm throwing just as hard as I ever did, but it doesn't seem to get there as fast as it used to.

— Lefty Grove

All five members of the Sweet nuclear family were expected to come together at the "family altar" twice daily (first thing after brushing one's teeth in the morning, last thing after brushing one's teeth at night) for family prayer. Our family altar did not boast a kneeling bench or elaborate room station, as some (especially middle-class) evangelical households did. We were too poor, and our customs too Appalachian, for that. What made our space sacred, what set apart the place for our ritual of family devotions, was the religious artwork on the walls.

The walls of evangelical homes are often decorated with religious art. Indeed, evangelicals have envisioned a role for the artist in society similar to that of the clergy. They have even called art "the fifth evangelist."[1] The three pieces of "art" that evangelized me growing up were a print of a painting, shellacked on wood, depicting a brother and sister crossing a deep chasm on a rickety suspension bridge, all the while unknowingly guarded by the most beautiful angel I had ever seen; a marbled, plaster-of-paris wall hanging of the Bible verse (the first verse I ever knew "by heart") "Thou wilt keep him in perfect peace, whose mind is stayed on thee" (Isaiah 26:3); and an engraved version of Thomas Cole's *Youth*, the most popular painting in *The Voyage of Life* series.

Actually, the latter's fuse was longest in my consciousness. It was not until I pastored a church that sat alongside the banks of the Genesee River in the "burned-over district" of western New York that I retrieved from memory the image of Cole's painting. At that point its "magic influence" (as one nineteenth-century pastor called it) made itself felt in my spiritual journey. For this was the same rural church where Frank Charles Thompson settled in as pastor and found the time to work on his famous *Chain Reference Bible* (1908), so beloved by evangelicals even today. This was also the area — Geneseo, Canandaigua, Portageville, Letchworth — that inspired Thomas Cole during the summer of 1839, when he made studies and sketches for the *Voyage* series as he traveled along the Genesee River.

Thomas Cole (1801–48) was celebrated as the foremost American artist of his day. Certainly he stands as America's first truly great landscape painter, and his belief that colors affect the mind in the same way sounds do still receives insufficient attention. *The Voyage of Life* series, for which he is best known, was commissioned in 1839 by evangelical banker Samuel Ward, father of Julia Ward Howe. Ward wanted Cole to paint an American version of *Pilgrim's Progress*. Ward planned to use Cole's oil paintings as artwork for the four walls of the "meditation room" in his New York home.

Cole kept a Bible open in his studio for inspiration and direction as he reflected on the spiritual significance of and encounter with the American landscape. What Cole ended up designing for Ward, who died before the series was completed, was a visual sermon-poem that would treat in an allegorical and theological way what we call today "passages" but then was called the "stream of life" or the "changing seasons of life." Instead of Bunyan's path or road, Cole chose a river to carry his cargo of messages and motifs.

So popular an expression of the evangelical soulscape was this series that half a million Americans (out of a total population of seventeen million) stood in line to see the four imposing pictures (each at least six feet long). In fact, *The Voyage of Life* series became a backdrop for the domesticated spirituality of Victorian-era evangelicalism, especially evangelicals gathered for family devotions. Thanks to James Smillie's printed editions of the series, by the 1850s it had replaced in popularity engravings of George Washington for evangelical parlors. It still can be found as wall decorations in many evangelical homes.

In *Childhood*, a laughing voyager emerges from a mysterious womblike cave onto the River of Life, with a guardian angel at the helm of the boat. Everything about the painting suggests a cozy, secure, joyous, wonder-filled journey. In fact, in his notes for the series Cole proposed putting the following inscription in the rock over the mouth of the cave: " 'Life issues from the womb of dark oblivion' or something to that effect. There might be added 'And Angels guide and watch it through the vale of earth.' Or 'From dark oblivion's gulf — the stream of life proceeds. Angels protect and guide the human voyager when first his boat is launched.' "[2]

In *Youth*, the landscape becomes diversified and lush; the narrow stream now opens into a wide, clear riverbank. Released by the guardian angel to the perils of life's course, the young man confidently steers the boat by the powers of his own reason, pursuing the lofty dreams that mushroom cloud-like before him in a distance. Ahead, unbeknownst to him, the beautiful stream suddenly bends into a rocky ravine. In his notes Cole proposed to inscribe in a rock on the riverbank, "When boyhood's illusion is past — reason must guide while guardian spirits watch."

*Manhood* is a scene of rushing rivers, dark ravines, steep canyons, precipitous gorges, threatening skies, and hovering demons (symbolizing intemperance, suicide, and murder). The rudder has broken off the embattled boat, and the middle-aged voyager, swirling in peril, must navigate around this trouble and temptation with the aid of moral discipline, faith, and providence. Cole proposed another inscription on a neighboring rock: "The prime of life is trouble and unrest and pain. But the Guardian Spirit still is near though hidden to human eyes."

In *Old Age*, a bald, white-bearded voyager faces expectantly the ocean of eternity spreading before him. There is now not only no helm but no greenery — only black clouds and a dark ocean lie ahead. For the first time the Guardian Angel is visible to the voyager, pointing toward a golden city of lights. Whereas Youth's vision was an illusion, the Aged's vision is divine. On a rock Cole wanted to inscribe: "Pass on ye Voyagers of Life's wild stream / Before ye opens mysterious gates / Of the great haven of the soul."[3]

Cole's *Voyage of Life* series freeze-frames quite effectively a host of evangelical attitudes in mid-nineteenth-century America. Life's journey is a solitary one. One has to go it alone in the boat of life. Although evangelicals saw life's major turning points as milestones in one's deepening commitment to the faith community and its social relationships and responsibilities, evangelical spirituality is at the same time deeply personal. Individual decisions determine whether bends in the river are successfully passed or not, and whether one's life will be placed in the hands of the only one who can see us safely through to the end. Cole's series portrayed this individualistic dimension of evangelical faith memorably.

What Cole's series also portrayed was the evangelical idealization of childhood, youth, and old age. In the words of historian Thomas R. Cole, "childhood, youth, and old age appear to be immune from life's vicissitudes. Childhood is protected and joyous rather than vulnerable and fallen. Youth is brightly optimistic about the future. Old age, beyond the storms of life, is dead to this world and only waits to ascend into heaven. All the cares, trials, and dangers of life are collapsed into the turbulence of manhood."[4] In an early testament to mid-life crises, the artist Cole demonstrated how the soul's journey through life is most sorely tested and tried in the middle-age period.

# I

"How old are you?" The young are apt to respond to this question with unembarrassed frankness and even fair-play turnabout: "How old are *you*?"

"How old *are* you?" The middle-aged are apt to reply in wily ways, responding with something flip — "Old enough to know better" or "That's for me to know and for you to find out" — or an authoritative posturing, "Old enough to be your mother/father." But to this is usually added some rider about not feeling as old as one looks or "You're as young as you feel" — almost as if one had asked them "How *young* are you?"

"How *old* are you?" The old are apt to reply in myriad ways. Some will be silent in embarrassed fatalism, or break silence in total bluntness: "That's none of *your* business." Others will respond self-consciously and defensively, as if one had asked them about their sex life. Others will smile with the playful challenge: "How old do you think I am?" Whereupon we venture a glaring understatement that is obviously short of the mark, followed by some haggling upward until the nervous comedy closes in laughter, mock surprise, and some expression complimenting them on how they carry their age, which is really a compliment on how they hide their age.

"*How* old are you?" Evangelicals' answer to that question reveals a great deal about the church, and even more about evangelicalism. It helps us see why the church has been, as David O. Moberg reminds us, "the best institutional friend outside the family the elderly have ever had."[5] Even when others deserted the aged, the church stayed with them. Evangelicals founded hospitals, nursing homes, retirement centers, hospices. The church has provided the aged with pastoral care, elected them to church offices, organized them into clubs, and surrounded them with surrogate families.

But more than anything else, evangelicals' answer to the question "How old are you?" reveals some of the hidden truths about the social and cultural meaning of old age, how it has changed over time, and why it is so problematic today. It also reveals why theology has not provided satisfactory answers to questions of aging or satisfactory sanctions and incentives, role models and norms, for entering "the third age" of life.[6]

In a multitude of ways our society hounds us to be young — in our clothes, our looks, our interests, our attitudes. The pressure is immense to hold back the passage of hours (lifetime average 660,000) and days (lifetime average 27,000) and to find some elusive fountain of youth. Evangelicals made smaller and smaller room for what psychiatrist Otto von Mering characterizes as the three s's of old age: sleeplessness, solitude, and silence. One can still find in evangelical culture the subtle ageism that asks its older members to define themselves in terms that disparage aging and elevate youth: "Young at Heart" groups and "Just Older Youth" (JOY) groups.

Modern lives do not come alive with the thought of getting older. Modern values do not cherish the aging of the mind, body, and spirit. Modern religion does not offer much moral endorsement or meaning to growing older. Modern evangelicals do not always follow the biblical instruction to "rise in the presence of the aged, show respect for the elderly and revere your God" (Leviticus 19:32). How has old age become the shabbiest part of life's story?

Age as a dragon that gobbles up the white swan of youth, as Ray Bradbury portrayed it in his novel *Dandelion Wine*, is an illustration of the "modernization of the life-cycle" that Gerald Gruman has described so brilliantly.[7] Modern thinking has emphasized age by elaborating the stages of life in age groupings. Known today as childhood, adolescence (youth), middlescence (adulthood), and elderescence (old age), each "escence" is seen as having its own essence of meaning and agenda. (The word *teenage* to designate adolescence entered the English language in 1945; in 1932 *teenage* was listed in Webster's dictionary only as "brushwood used for fences and hedges.")[8]

The equation of elderescence with senescence, and all that such an identification of old and obsolete entails, reveals the absence of what historian Thomas R. Cole calls an "age-integrated society," or "a balanced vision of the life cycle — in which each age is infused with socially valued characteristics."[9] Evangelicals have perceived and treated childhood, adolescence, middlescence, and elderescence differently in different eras of its history. Evangelical estimates of the elderly's role and worth have changed significantly through the course of American history; they can only be intimated here.

In the Puritan era, as studied by Thomas R. Cole and David Hackett Fischer, a "dialectic" of "decline" and "fulfillment" prevailed in which aging was pitied but the aged were venerated through rituals, beliefs, social conventions, and symbols. Reformation Protestants, especially Calvinists, faced squarely what they called life's "losses and crosses," including mental decline and deteriorating body parts, while at the same time they treated those few receiving the "distinguishing favor" of old age as holy beings and "visible monuments of sovereign grace."[10] It is too severe to call Puritanism "the negation of youth erected into a system." Advanced years was not something that one aimed at or held up as an achievement. It was rather a special gift from God that brought with it special responsibilities — such as imparting to the young wisdom about faith within life and hope beyond death and preserving for the culture memories and traditions. In the complex Puritan calculus of providence and suffering, bad old age could be seen as punishment for wasted life or unredeemed sin. Good old age was an act of grace or a sign of election.

Puritans did not try to hold back the mysterious and unmanageable passage of time. Life was not just for the young. Indeed, life was a pilgrimage, a spiritual journey of growing a soul, of turning water into wine. In other words, life takes time. It can get better with age. Even though at the extreme ends wine begins to turn to vinegar, still the most aged and decrepit pilgrim had an indispensable role to play. Some Puritans can be found perpetuating the medieval designation of the dying as *pellerin:* pilgrims whose advanced standing in their pilgrimage and proximity to the other world deserved awe and respect. Puritans accepted the decay of aging as part of God's inscrutable plan, and they encouraged people to live within their limitations and renunciations. Aged pilgrims lived a life with enhanced, not reduced, meanings. Puritans had important business to attend to in growing old.[11]

In the Puritan-evangelical transition and evangelical eras, the pilgrimage motif was preserved but significantly modified. Thomas R. Cole has explored evangelicalism's "phenomenology of aging" by reading nine hundred sermons on aging by twelve evangelical ministers between 1800 and 1900. The controlling Puritan metaphor of a spiritual journey, voyage, or pilgrimage was continued. But nineteenth-century middle-class evangelical culture after the 1830s made old age something psychological rather than physiological, a cultural meaning to aging which dominated American society from the 1830s to World War I.

Cole admits that in beginning his study he "underestimated the richness and depth of its [evangelicalism's] tradition of advice, inspiration, and consolation" to the aged.[12] It was this tradition, however, that made old age's reputation extremely various, even contradictory, and that made aging take on a considerable cargo of prejudice that helped build today's ageist society.

It was evangelicalism, in other words, that started American society's lusty youthfulness and lifelong sulk against getting old.

First, evangelicalism introduced into American culture the "cult of youthfulness." If old is not a four-letter word, as Jean Abernethy put it in her sprightly study of the Christian response to aging,[13] what kind of word is it? Evangelicals did not find it a happy word, but neither was it an unchristian word.

In the youth culture created by industrial America, however, there was one kind of word it was not — old was not an American word. Youth became the American word. "There is no country in the world where age is so little reverenced and youth so much respected as the United States," wrote George A. Beard in his influential 1873 address to New York's Medico-Legal Society.[14] Evangelicals built a youth-oriented culture that valued achievement, productivity, mobility, and activity. Asked how he would spend the intervening time if he were to die at midnight the next day, John Wesley replied, "Why, just as I had intended. I should preach tonight at Gloucester, and again at five tomorrow morning. After that, I should ride to Tewkesbury, preach in the afternoon and evening. I should then repair to friend Martin's house, retire at ten o'clock, and commend myself to my heavenly Father, lie down to rest, and awake in glory." A good old age came to mean youthfulness, usefulness, piousness, and self-reliance. A bad old age came to mean physical dependency, irreverence, and irrelevance.

The idealization of childhood and youth in the evangelical vision of life as a voyage, coupled with the need for preparedness to chart successfully the raging waters of middle age, meant that great amounts of energy were expended in the nurturing processes of training children and youth in the temperate habits of "the way they should go" (Proverbs 22:6). Child-related passages (for example, Matthew 18:1–11; Mark 10:12–16) have been some of evangelicals' most beloved and memorized Bible verses.

There is much opposition to home influences wherein there is "the child left to itself" (in a striking phrase from Proverbs 29:15). Evangelicals believe parents are responsible for the religious training of children, and the evangelical tradition has given rise to an extensive library of child-rearing manuals written for Christian parents. Susanna Wesley's "Rules," more formally known as *On the Education of Her Family* (1732), set the pattern and pace for other evangelical parents to follow in their own child-rearing practices and recipes for good old age.

The family and the church, evangelicals believe, are the two earthly institutions founded directly by God. But the holy of holies is the home. A lot of houses are inhabited. Not a lot of houses are homes. Evangelicals aspire to homemaking, and the sacredness of home life is attested everywhere. Family worship in both the home and church occupies a central place in child-hood and youth. The family is the church in miniature. Church life began in homes, and it is strong only when it is sustained in home life.

This is why the Sabbath becomes so important in evangelical households. It is family day, and there is constant concern throughout the evangelical tradition that the balance between family life and church life is kept and properly proportioned. Voices are raised in every generation questioning whether evangelicals are spending too much time running to and fro — to revivals, to committee meetings, keeping up with public services — at the expense of family worship and home religious education.[15]

It is the faith of the family that can put Christian children in a dif-ferent relationship to Christ than non-Christian children until their "age of accountability." In other words, evangelicals believe that children of Christian parents are accounted by God as Christians from birth until old enough to commit themselves on their own to love and serve God (Acts 16; 1 Corinthians 7:14). Conversion thus is both literally and symbolically a family affair.

The founder of "Focus on the Family," psychologist James Dobson, is the reigning evangelical expert in child management. The evangelical version of Dr. Spock, Dobson believes that the family is the key to the moral fiber of the social order. Parenting is not for cowards, he counsels. Parents must commit themselves to the task of child-rearing with deep dedication and dis-cipline. If the home is a "school," both parents are its principals, although the mother has been most often credited as the primary care-giver and de-veloper of a close family circle. Interestingly enough, evangelical nurture literature increasingly elevates the father's role in the home as more than a disciplinarian. What evangelicals fail to appreciate is that the kind of fam-ily structure they take for granted is fast disappearing in postmodern life, where many marriages are held together by telephone lines as much as by dinner tables.

Education in moral development is primarily a parental responsibility in evangelical communities. Believing that the child is a "clean slate" upon which one writes morality, a "dry sponge" ready to absorb all the "moral moisture in the air 'round about,"[16] evangelical nurture literature has stressed the relational foundations and fountains of healthy moral behavior — rela-tionships with God, with parents, and with oneself. Quick to point out that the words *discipline* and *disciple* come from the same root, evangelicals have stressed that parental indulgence can be as damaging as authoritarian harshness. Children need discipline, especially that discipline directed to the preventative more than the punitive.

Arguments that child-beating and other forms of physical abuse correlate with evangelicalism more often than other religious traditions[17] fail to take into consideration the varieties of social meanings attached to corporal discipline throughout American history, as well as the diversity of opinion among evangelicals about the advisability of taking children to the woodshed. While for most evangelicals corporal punishment (usually spanking) is deemed acceptable until adolescence, this is not always the case, especially in the current prescriptive literature.[18]

Praise rewards and rational discussion are the favorite means of behavior control. Surprisingly, the behavioral sciences provide major sources of insight and authority in evangelical nurture literature.[19] Forming healthy sexual attitudes is of prime importance to evangelicals, who are not opposed to sex education in the schools, only sex education that instructs in sexual irresponsibility.[20] Indeed, the very first day a child has been taught to feel good about his or her body, and to trust life itself, evangelicals have insisted, sex education has begun.

If the Christian home is the chrysalis within which a child is transformed into an adolescent, a key question becomes how one launches children with integrity in an age of promiscuity and moral decay. According to Donald Joy, raising healthy adults requires five things.[21] First, there must be healthy family systems in which adolescents are provided with constructive role models by parents who will spend quality time with their kids. But more importantly, since role identification is less focused on parents during adolescence, young people also need positive role models in the church and school and community. Second, there must be competency teaching, and an inculcation of the thrill of being productive. The third requisite is a chain of intergenerational and multicultural relationships instilled by bonding rituals (birthday parties, anniversaries, and the like) at church and home. Fourth, adolescents must feel some power over their future, learning the difference between instant gratification and deferred gratification. Finally, there must be self-discipline, in many ways the product of the foregoing developmental disciplines.

These five indicators — role identity, a sense of competency, a feeling of connectedness, the grasp of leverage, and self-discipline — Joy calls "risk-proofing your kids." And it is kids who evangelicals believe are most at risk in the world today. Evangelicals denounce easy ways of parenting, or giving simplistic answers to the complex world of teens today. Evangelicals also denounce a moral climate where everything is permissible so long as there is no pregnancy, or baby, or disease.

In the first quarter of the nineteenth century evangelicals developed what Cole calls a "civilized morality,"[22] the result of an alliance between revivalists, health reformers, and social reformers (especially temperance advocates) who were contending with the decline of hierarchical and communal authority. Evangelicals fashioned in place of the social control of inherited authority "an especially rigid form of moral self-government," as Cole phrases it. Imposing a self-denying ordinance on all of life, evangelicals internalized control and accented the harnessing of one's energies, the discipline of one's passions, the sanctification of everyday life.

Evangelicalism's doctrine of usefulness was critical to the development of this ethic of self-control, deferred gratification, democratic individualism, and voluntarism.[23] The evangelical definition of *virtue* is illuminated by the German word for virtue, *Tugend*, which comes from the verb *taugen*, meaning "to be of use, to be good for."

Charles G. Finney was once asked if it were wrong to pray for happiness. Finney replied that even the devil could pray that prayer. Quoting the psalmist — "Uphold me with thy free spirit. Then will I teach transgressors thy ways, and sinners shall be converted unto thee" (Psalm 51:12) — Finney replied, "See...the Psalmist did not pray for the Holy Spirit that he might be happy, but that he might be useful."[24] Slackness of mind, flabbiness of body mocked evangelicalism's doctrine of usefulness, which provided religious support for entrepreneurial capitalism's measuring of human worth in terms of market productivity. As evangelicals looked balefully on the debilitating effects of aging, the old venerables became the new contemptibles.[25]

Disease and suffering were the result of human sin and transgression — the proofs of disobedience to God's natural laws. The handrails of life (obedience to God's natural laws of health and hygiene) and the guardrails of faith (obedience to God's spiritual laws of salvation and perfection) could usher one into a state of healthy longevity and activity never before imaginable. Metaphors began shifting from a pilgrimage through life to a crusade against time. Time was the one thing evangelicals never had enough of, but which always seemed to have too much of them. Aging was now something to be mastered and controlled rather than something for which one prepared and which one accepted.[26]

The hostility toward old age resident in evangelicalism's doctrine of usefulness had been muted by Romanticism's religion. In poets William Wordsworth and Robert Browning, evangelicals found a vision of the "last of life, for which the first was made" in which old age became "a final eminence" of "awful sovereignty."[27] But evangelicals' fight against time manifested itself in various guises, and in increasingly virulent forms, after the Civil War. Nineteenth-century Methodists used to say that "superannuated" or "worn-out" (that is, retired) preachers were "more welcome guests in heaven than on earth."[28]

One of the biggest gifts the aged gave to early evangelicals was the reminder of the finality and fragility of life. Now that gift became the aged's biggest curse. Optimism about health and long life meant that, at best, figures of aging were simplified into silhouettes or congealed into stereotypes. Some aging evangelicals even found themselves having to cry out in the words of the seventy-first Psalm: "Do not cast me away when I am old" (Psalm 71:9). Charles S. Porter's sermon on aging in 1842 demonstrates how patterns of patronizing the elderly were becoming established in antebellum culture:

> Let your intercourse with them be characterized by great respect, patience and tenderness, remembering that the cup which you put into their hands, your children may mete out to you. And if they are Christian, who can tell what blessings may descend and rest upon you and yours in answer to their prayers, when they shall be with God? Anticipate their wants — relieve, if possible, their necessities, and tenderly guard their second childhood, as they did you, when first your steps commenced threading the mazes of this mortal life.[29]

An aging Dwight L. Moody, who chafed when a newspaper referred to him as "old Moody," could still be heard on the last day of his life declaring "I am not old." Reflecting medical beliefs that equated old age with disease and dependence, he admonished evangelicals in their relationships to parents and the truly old to "treat them kindly. Do all you can to make their declining years sweet and happy. Bear in mind that this is the only commandment ["Honor thy father and thy mother"] that you may not always be able to obey."[30]

Evangelical culture in the late nineteenth and early twentieth century tried not to make the aged feel like useless outcasts. Evangelical youth got accustomed to listening to "scrub and lecture" sermons from the elderly, who got out the soap and Ten Commandments in decrying everything wrong with the world. But resentment of the aging body — its cardiac constraints to usefulness, and the corporeal cage that inhibited "dynamic Christian living" of the "higher Christian life" — had to surface. It did so in negative ways that eroded the force of evangelicalism's traditional acknowledgment that life has limited duration (1 Peter 1:23–25); that death is the outcome of living (Hebrews 9:27) but not the end of life (1 Corinthians 15:21–22); that life is more than an accumulation of days; that old age has its own usefulness and meaning.

By the twentieth century, as Cole frames the issue, "old age emerged as the most poignant — and most loathsome — symbol of the decline of bourgeois self-reliance."[31] Old age meant "no longer of use." Older evangelicals changed their lament from "I have outlived my generation" to "I have outlived my usefulness."[32] Americans began to see the period beyond the age 65 as a debilitated stage of life. Americans also began to see the person beyond 65 as disposable (if you're not "good for something," the saying went, you're "good for nothing") and to fear this "fixed period" of life, for some an ogre, for others a ghost.

In short, self-mastery, self-reliance, and natural hygiene did not prevent the unsparing, unerring accuracy with which aging's deputies of death acted out their mortal errand. At the same time the cultural dominance of a consumption ethic, corporate capitalism, bureaucratic forms of management and organization, and professional ideologies (reflected by the medical and social science professions) reshaped public definitions of old age by reducing the emphasis on what the individual could do unaided and without "professional" help to solve what was now referred to for the first time as "the problem of old age."

An entire age group had now been "scientifically" categorized and classified as "superannuated." No longer did someone like the early Baptist preacher Isaac Backus walk almost imperceptively in his working life toward inactivity, from preaching 153 times and traveling 1,145 miles during his forty-seventh year of ministry (1794), to 130 and 853, respectively, during his forty-eighth (1795), to 122 and 629 his fiftieth (1797), to 112 and 336 his fifty-second (1799), to 113 and 121 his fifty-third (1800), to 73 and 187 his fifty-seventh (1804), and — the year before his death at age 86 — to 58 and 189 during his fifty-eighth year of ministry (1805). Evangelicals increasingly found themselves performing valuable service one day under what Backus called the "showers and shines of Heaven" and the next day not working at all.[33]

By 1935 aging had became, in the medico-nursing jargon, "a management problem," best addressed through bureaucratic solutions. Old people were systematically segregated from adult society once they reached the same age Chancellor Otto von Bismarck chose when he launched the first social security system in 1881, after consulting his actuaries for the age beyond which few Germans lived. An aging industry grew up around geriatric medicine, old-age homes, mandatory retirement, and pension laws and programs enacted by corporate and government bureaucracies and based strictly on chronological age. A cluster of complex factors and simultaneous forces at work culminated in the Social Security Act of 1935, which symbolized how the concept of superannuation changed from the plight of a few to the condition of all people "beyond sixty-five." As anyone can attest who has read the chronicles of the aging during this period — they are more drearies than diaries — the degenerative disease of old age drenched their days and shrouded their spirits. To grow old was to walk into decay, grief, cancer, loneliness, worthlessness, dependency, and death.

Seeing America as a society that buried its aged before they were dead, older Americans felt consigned either to the scrap heap as useless goods or to attic shelves as so much surplus, superannuated stock. Doctors viewed old age as an illness that contained its own pathology and required its own special treatments. Only professional expertise and scientific knowledge could abolish its symptoms or delay its progress for as long as possible. Neither God nor nature was an ally in the task as before. Indeed, nature became the particular culprit that science would countermand.[34]

Richard B. Calhoun's study *In Search of the New Old: Redefining Old Age in America, 1945-1970* has demonstrated the emergence during those years of a genial "senior citizen," "Geritol generation," which the modern American welfare state made to feel dependent, in need of services, and incapable of leading real lives like those of the "Pepsi generation."[35] Encouraged by social scientists, management, and unions to move from a work ethic to a retirement ethic, embodied in national policy by the Older Americans Act (1965), a graying population was expected to get out of the work force even before age 65 and move to some happy, "adult" (that is, no children allowed) retirement village in Florida, Arizona, or California.

Second best was to stay at home and develop time-consuming hobbies. Unforeseen was the restlessness, resentment, and depression that cropped up from suppressed notions about idleness being the devil's workshop and repressed fears of being no longer a productive member of society. Billy Graham counseled retirees "with an old head and a young heart" that "sunsets are always glorious." Retirement can provide "some of your most useful and happy years," especially since "your busy pastor has many little tasks that are really important in themselves to which he can assign you."[36] Thanks to the church, the old were not as alienated and abandoned in evangelical culture as in the wider culture, where their presence reminded Americans of the fact of their own ugly, unmentionable deaths.

The social disease of ageism persists into the 1990s, but it is gradually being dismantled. Intergenerational relations are getting better; the neuterdom of the nursing home is less offensive, with healthy regard for the full range of the elderly's needs, constraints, and ambitions; chronological boundaries of old age are getting fuzzier; the old are getting more fully integrated into society than at any time since the Puritan era.

Today's enlightened view of old age and its ethic of activism or "the third age" — preserve health and usefulness and independence for as long as possible — is a reminder of evangelicalism's lingering legacy. André Maurois summed up this ethic succinctly when he said that growing old is no more than a bad habit that a busy man has no time to form.[37] Or in Casey Stengel's immortal words, "The trick is growing up without growing old." We admire most those who never seem to grow old. Even the new conceptions of "retirement" are defined in terms of its increased opportunities for usefulness and creativity.

There is great danger in this reborn activist mythology, however. For one thing, as Abraham Heschel has prophesied, "Old age is a major challenge to the inner life....Old age involves the problem of what to do with privacy."[38] For another, the greatest offense of the aged is not that they are not useful, but that they are not beautiful. For another, Cole warns that "the contemporary attack on ageism originates historically in the same chorus of cultural values that gave rise to ageism in the first place." The new "enlightened perspective," in other words, creates a "perpetual middle age, legitimized by the illusory promise of scientifically retarding or abolishing biological aging."[39] Almost alone among the people who write on one of the four "devil words" of the day (sexism, racism, ageism, and handicapism), Cole warns that "in repudiating myths of dependence, decay, and disease," the attack on ageism represents "a new mythology of older people as healthy, sexually active, engaged, productive, self-reliant," a mythology that can be as "politically and ethically dangerous" as the ageist one since it "shows no more tolerance or respect for the intractable vicissitudes of aging than the old negative mythology."[40]

Evangelicals are beginning to rethink the moral and spiritual significance of aging and offer a workable conception of growing old. They are starting to point out to American culture ways in which the different parts of our life stages can fit together meaningfully and realistically. Like never before, they are facing up to the natural fact that we do age; our bodies wear out. One cannot fight gravity and win.

To cite but one example, William L. Hendricks's elaboration of a Southern Baptist theology for senior adults argues that there is value in life, even late-life experiences that pass through the jamming and static of old age.[41] Evangelicals need to listen more intently to Eugene C. Bianchi's call for persons in mid-life "to make their lives more contemplative within the context of active worldly endeavors" and for those in elderhood to participate more fully "in the great concerns of humanity."[42]

Like the silent, withdrawn biblical character named Lazarus, who did nothing to contribute to his community except be there for Jesus, we too serve and honor God not only by what we do and give but by what we receive and allow to happen to us. John Redhead describes an old man in this fashion: "His face was like an ancient chapel with all the lamps inside lighted up for evening worship."[43] Each age has a contribution to make to life: the season of twilight is as important and vital a part of life as the season of dawn. The birthright of youth contributes freshness and daring to a society. The crown of old age contributes memory and wisdom to a society. We can ill afford to reject either contribution.

Erik Erikson has argued that the last years of life are designed precisely for the integration of previous experiences and wisdom; that old age is the best time for exploring the ultimate meanings of life; that the mind and spirit grow more slowly than the body.[44] In a physical sense, then, a decaying exterior can sheathe a blossoming interior. In a religious sense, downsizing may be in some mysterious, metaphysical balancing relationship to upgrading.

Life does not age. Life does not grow old. Life does not die. Life is a dynamic, ever-changing stream that is not dammed, or damned, by age. The flow of life does not give itself to us quickly. It requires rather that we learn both how to rush and when to amble along.

Long life is not a matter of length of years, but of going with the flow... the flow of God's life and spirit.

# ·9·

# Deathbeds and Graveyards: "The Strange Madness of Our Joys"

> O what a soul-transporting sight
> Mine eyes to-day have seen,
> A spectacle of strange delight
> To Angels, and to men!
> Nor human language can express,
> Nor tongue of angels paint
> The vast mysterious happiness
> Of a departing saint!
>
> — Charles Wesley

> Come, see how Christians wail their dead;
> Come, share in our mysterious bliss;
> On Satan, sin, and death to tread,
> O what an happiness is this!
>
> Though once ye intermeddled not
> With the strange madness of our joys,
> Ye all may be to *Eden* brought
> And heighten our triumphant noise.
>
> — Charles Wesley

George Pickering lay dying. At age 77 he was celebrated as the oldest active Methodist preacher at that time (1846). A delegation of fellow itinerants dutifully visited his sickroom. The strict protocols of the sickroom were customarily observed. An attendant dressed in black luster (silk rustled and was expensive), fitted closely at the waist and short enough not to trail the floor, moved quietly to the door. The soft shoes and jewelryless apparel made the nurse's movements almost imperceptible. The unadorned hand that extended its greeting also made a "shh" sound with a short-nailed index finger — not

177

to impose a gravelike silence as did some nonevangelical families, but to remind the visitors of the sickroom's disciplines. The itinerants were invited to gather around the bed, but asked not to whisper or tiptoe — surefire methods of making floorboards creak and sounds reverberate, disturbing joyful spirits.[1]

Because the near-death experiences of evangelicals were prized as communal rites of passage, Pickering welcomed his guests immediately to his deathbed, although he was too weak to address them individually. The customary interrogation into the state of his soul began when one itinerant was respectfully designated as spokesperson.

> "Beloved father, a number of your ministerial brethren are present, and have requested me to express to you their Christian affection and sympathy."
>
> He replied, with strong emphasis and tears, "I thank you; you all have a high place in my affection."
>
> "They are happy to learn that in this your extremity, you still rejoice in hope of the glory of God."
>
> "Yes! O yes!"
>
> "That you feel the sting of death is extracted?"
>
> "Yes! O yes!"
>
> "And that you can resign yourself fully into the hands of your Lord?"
>
> "Yes, O yes; glory be to his name!"
>
> Grasping the hand of the brother addressing him with still firmer hold, he then, with tears and sobs, exclaimed: "You all have my high esteem and affection. Tell, O tell the brethren, to preach Christ and him crucified — an all-able, all-powerful, all-willing, all-ready Saviour — a present Saviour, *saving now.* Preach, 'Now is the accepted time, now is the day of salvation.' O, tell them to preach *holiness;* holiness is the principal thing. God enable you to preach holiness!"

With this Pickering broke down, vainly trying to say more but overcome with weakness and emotion. The delegation gave the veteran itinerant their corporate blessing, spoke their individual benefactions, and gathered in the downstairs parlor where they sang a final benediction:

> On Jordan's stormy banks I stand,
>     And cast a wishful eye
> To Canaan's fair and happy land,
>     Where my possessions lie.
>
> O the transporting, rapt'rous scene
>     That rises to my sight!
> Sweet fields array'd in living green,
>     And rivers of delight![2]

# I

Deathbed scenes like these were early evangelical equivalents to the obligatory sex scenes of today's slick-sick paperbacks and mass-media productions. Death is the oldest and most talked about topic in the world. If one-half the world's literature deals in one way or another with the subject of death, as some have calculated, evangelicals at least kept up their part of the percentage. Revivalists frequently used deaths of young people (12–23 years of age) as *memento mori*, reminders of death and lessons of life's transitoriness — *sic transit gloria mundi* (thus passes the glory of the world).

Indeed, the Pickering story is one of many taken from a book prepared for youth contrasting the terrible deaths of the impious with the evangelical tradition of "triumphant dying."[3] *The Dying Hours of Good and Bad Men Contrasted* instructed evangelical youth in how to "prepare to live and die right." By neglecting true religion, the wicked "met a dreadful end." Infidels like Voltaire feared death, fought death, and failed the dying hour. "Rage, remorse, reproach, and blasphemy, all accompany and characterize the long agony of the dying atheist." The moral was unforgettable and, in chapter after chapter, unrelenting: "see how unbelievers and apostates die"; see also "the power of the Christian religion to comfort and sustain in nature's last conflict."[4]

Evangelicals feared death less than they feared death terminating life without conferring meaning to the living. Behavioral scientist A. Gregory Schneider calls this "the ritual of happy dying."[5] No evangelical, no matter how prominent, was spared the scrutiny of death's "honest hour." Even the great Methodist theologian and successor to John Wesley, John Fletcher, unable to speak or move, was visited less than twenty-four hours before his death by a colleague who insisted: "'My dear creature, I ask not for myself — *I know thy soul* — but for the sake of others; if Jesus be very present with thee, lift up thy right hand.' Immediately he did. 'If the prospect of glory sweetly opens before thee, repeat the sign.' He instantly raised it again, and in half a minute a second time."[6] Every dying built family and faith among the living. Those who had one foot in the next world were looked to for wisdom and advice on how to walk in this world. As the "smile of joy lit up the brow of death," in the words of more than one deathbed account, and even as the dying sometimes "got happy" and "shouted for glory," evangelicals found the confirmation, encouragement, and exhortation to continue taking up the cross and following Jesus into that "O Happy Day."

Indeed, evangelicals so integrated a living death into their dying life that evangelical religion can be seen, in Schneider's marvelous way of putting it, as "an effort to steal a march on death, a strategy for conquering death by living a dying life," which one entered at one's conversion when one "died to the world" and lived to Christ.[7] Irene Quenzler Brown's study of evangelical memoirs, particularly those of missionary wife Mary Hawes Van Lennep (1821–44), reveals an evangelical culture of friendship where the disciplines of both bonding and separation were linked in death — "where the circle will be unbroken." Evangelicals were pregnant with their own deaths, as manifested in their early "coffining" of the consciousness ("Resolved to think much on all occasions of my dying") and their daily death-in-life existence ("Resolved that I will so live as I shall wish I had done when I come to die").[8]

Even though by the late 1800s evangelical leaders were less inclined to recline mentally in their coffins, the tradition of "living a dying life" lingered on, even translating itself into terms of preparedness for living as well as preparedness for dying. This has put evangelicals at serious odds with prevailing attitudes, especially those shaped by Elisabeth Kübler-Ross, Raymond A. Moody, Jr., and other death therapists and death defenders.

At issue is more than the fact that the literature of deathbed scenes for children and youth, so common in earlier evangelical culture, is virtually extinct. In fact, the death of a child is now so rare that funeral directors have stopped stocking caskets for children; instead they place special orders when the occasion arises. America's children and youth have no idea what it was like to have been bombarded constantly with reminders like these: "That youth, health, and beauty, with all the charms of natural and acquired accomplishments, together with the most flattering earthly prospects, are liable to be blasted in the head, and swallowed up in death."[9]

The real problem is that, contrary to what is read in books, seen at the movies, heard on late-night talk shows, and even sung in hymns ("Rescue the Perishing, Care for the Dying"), Americans are now living in a culture that denies the reality of death as firmly as almost any other culture in history. "Our own era simply denies death....The individual is forced to repress it....Thus the fear of death...remains alive in spite of the attempt to deny it."[10] Woody Allen is more honest than most: "I don't want to achieve immortality through my works; I want to achieve immortality by not dying."

It is hard for people to see what evangelicals are pointing to because the new modern form of death's denial is a very deceptive one. Critics of our culture's attitudes toward dying have pointed this out in various forms. Lutheran pastor H. Paul Santmire calls it "the death and dying movement." Novelist and critic Ron Rosenbaum refers to it as the "pro-death movement." Reformed Church minister Robert Gram has christened it "the myth of meaningful death." Methodist ethicist Paul Ramsey fashions it "the indignity of 'death with dignity.'"[11] One might even call it the cult of St. Thanatos, or the offense of disposable death.

How craftily even Christians have learned to deny death by making it "meaningful" and "beautiful" became apparent to me one day as I was amiably chatting with the resident pastor prior to our co-officiating at a wedding service. On an endtable by the couch in his office, I noticed a picture of his wife and four daughters. Complimenting him on such an attractive family, I asked how long he had been married. "Seven months," he replied. He enjoyed my nervous bewilderment for a moment and then explained that a little over a year earlier his first wife had died of cancer, leaving him with four children ranging in ages from twelve to three.

My first reaction was to ask how his daughters were doing. He quickly, too quickly, replied, "Fine." I then asked how he was doing. Again I got a surprisingly enthusiastic "Wonderful." Not satisfied with either response I probed further, remarking that the walk through this valley must have been one of the most arduous pilgrimages of his life. "Not at all," he replied too sharply. "It was actually one of the most beautiful and meaningful experiences of my life." As my mind pondered this response uncharitably, his purring continued: "My first wife and I shared the five stages together, and I am today a much better pastor because of it." Feeling rather protective of the interests of the deceased wife, and disturbed by the seeming insignificance of her life as measured by any deep sense of loss and grief, I asked if I could see a picture of her. "I do not want the kids to live in the past," he explained with much fidgeting, "so I got rid of them all. We have a new life now." At least two things were going on here. First, conditional love has become the norm for American culture, leading to terminal arrangements celebrated in all sectors of our social life, from marriage ceremonies to memorial services. Behind "I will love you 'til death do us part" can lie an undraped version: "I will love you so long as you meet my needs." Even Elisabeth Kübler-Ross has lectured in recent years on the need for modern culture to rediscover the meaning of unconditional love if its institutions are not to crumble further. Evangelicals' sensitivity to this issue is one reason why termination-of-treatment decisions are so difficult for them.

Second, as psychoanalyst Kurt Eissler has suggested, Americans have a way of coming to terms with the unpleasant by calling it pleasant. We integrate the ugly by making it pretty; we confront evil by renaming it good. If we can persuade ourselves that dying is one of life's natural and satisfying experiences, then it fits snugly into our hedonistic life-style, and we can go pleasurably and fearlessly into that dark night. By demystifying the ultimate mystery and making death meaningful, we have blurred the boundaries between life and death. We can say, with clinical matter-of-factness, death is a normal, natural, meaningful part of life, the "final stage of growth." Huddled in America's twenty-one thousand hospices, reading near-death visionaries, we can encourage each other to experience fully and completely what generic death has to offer: "I'm in the acceptance stage. Which stage are you in?" The problem with this frivolous and cozy view of death for evangelicals is that the Bible knows none of it. Death is "the last enemy." Death came to earth as the result of the apostasy of sin, evangelicals believe. Even the mid-nineteenth-century layman who created a furor in the pages of the *Methodist Quarterly Review* by arguing that death was originally "a merciful dispensation" and "peaceful messenger" of the Creator ended up at the same place with the rest of the evangelical community: because of sin, death became our "mortal enemy," an "appalling foe, armed by sin with a poisonous and deadly 'sting.'"[12]

Paul names death as the final force of destruction, along with "all dominion, authority, and power," that Christ is working to overcome (1 Corinthians 15:24–26). Death is not just pleasant dreams or an appointment with a friend. Even those nineteenth-century evangelicals who lived through what David Stannard calls the "self-indulgence, sentimentalization, and ostentation" of Romanticism's attitudes toward death and dying could never fully equate death and beauty into their elaborate mourning practices and rituals.[13] Death's "sweetness" and "beauty" in this "Age of Beautiful Death," as French historian Philippe Ariès calls it,[14] was for evangelicals both a birthday in eternity and the power of faith to wrench meaning and purpose out of something as bitter and ugly as death. It was never the romantic notion that love can find true consummation only in death.

"Death is an insult," a respected physician writes in an influential medical journal: "the stupidest, ugliest thing that can happen to a human being." Pointing out that the first death in history was a murder of a brother by a brother, the Jewish writer Elie Wiesel contends that "every death is a murder. We must fight death. We must never be on the side of Cain, but always on the side of Abel."[15]

In many ways the fierce resistance against death that occurs every day in hospitals is more on the side of Abel, and the blissful resignations and beatific meditations that characterize many funeral services more on the side of Cain. "One night after a long, unsuccessful fight to save a patient," Elisabeth Kübler-Ross tells us, "a nurse overheard the family priest say to the relatives, 'Well, it was God's will.' The nurse blew up and stormed out of the department."[16] God does not wish that any should die any more than God wishes that any should suffer.

Death's throttling question — "Why, God?" — refuses to be exorcised by waving styrofoam crosses that represent death as a natural part of life, or dying as a beautiful, even transcendent experience. To be sure, to someone being eaten alive from the inside out by a carcinogenic cannibal whose appetite cannot be curbed, death is the final healing act. "O the pain, the bliss of dying" were the last words of Elijah R. Sabin, a Methodist itinerant who died in 1818. But the beauty and bliss is in the healing, not the death. Jesus prayed in the Garden, "Let this cup pass from me" (Matthew 26:39). Evangelicals do not see it as a sign of faltering or infirm faith if, when the cup is passed our way, we too want to say, "I'll pass."

But each of us must one day take a large draught from the bitter cup. Nothing can make it sweet and welcome — not even those newfangled near-death experiences that evangelicals have been conspicuously and stubbornly reluctant to embrace. Christians should always fight having to taste death; they must never greet death as friend.

For the evangelical the only thing that removes the fear of dying — nineteenth-century evangelicals called it "stingless death" — is the resurrection of Jesus Christ. Death is "the humiliation that precedes enthronement," one evangelical minister wrote in 1868.[17] The great Congregational preacher, Henry Ward Beecher, in his early evangelical days captured truly this bifocal orientation in his simultaneous affirmations that the resurrection meant that "a Christian ought not to be afraid of his Father's Garden" and that "nowhere on earth is death more solemn than in New England, nor the remembrance of the dead more ineffaceable. Nowhere else is man valued so highly, or his loss more universally felt."[18]

The hope that brings courage and calm is based not on some death-denying transcendent experience or out-of-body journey, not on some resigned acceptance of the biological inevitability of death, but on that first Easter Sunday when despair took a day off. The Easter event demonstrated even the grave's powerlessness to bury God's love and presence. The last poem in the *Oxford Book of English Verse* (1900) contains this eloquent statement of the evangelical perspective:

> When the will has forgotten the lifelong aim,
> And the mind can only disgrace its fame,
> And a man is uncertain of his own name —
> The power of the Lord shall fill this frame.[19]

Easter makes death a "defeated enemy," as the Welsh evangelical preacher R. Maurice Boyd puts it. "Once your enemy has been defeated, you can make him a friend."[20]

Death's ultimate power over us has been conquered by the resurrection. When Dr. B. W. Hinson was told by his physician that he had fallen victim to an incurable disease that would soon bring death, he attested:

> I walked out to my home five miles from the water of the city [Portland, Oregon]. There I looked at the rivers and the mountain which I love, and then — as the twilight deepened — as the stars glimmered in the sky — I said to them, "I may not see you many more times. But river, I shall be alive when you have ceased running to the sea. Mountain, I shall be alive when you have sunk down into the plain. Stars, I shall be alive when you have fallen in the ultimate disintegration of the universe.

In place of a "meaningful death," evangelicals plan for a declarative death. A 1741 funeral hymn by Charles Wesley, written first for Elizabeth Hooper and used thereafter in numerous eighteenth-century evangelical funerals, refers to death in this fashion: "Accomplish'd is our sister's strife."[21] Death should be an act we personally perform, not an experience we endure. The poet evangelicals like to quote most, Emily Dickinson, wrote about "the overtakelessness of those / Who have accomplished Death."[22] Death is not something you evade or stumble into. Death is something you accomplish, a positive achievement. Death is not just a physical event; it is also a spiritual event.

The best of the evangelical tradition would argue that this view of death be taken one step further — that death be seen as both a personal and a communal act, a spiritual experience to be shared, and as a shared experience one which others can live partially before their time. The communal aspect of death is so foreign to our experience that those cultures that have retained its rituals and artifacts appear oddly out of time and inevitably suffer social opprobrium.

Strong Memorial Hospital in Rochester, New York, one of the nation's leading research-teaching hospitals, has still not recovered from the experience of the death of a gypsy some years ago. A member of a traveling gypsy community was hospitalized at the terminal stages of an illness, and the entire gypsy camp moved into the lobby of the hospital to be as near by as possible. The leaders of the gypsy colony refused to be budged from a twenty-four-hour bedside death vigil, replete with black candles, charts, incantations, and a steady procession of loved ones going in for their parting words with the dying. How many congregations would stubbornly insist on retaining their rituals in the face of frowning bureaucratic regulations, much less even consider gathering the whole congregation in the hospital lobby as a final act of solidarity and love for the dying person?

Whereas in "meaningful" death we end up speaking on behalf of death, in declarative death, death ends up speaking on behalf of us. John Wesley observed that "our people die well." By this he meant more than resignation to death:

Thus may we all our parting breath
Into the Saviour's hands resign:
O Jesu, let me die her death,
And let her latter end be mine![23]

He also meant by this the fact that evangelicals declared through their dying the values and ideals of their living. For this reason living wills, transplants, and organ donations have not posed serious problems for evangelicals. "It seems to me to be in the spirit of Christ for a person to 'will' his eye, or heart to someone else," Billy Graham responded in the 1950s to a question about the ethics of transplanting human body parts.[24] What better way for Christians to offer gifts of life in their deaths?

The one thing evangelicals want people to be able to say about their dying is that they did it well — with grace, humor, and trust in God, and within the context of a community. How we die, where we die, with whom we die, even when we die, speak volumes about Christian faith and discipleship. In the words of Carl F. H. Henry, "Can evangelical deathstyle perhaps witness to this generation about God as much as evangelical lifestyle?"[25]

On New Year's Day, 1790, an eighty-seven-year-old John Wesley described himself as "an old man, decayed from head to foot. My eyes are dim; my right hand shakes much; my mouth is hot and dry every morning; I have a lingering fever almost every day; my motion is weak and slow. However, blessed by God, I do not slack my labor. I can preach and write still."[26] One of Wesley's early biographers, Henry Moore, was in the house with him when he wrote these words and could scarcely believe his eyes when later he read what Wesley had written.

> I knew it must be as he said; but I could not imagine his weakness was so great. He still rose at his usual hour, four o'clock, and went through the many duties of the day, not indeed, with the same apparent vigor, but without complaint, and with a degree of resolution that was astonishing. He would still, as he afterwards remarks, "do a little for God before he dropped into the dust."[27]

What made truth terrible for the impious, triumphant for the Christian? There was the same amount of pain for both. Believers were not spared the cussed ironies of existence. George Pickering was no more protected from death's suffering and anguish than Thomas Paine or Voltaire. The difference was in the remorse, fear, and horror of the end that characterized the dying of infidels and the joy, courage, and serenity that characterized the dying of Christians. With soaring spirit from a sinking body, Christian death could declare the glory of God.

To live life to the end, Boris Pasternak wrote in one of his poems, is not a childish task.[28] For some, like the world-renowned Methodist missionary and evangelist E. Stanley Jones, a declarative death will take the form of perseverance in the face of pain and brokenness. After suffering a paralyzing stroke at age 87 that left him unable to write and hardly able to see or speak, Jones lived for fourteen more months, determined that God was calling him to write one more book, his twenty-ninth. *The Divine Yes* (1975), a book dictated fitfully into a cassette recorder, stands as his last will and testament to a compassionate and loving God.[29]

## II

Of course, we can hold on to life too tightly. Evangelicals have been taught that they are, after all, more at home in heaven than on earth. That is why a declarative death will sometimes take the form of a human "No!" a firm opposition to all heroic measures to extend the quantity but not the quality of life. The critic Alexander Woollcott, who suffered a series of heart attacks, complained bitterly in his last illness that doctors wanted to keep him alive, but he wanted to live! Sometimes being alive and living are two different things.

Declarative death decisions need to be made within the context of a covenantal understanding of community and a willingness to admit the perspectives of family and friends into one's definition of declarative. But for all who are truly taught of the Spirit, a declarative death will praise God for the gift of life both on this side and the other side of death. In the magnificent words of an entry found in the journal of Danish philosopher-theologian Søren Kierkegaard:

> What pleases him [God] even more than the praise of angels is a human being who in the last lap of this life, when God seemingly changes into sheer cruelty and with the most cruelly devised cruelty does everything to deprive him of the zest for life, nevertheless continues to believe that God is love, that God does it out of love. Such a human being becomes an angel....Like a man traveling around the whole world with the fixed idea of hearing a singer with a perfect tone, God sits in heaven and listens. And every time he hears praise from a person whom he has brought to the extremity of life-weariness, God says to himself: This is it. He says it as if he were making a discovery.[30]

Death as much as life is a far from immaculate business. Death can be as unpredictable, untidy, and clumsy as life itself. The issue of euthanasia illustrates this point. Only the moral issues of abortion and homosexuality can

generate such uneasy emotional reactions among evangelicals as does euthanasia. Actually, the Christian tradition concerning euthanasia is far more
complex than evangelicals admit. Medieval Christians were known to practice "Christmas euthanasia" based on folk superstition that if one died on
Christmas Eve, one could escape having to pass through the portals of pur-
gatory.[31] St. Thomas More applauded euthanasia in his *Utopia* (1516), and in
*Out of the Silent Planet* (1938), C. S. Lewis included euthanasia in his utopia,
albeit with modified forms and intentionalities.

The anguish and ambiguity of evangelical responses to this preference
to die well rather than to live ill is reflected in the language used to discuss euthanasia. For some the term translates literally as "good death," the
very putting of the two words together an anathema to those who believe
in the sanctity of life. For others it means "dying well" or "dying with dignity," a translation which permits Christians to make subtle but critical
distinctions between passive/negative euthanasia, active/positive euthanasia, assisted suicide, mercy killing, or the preferred term of Derek Humphry,
proponent of legalized euthanasia and founder of the Hemlock Society,
"self-deliverance."

"Passive euthanasia" rarely poses a problem for evangelicals because they
deny it is euthanasia. Life and death belong in the hands of God. The evangelical mind repudiates the notion that the question of means is a nonmoral
issue. It has refuted to its own satisfaction Kant's argument that if one accepts the end, one accepts the means. There is a necessary, indeed absolutely
central, moral distinction to be made between killing and allowing to die.
In the words of one evangelical declaration on euthanasia, "always to care,
never to kill."[32]

Morally speaking, there is a vast difference between what others (often
dubbed secular humanists) call passive and active euthanasia. The difference
revolves around the question of intentionality. Passive euthanasia — allowing a dying person to die without resorting to drastic, "heroic" measures
that might maintain vital signs — is not legally or morally wrong, nor is
it even properly called euthanasia according to the National Association of
Evangelicals.[33]

Active euthanasia, which evangelicals call mercy killing, intends the final
act of death and thus is theologically contemptible.[34] Terminal care, which is
designed not to terminate life but to relieve suffering (morphine, for example, may hasten death), intends life and does not prolong death. Withholding
or even withdrawing life-prolonging treatment can be justified where the
benefit is insufficient to outweigh the harm. Just as humans have the right
to life, evangelicals insist, they also have the right to death. When does that
right come into effect? Increasing numbers of the evangelical community

assent to the whole-brain-death criterion (not the higher-brain-death criterion of irreversible loss of consciousness) to determine when the death of a person takes place.[35]

Evangelicals have not tried to tell medicine when to stop except when "meddlesome medicine" takes extraordinary measures to keep the dying alive, thereby preventing them from being with their Lord. The measure of a life's contribution, as Peter Marshall phrased it, is in terms of one's donation, not one's duration.[36] Decisions about withdrawing or withholding treatment in terminal illnesses are usually entrusted to physicians as long as suffering is relieved without life-taking measures. Evangelicals have not been driven to hysteria like some other religious and social groups by the fact that 70 percent of all hospital deaths, according to the American Hospital Association, occur when a decision is made to stop some life-sustaining machinery or technology. Evangelicals have no problem with Arthur Hugh Clough's couplet commandment: "Thou shalt not kill; but needs't not strive / Officiously to keep alive." As Sir William Osler, the great Canadian physician, phrased it during his final illness, "I am so far across the river; if anything happens, don't try to bring me back."[37]

Evangelicals reject voluntary, active euthanasia on a multitude of biblical and theological as well as nonreligious grounds. First, there is the biblical perspective of the sacredness of human life, which has been created *imago dei* and thus must not be violated. "Because man bears the image of God, his life is sacred in every state of its existence, in sickness or in health, in the womb, in infancy, in adolescence, in maturity, in old age, or even in the process of dying itself."[38] Every life has some worth. Closely tied to this is the biblical principle of the sovereignty of God. Active euthanasia is a human invasion of the absolute and exclusive dominion of God in human life. God gave life. It must be God who takes life away.[39]

Second, a faith that would accommodate euthanasia is a faith without faith—either in God's healing powers, or in God's promise of life after death. The Bible records eight cases of resurrections from death itself, not to mention the numerous accounts of healings and of the prayer of faith that can save the sick.[40] Medical breakthroughs may occur that can spare the life of the patient, not to speak of miraculous interventions.

Belief in life after death provides evangelicals with what Antony Flew has termed "the most powerful moral reason against helping euthanasia in any way." To die without God is to spend eternity without God. To end human torment in a hospital may be to send someone to eternal torment in hell. Millard J. Erickson and Ines E. Bowers develop this position most fully: "If we believe that there is both a personal heaven and a personal hell beyond this life, then perhaps euthanasia is not mercy-killing at all. It is sending a person from a bad condition to a worse one."[41]

Third, active euthanasia ignores the biblical perspective on suffering. God puts purpose into suffering and can use suffering redemptively. Indeed, a prime way of growing wings in life, of learning to fly spiritually, is through trials and temptations. It must be admitted, however, that evangelicals have not always been clear whether there is ever a point where suffering becomes so extreme that some form of active euthanasia becomes tolerable.

Finally, advocacy of euthanasia represents a failed "test of love." The sick, even the limbless and virtually lifeless, develop virtues in those that attend them, virtues without which no community can be considered civilized. From a sociological perspective, euthanasia is an easy escape from a difficult social and economic problem. From a theological perspective, it takes epic amounts of courage and faith to walk through every day with one's handicapped child, more than if one relieved oneself of the handicap. Evangelical theologian John Jefferson Davis admonishes Christians to be "shining lights to a world of darkness," choosing life and "offering to the dying not deadly poisons, but rather neighbor love and the hope of life eternal."[42]

Evangelical ethicist Lewis B. Smedes has identified three basic attitudes toward the morality of suicide: it is a sin; it is a moral option; it is a tragedy, not to be summarily judged.[43] All three can be found within the evangelical community, although the last one is the most prevalent.

First, suicide is a sin. There are five accounts of suicide in the First Testament: Samson (Judges 16:29–30), Saul (1 Samuel 31:4), Abimelech (Judges 9:54), Ahitophel (2 Samuel 17:31), and Zimri (1 Kings 16:18). There is one suicide in the Second Testament: Judas (Matthew 27:5). "When we look for Biblical evaluations of suicide," two evangelical theologians lament, "we are disappointed."[44] None of the passages prohibits suicide; nowhere is it condemned. In fact, Samson is given a decent burial (Judges 16:31), and the writer of Hebrews cites him as a hero of the faith (11:32). It was Augustine who helped antagonize the church to suicide, making it what John Wesley would later call "self-murder," a violation of the commandment against homicide. Thomas Aquinas went further to make suicide a crime against God and a mortal sin; centuries earlier Aristotle had considered suicide a crime against the state. Dante influenced Christian theology more than anyone, however, placing in the seventh circle of the *Inferno* those who committed "self-murder."

Thanks largely to Augustine and Dante, extreme punishments for suicide have been conceived for both this world and the next. In Tudor England, the suicidal victim was interred in unconsecrated ground outside the church cemetery, and all earthly possessions were confiscated by the crown. Corpses of "self-murderers" were mutilated and publicly humiliated. Although evangelicals have not refused funeral services or burial in churchyards to suicide victims, a good number of them have associated suicide with the "unpardonable sin," for which one goes straight to hell. Evangelicals widely condemned as contrary to Christian morality the 1975 suicide pact between theologian Henry Pitney Van Dusen and his wife.

Life is a gift. It is a sin to desert one's post, a crime to end life voluntarily, and an arrogance to deny nature by placing death under one's own control. The moral stigma still attached to suicide is reflected in the fact that as late as 1964, nine American states still had statutes against the "crime" of suicide.

Second, suicide is a moral option. John Donne's *Biathanatos* (1608) was the first defense of suicide in English. After admitting "I often have such an inclination," Donne made a strong case that the Bible, the church, and even theologians are at best ambivalent on whether suicide is a sin. Evangelicals have read the literature and pondered the arguments of contemporary theologians who say that suicide can be an act of Christian conscience, even a creative act, especially if it is a sacrificial death in a good cause.[45] Often evangelicals have come away with a less rigid formulation of their position on suicide.

The morality of suicide is an issue fraught with fever for evangelicals, even blasphemy, because at the heart of retelling the old, old story is an unsettling story of a person who freely chose to lay down his life to save others. Evangelicalism's atonement theology is one in which Jesus virtually designed his own death. In confronting suicide, evangelicals must face one of the most difficult questions raised by the gospel: What does one call it when someone takes a course of action that he has the power to prevent, and that he knows will end in his death, but takes it anyway? The distinction between suicide and martyrdom only partially helps out here. Jesus purposefully laid down his life to show the greatness of God's love and to save us from our sins. There is also the wobbling question of "shaded" or "partial" suicides, including overeating, undereating, underachievement, overachievement. The risk-taking adventure of dangerous living for righteousness' sake is more the evangelical ideal than playing it safe or not running risks.

But arguments for the morality of suicide are widely unfamiliar in popular evangelical culture, which increasingly lines up behind the third moral perspective on suicide: suicide as a tragedy. Evangelicals have tended to treat suicide less as a rational act than as the product of spiritual disease or a deranged mind. Evangelical leaders can now be heard calling the church to resist judgment, show compassion, and allow for the possibility that some suicides may not be a rejection of God so much as a "tragically misguided attempt at saying 'yes' to God."[46]

Evangelicals have come into closest, no longer closet, connection with this position, partly because American society is producing suicides like no other nation on earth. Indeed, sociologists now conclude that the influence of religion has sunk in the wider culture to the point that there are declining correlations between religion and suicide.[47] Hundreds of suicide prevention centers have been established within the past two decades, and there has been widespread acknowledgment of the proposition that every human being, at one time or other, has done more than simply think, "I wish I were dead." Evangelical psychologists and psychiatrists have been educating their constituency in the fact that suicidal impulses are a normal, natural reaction to stress.

To appropriate Durkheimian categories, when "egoistic" feelings of wearisome loneliness (suicide is the ultimate act of loneliness, and evangelicals track suicide to its lair in loneliness) or "anomic" shock (from losing a job or loved one) break upon the human psyche, we are not sinning or going crazy unless we refuse to confront these feelings and what they speak to us. The best way to cope with these moods is prayer and patience: "This too shall pass." Or, as the poet and hymn writer William Cowper, who himself fought impulses to end his life and almost lost, wrote in the eighteenth century, "Beware of desperate steps; the darkest day, lived 'til tomorrow, will have passed away."[48]

## III

If the myth of meaningful death has taught us that we have no need to fear death, the myth of the disposable person has taught us that we have no need to mourn death or dwell on it. Technological society values efficiency and utility above all else, and those that can no longer produce as much as others are shunted to the side and scrapped as so much excess weight and worry. The myth of the disposable person has been taken one step further in recent years as the worth of people is beginning to be classified not according to how useful and efficient they are but according to the technological value of what they are useful and efficient at.

Evangelical sensitivity to the myth of the disposable person has made disposal of the dead body somewhat problematic. Yet evangelicals have not thought their way through the issue of what are the authentic biblical and theological methods of returning "dust to dust" as fully as one might suspect. Of the over thirty methods of disposing of the human body, the choice for evangelicals has been either burial or cremation. The latter did not even become an option until the late nineteenth century, however, as America's first crematory was not built until 1876, in Washington, Pennsylvania.

Evangelicals initially opposed the practice of cremation as a dishonorable disposal, undignified and undeserving of the respect due a disciple of Christ and a "temple of the Holy Ghost." No Christian, the argument went, deserves such irreverent and cheap treatment. Evangelical arguments against cremation have had more to do with cultural than theological "appropriateness." The theological objections that evangelicals have raised revolve around the doctrine of the resurrection of the body and the biblical injunction that we are not free to do with our bodies as we please (1 Corinthians 6:19-20).[49]

Besides violating the sacred memory of the believer, cremation was also seen as a custom that originated in ancient heathen lands. Cremation was associated in the evangelical mind with pagan idol worship. It was the choice of criminals and haters of the church, the burial preference of the biblically unenlightened at best, the ungodly, immoral, and evil at worst — people like Adolf Hitler, Adolf Eichmann, and Joseph Stalin.

Gradually, however, evangelical voices were raised that put the matter into larger historical, cultural, and theological perspectives. Some evangelicals observed that burial as well as burning was of pagan origin and pre-Christian. One evangelical etiquette manual pointed out that since the evangelical community accepts with equanimity autopsy and embalming, not viewing these practices as mutilations of the dead, why does it trouble itself with cremation? Cremation "is only a rapid way of accomplishing what nature, through putrefaction, will do in a longer period. In earth-burial it is 'dust to dust'; in cremation it is 'ashes to ashes.'"[50] Others have argued that, at a time when many American burial practices are pagan, to focus on cremation is an exercise in theological obfuscation.[51]

For all these reasons contemporary evangelicals by and large do not expressly forbid cremation. Ordinarily they will find inhumation preferable to cremation. But the choice is not a matter of evil and sin, right and wrong. Disposal of the body must be a matter of dignity and honor and respect, and following in the footsteps of Christ.

## IV

The myth of the disposable person comes in both conservative and liberal religious varieties. The conservative variety was illustrated in the reaction of one of radio's fundamentalist auctioneers of the Almighty to the tragic deaths of eight Houghton College seniors, the entire homecoming court, who were crammed into a car en route to pick up their homecoming suits and dresses when they were hit by a truck. Professing not to be able to understand why everyone wants to go to heaven but no one wants to die, the radio evangelist declared that all the weeping and mourning for these Wesleyan coeds was an embarrassment to the faith and an affront to God. God had called them to a higher homecoming celebration than that of their college, and Christians ought to rejoice with them and their families that they were spared the anguish of living in these latter days and were instead ushered into God's presence at the very prime of their lives.

The liberal expression of the myth of the disposable person takes the more subtle form of memorial services styled "celebration of a life." Instead of a service where both grief and gratitude are recognized and uplifted, the grief is denied and everything is upbeat praise to God for the deceased person's life. We have been blessed with this gift of life for as long as we've enjoyed it, and we ought to be satisfied with what we've received and not be greedy. Less a witness to the resurrection than a witness to reminiscences, these celebrations are increasingly held in churches without funeral reminders of casket, urn, or flowers. Everything about the service is geared to enable us to pay our respects without undue sentimentality or delay. We are applauded for "taking it well" and encouraged to prepare for the future with decent dispatch. After all, life must go on.

The commonalities in both the liberal and fundamentalist varieties are obvious. In both, the hurt and grief are largely missing from the community's rituals. While the Bible teaches us to "mourn not overmuch" or not "grieve like the rest" (1 Thessalonians 4:13), it still makes room for mourning. An entire book of the Bible (Lamentations) is devoted to it. The old-fashioned parading of grief by the "renting of garments" has sometimes been replaced by a newly fashionable parading of transcending grief as we compliment each other on how well we are doing and taking it all. The idea that the word *death* should have no meaning for the Christian stems precisely from this surrender to death and the sad fact that many Americans lack a theological language and shared biblical interpretations to deal with it. With all the pressure not to mourn and not to "dwell in the past," one can understand how human love becomes all too often a love that dies with the grave.

Both liberals and fundamentalists also have a common perception of death as a "blessing," for fundamentalists a blessing that relieves one of the traumas of living in the world, for liberals a blessing that relieves one of the trauma of not being able to live in the world. Only in a theological sense can death ever be defined as a blessing. The resurrection of Jesus Christ, John Wesley wrote in his notes on 2 Timothy 1:10, has "taken away its sting, and turned it into a blessing."[52] Or, in the words of Charles Wesley, commenting on the death of one of the earliest British lay preachers, "Can we weep to see the tears / Wiped forever from his eyes?"[53] But our references to the "blessing" of death are mostly sociological, seldom theological. "Surely his death is a blessing" is especially said of "4b" types (bifocals, bridges, baldness, and bulges), for we live in a society that buries its aged before they are dead. But it can also frequently be heard bandied about the caskets of the handicapped and bedridden of all ages.

If ever a phrase were a deserving candidate for verbal euthanasia, it is this one. "It's a blessing" is the obverse side of the "premature death" lament, as if there were a mature and proper time to die. Is there a decent age to die? Is there a proper time to die? If people in the childhood, youth, and young adult stage can find life in every moment, why can't those in the "you look wonderful" stage?

I shall never forget standing alongside my father's open casket and listening to a relative rehearse the heart attacks and strokes that preceded his death two weeks before I was to graduate from seminary. She then fixed her eyes on my face and smiled comfortingly, "Who would wish him back?" Who would wish him back? I mumbled under my breath angrily, "Me!" There is nothing sorrier than sentiments that try to rationalize death on account of life's longevity ("She lived a long life"), the hideousness of pain ("He's not suffering anymore"), the dreadfulness of a deathless world ("A world without death would be a dead world"), the "charm" of mortality (we can cope with being 70, or even 100 years, but with a thousand?), or the need to move over so that there can be room for another generation to move in. Life is never long enough for those you love, and for those who love life.

Death is more than a biological shutdown or a spiritual breakthrough. Here lies the tragedy and finality of death: an absolutely irreplaceable, nonrepeatable human being has been lost forever. And even though there is a difference in the sense of loss that attends the death of an old person whose potential has been lived out after a rich, full life and the death of a young person whose promise is snuffed out, the grief is as acute for the loss of a ninety-year-old patient in a nursing home as it is for a two-year-old child in a crib.

For underneath this decaying body is a uniquely beautiful human being— a person whose hands changed diapers and wiped tears, whose ears turned red and thrilled to Mozart, whose stomach craved strawberries and cringed at squash, whose arms embraced the strong and carried the weak, whose eyes loved sunrises and deserts of snow, whose fingers cracked noisily and gently caressed the face of a friend, whose feet hiked through the woods and trekked through umpteen every-member-canvasses, whose lips kissed lovers and prayed "Thy Kingdom Come." God cannot make another her. She is lost to the world forever.

When my second son reached two, I took him to visit the grave of the grandfather he had never seen. As we plodded through the grass to the simple marker that identified his grave, I explained to Justin that his grandfather's body was buried in the ground, but his spirit was with God. After I read the inscription on the gravestone for him, Justin bent down as only a child can, his head scissoring his ramrod legs and protruding posterior. He knocked on the stone with his pudgy fist and called out: "Grandpa Sweet, you come out of there." Because of Jesus Christ, evangelicals believe he already has. The grave is not a matter of life and death, but life and life. But evangelicals do not get past Good Friday to Easter Sunday too quickly.

This chapter ends where it began: with a book for youth. No twentieth-century thinker has had a greater impact on the evangelical mind than C. S. Lewis. When evangelical children go to bed, their parents often read them *The Chronicles of Narnia.* Lewis closes the stories of Narnia after the children and their parents have been killed in an accident. Tenderly telling them that they are dead, Aslan the Lion calls them to awaken from the dream, for now it is morning and the holidays have begun. Lewis then signs off with this hope:

> And for us this is the end of all the stories, and we can most truly say that they all lived happily ever after. But for them it was only the beginning of the real story. All their life in this world and all their adventures in Narnia had only been the cover and the title page: now at last they were beginning Chapter One of the Great Story, which no one on earth has read: which goes on for ever: in which every chapter is better than the one before.[54]

# Notes

## Introduction: "There Is a Balm in Gilead"

1. Waterman Sweet, *Views of Anatomy and Practice of Natural Bonesetting by Mechanical Process, Different from All Book Knowledge* (Schenectady, N.Y.: I. Riggs, 1843).

2. Quoted in Frances Vaughan, *The Inward Arc: Healing and Wholeness in Psychotherapy and Spirituality* (Boston: New Science Library, 1986), p. 6.

3. For an extensive definitional treatment of evangelicalism that features the doctrines of conversion, usefulness, commonsense realism, and millennialism, see my entry "Nineteenth-Century Evangelicalism" in *Encyclopedia of the American Religious Experience*, ed. Charles H. Lippy and Peter W. Williams (New York: Charles Scribner's Sons, 1989), 2:875–99.

4. *Religious Telescope*, 19 November 1851, p. 45.

5. As quoted in *U.S. News and World Report*, 4 April 1994, p. 53.

6. Theodore Roosevelt, as reported in the *Chautauqua Assembly Herald*, 12 August 1905, p. 3. A Chautauqua gathering "is typically American in that it is typical of America at its best."

7. Ivan Illich laments the "medicalization of life" in *Limits to Medicine: Medical Nemesis, the Expropriation of Health* (London: Marion Boyars, 1976), pp. 39–124, 271–75. See also Mark A. Noll's guest editorial "To Your Health," *Christianity Today*, 12 June 1987, pp. 14–15.

8. A. M. Daniels, as quoted in Martin E. Marty's *Context*, 1 April 1992, p. 4.

9. Daniel E. Fountain, *Health, the Bible, and the Church: Biblical Perspectives on Health and Healing* (Wheaton, Ill.: Billy Graham Center, 1989), p. 1.

10. Mark A. Noll, "Body and Soul: Perspectives on Health," *Second Opinion* 3 (1987): 110.

11. George Eldon Ladd, *A Theology of the New Testament* (Grand Rapids: Eerdmans, 1974), p. 76. Ladd consistently discusses "healing" under the heading of "salvation." See also Ladd, *Jesus and the Kingdom: The Eschatology of Biblical Realism* (New York: Harper and Row, 1964), pp. 203–9.

12. Russell L. Dicks, "The Place of Religion in Modern Medicine," *Pastoral Psychology* 8 (October 1957): 24.

13. See Meredith B. McGuire and Debra Kantor, *Ritual Healing in Suburban America* (New Brunswick, NJ.: Rutgers University Press, 1988), esp. pp. 3–14.

14. Mark A. Noll, "Constructive Steps toward an Evangelical Theology," unpublished manuscript, p. 5.

15. See Ellen Goodman's syndicated column, "New Commandments," *Boston Globe*, 3d ed., 2 February 1989.

## Chapter 1 / Fearing and Believing

1. For example, see *Charles Hodge: The Way of Life*, ed. Mark A. Noll (New York: Paulist Press, 1987), p. 210.

2. Phillips Brooks, *The Light of the World and Other Sermons* (New York: E. P. Dutton, 1896), p. 229.

3. As cited by David F. Wells, "Conversion: How and Why We Turn to God," *Christianity Today*, 14 January 1991, p. 31.

4. William V. Kelley, "A Doctor's Confession," *Methodist Review* 90 (September 1908): 788.

5. William A. Alcott, *Letters to a Sister; or, Woman's Mission* (Buffalo: George H. Derby, 1850), p. 39.

6. John Atkinson, *The Garden of Sorrows; or, The Ministry of Tears* (New York: Carlton and Lanahan, 1868), p. 57.

7. Harold John Ockenga, *These Religious Affections* (Grand Rapids: Zondervan Publishing House, 1937), p. 135.

8. Worthington Hooker, "The Mutual Influence of Mind and Body in Disease," *New Englander and Yale Review*, October 1845, pp. 493–509, esp. 495, 496.

9. Charles E. Rosenberg, "Body and Mind in Nineteenth-Century Medicine: Some Clinical Origins of the Neurosis Construct," *Bulletin of the History of Medicine* 63 (Summer 1989): 194.

10. *Emotionology* is the term introduced by Peter N. Stearns with Carol Z. Stearns in their pioneering study "Emotionology: Clarifying the History of Emotions and Emotional Standards," *American Historical Review* 90 (October 1985): 813–36.

11. "The Mind, the Body, and the Immune System: Part II," *Harvard Mental Health Letter* 8 (February 1992): 1–3.

12. Ludwig Wittgenstein, *Philosophical Investigations*, 3d ed., trans. G. E. M. Anscombe (New York: Macmillan, 1958), p. 178.

13. *Charles Hodge: The Way of Life*, p. 232.

14. Harold Lindsell, *When You Pray* (Grand Rapids: Baker Book House, 1975), p. 108.

15. E. Stanley Jones, *A Song of Ascents: A Spiritual Autobiography* (Nashville: Abingdon Press, 1968), p. 337.

16. For a current statement of this position from a nonevangelical source, see Robert C. Solomon, "Emotions and Choice," *Explaining Emotions*, ed. Amélie Oksenberg Rorty (Berkeley: University of California Press, 1980), pp. 251–81.

17. These recommendations were passed along from Dr. Benjamin Rush by the anonymous author of "The Tear — Its Philosophy," *Quarterly Review of the Methodist Episcopal Church, South* 3 (October 1849): 625.

18. See Calvin D. Linton, "How Are You Feeling?" *Christianity Today*, 11 October 1974, pp. 6–8.

19. Edgar Lee Masters, *The Serpent in the Wilderness* (New York: Sheldon Dick, 1933), p. 75.

20. Régis Debray, "When God Fails, Russia Remains," *New Perspectives Quarterly* 5 (Winter 1988–89): 33. Debray was a chronicler and confidant of the great political saints and martyrs of the Third World: Salvadore Allende, Che Guevara, and Fidel Castro. After serving as a political prisoner in South America he returned to France where he became an adviser on foreign affairs to François Mitterand.

21. For "scared-saved evangelism" see my *Quantum Spirituality: A Postmodern Apologetic* (Dayton: Whaleprints, 1991), 203–5.

22. *Minutes of the Methodist Conferences, from the First, Held in London, by the Late Rev. John Wesley, A.M. in the Year 1744* (London: Conference Office, 1812), 1:23–24.

23. See, e.g., William B. Sprague, *Lectures on Revivals of Religion*, 2d ed. (New York: Daniel Appleton, 1833), p. 32.

24. Ronald L. Numbers and Janet S. Numbers, "Millerism and Madness: A Study of 'Religious Insanity' in Nineteenth-Century America," *Bulletin of the Menninger Clinic* 49 (July 1985): 294, 289–320.

25. See Mary Ann Jiminez, "Madness in Early American History: Insanity in Massachusetts from 1700 to 1830," *Journal of Social History* 20 (Fall 1986): 25–44). See also John F. Sena, "Melancholic Madness and the Puritans," *Harvard Theological Review* 66 (July 1973): 294–309.

26. Numbers and Numbers, "Millerism and Madness," p. 313. Millerism, one of the nineteenth century millennial groups, derives its name from William Miller (1782–1849), the founder of the Adventist Church. By interpreting biblical chronology Miller, a Baptist lay minister, set a March 1843 date for the Second Coming of Christ. His revival and camp-meeting preaching attracted a large following, some of whom remained faithful even after his 1843 and two 1844 predictions proved to be incorrect.

27. In the minds of asylum superintendents, spiritualism replaced Millerism in the 1850s as the chief cause of insanity. See Numbers and Numbers, "Millerism and Madness." For examples of evangelical ministries to the "insane," see W. Lee Spottswood, *Brief Annals* (Harrisburg, Pa.: Publishing House of the M. E. Book Room, 1888), p. 52. Spottswood had a regular appointment at an asylum in the Maryland Hospital.

28. See Amariah Brigham, *Observations on the Influence of Religion upon the Health and Physical Welfare of Mankind* (Boston: Marsh, Capen, and Lyon, 1835), pp. 170–72.

29. "Observations on the Influence of Religion upon the Health and Physical Welfare of Mankind," review article by Ed. [Editors: James Walker and F. W. Greenwood], *The Christian Examiner* 19 (January 1836): 302–14, 310.

30. Charles G. Finney, *Lectures on Revivals of Religion* (New York: Fleming H. Revell, 1868), p. 11.

31. George Campbell, *Lectures on Systematic Theology and Pulpit Eloquence* (Boston: W. Wells and T. B. Wait, 1810), p. 326.

32. Finney, *Lectures on Revivals*, p. 11.

33. Barbara Sicherman, *The Quest for Mental Health in America, 1880–1917* (1967; reprint New York: Arno Press, 1980), pp. 88, 315.

34. C. Daniel Batson and W. Larry Ventis, *The Religious Experience: A Social-Psychological Perspective* (New York: Oxford University Press, 1982).

35. David Meredith Reese, *A Plain and Practical Treatise on the Epidemic Cholera, as it Prevailed in the City of New York in the Summer of 1832: Including its Nature, Causes, Treatment, and Prevention* (New York: Conner and Cooke, 1833).

36. See Gerald L. Klerman, "The Age of Melancholy?" *Psychology Today* 12 (April 1979): 36–42, 48.

37. For a sampling of evangelical treatments of depression in the popular literature, see marriage and family counselor Andre Bustanoby, "How to Cope with Discouragement," *Christianity Today*, 7 January 1977, pp. 396–98; psychiatrist Enos D. Martin, "Ministering to the Depressed," *Leadership* 2 (Spring 1981): 27–34; psychiatrist Armand Mayo Nicholi II, "Why Can't I Deal with Depression?" *Christianity Today*, 11 November 1983, pp. 38–41; Richard F. Berg and Christine McCartney, *Depression and the Integrated Life: A Christian Understanding of Sadness and Inner Suffering* (New York: Alba House, 1981).

38. "Christians are not altogether immune from depression," Billy Graham wrote early in his career. See *Billy Graham Answers Your Questions* (Minneapolis: World Wide Publications, n.d.), p. 144.

39. Some of the more severe manifestations of depression, of course, were carefully concealed. See, e.g., one of the most astonishing letters in church history, dated 27 June 1766, and written by John Wesley to his brother Charles with the bracketed words in Greek and cipher, signaling John's intent that it was "For Your Eyes Only": "I do not feel the wrath of God abiding on me, nor can I believe it does. And yet (this is the mystery) [I do not love God. I never did.]...And yet to be so employed of God! and so hedged in that I can get neither forward nor backward! Surely there never was such an instance before from the beginning of the world! If I [ever have had] *that faith* it would not be so strange. But [I never have had any] other [evidence] of the eternal or invisible world than [I have] now; and that is [none at all], unless such as fairly shines from reason's glimmering ray. [I have no] direct witness, I do not say that [I am a child of God], but of anything invisible or eternal. And yet I dare not preach otherwise than I do....I have no more fear than love. Or if I have (any fear, it is not that of falling) into hell but of falling into nothing." From *The Letters of John Wesley, A.M.,* ed. John Telford (London: Epworth Press, 1931), 5:15–16.

40. "Despondency, Its Cause and Cure," in J. Oswald Sanders, *A Spiritual Clinic* (Chicago: Moody Press, 1958), pp. 34–40.

41. *An Account of the Experiences of Hester Anne Rogers...* (New York: B. Waugh and T. Mason, 1832), pp. 28, 67–68.

42. Walter Trobisch, *The Complete Works of Walter Trobisch* (Downers Grove, Ill.: InterVarsity Press, 1987), p. 685.

43. Atkinson, *The Garden of Sorrows,* pp. 73, 83.

44. I was reminded of this song by Berg and McCartney, *Depression and the Integrated Life,* p. 90.

45. Quoted in Silvano Arieti, ed., *American Handbook of Psychiatry* (New York: Basic Books, 1959), 1:348.

46. Timothy Flint, *Recollections of the Last Ten Years Passed in Occasional Residences and Journeyings in the Valley of the Mississippi...in a Series of Letters to The Rev. James Flint, of Salem, Massachusetts* (Boston: Cummings, Hilliard, 1826), pp. 240–41. I first encountered this reference in James H. Cassedy, *Medicine and American Growth, 1800–1860* (Madison: University of Wisconsin Press, 1986), p. 75.

47. Edwards to Mrs. Esther Burr, 20 November 1757, as cited in *Jonathan Edwards: Representative Selections, with Introduction, Bibliography, and Notes,* ed. Clarence H. Faust and Thomas H. Johnson, rev. ed. (New York: Hill and Wang, 1962), p. 414.

48. Richard Baxter, *Preservatives against Melancholy and Overmuch Sorrow, or, the Cure of Both* (London: Printed for Joseph Marshall, 1716); George Miller, *Kurze Beschreibung der Würkenden Gnade Gottes bey dem Erleuchteten evangelischen Prediger Jacob Albrecht* (Reading, Pa.: Johann Ritter, 1811), pp. 20–21; Jesse Lee, *A Short Account of the Life and Death of the Rev. John Lee: A Methodist Minister in the United States of America* (Baltimore: John West Butler, 1805), p. 81; see also Leonard I. Sweet, *The Minister's Wife: Her Role in Nineteenth-Century American Evangelicalism* (Philadelphia: Temple University Press, 1983), pp. 147–48; *A Journal of the Travels of William Colbert, Methodist Preacher Thro' Parts of Maryland, Pennsylvania, New York, Delaware and Virginia in 1790 to 1838,* typescript of manuscript, Garrett-Evangelical Theological Seminary (1929), 27 May 1796, 2:95.

49. C. H. Spurgeon, *Lectures to My Students* (Grand Rapids: Zondervan, 1965), p. 155. For other discussions of ministerial proneness to depression, see "Despondency, Its Cause and Cure," chap. 4 of J. Oswald Sander, *A Spiritual Clinic: A Suggestive Diagnosis and Prescription for Problems in Christian Life and Service* (Chicago: Moody Press, 1958), pp. 34–40; and "The Dragnet of Discouragement," chap. 14 of Ralph Turnball, *A Minister's Obstacles* (Grand Rapids: Baker Book House, 1964), pp. 121–29.

50. Kenneth B. Wells et al., "The Functioning and Well-being of Depressed Patients: Results from the Medical Outcomes Study," *Journal of the American Medical Association* 262 (18 August 1989): 914–19.

51. Oliver Ransford, *David Livingstone: The Dark Interior* (London: John Murray, 1978).

52. Atkinson, *The Garden of Sorrows*, pp. 64–65.

53. David Allan Hubbard, *How to Face Your Fears* (Philadelphia: A. J. Holman, 1972), p. 27.

54. William James, *The Principles of Psychology*, vol. 8 of *The Works of William James* (Cambridge: Harvard University Press, 1981), 1:281.

55. Philip Roth is quoted by Lorna Sage, "The Periodicals, 26: The Paris Review," *TLS*, 29 March 1985, p. 344.

56. Vernon Scannell, "Drinking Up Time," *Funeral Games and Other Poems* (London: Robson, 1987), p. 52.

57. Ruth Bordin, *Woman and Temperance: The Quest for Power and Liberty, 1873-1900* (Philadelphia: Temple University Press, 1981), p. 99.

58. Frances E. Willard, *Woman and Temperance; or, The Work and Workers of The Woman's Christian Temperance Union* (1883; reprint New York: Arno Press, 1972), p. 42.

59. Willard, *Woman and Temperance*, p. 254.

60. See Herbert Fingarette, *Heavy Drinking: The Myth of Alcoholism as a Disease* (Berkeley: University of California Press, 1988). Lloyd H. Steffen alerted me to this book in his excellent article "Rethinking Drinking: The Moral Context," *Christian Century*, 19–26 July 1989, pp. 684–86.

61. See Leonard I. Sweet, *The Lion's Pride: America and the Peaceable Community* (Nashville: Abingdon Press, 1987).

62. Richard K. Curtis, *They Called Him Mister Moody* (Garden City, N.Y.: Doubleday, 1962), p. 229.

63. *Trials and Triumphs (for Half a Century) in the Life of G. W. Henry... Together with the Religious Experience of His Wife....*(Oneida, N.Y.: Published by the Author, 1859), p. 216.

64. Charles G. Finney, *Sermons on Gospel Themes* (New York: Fleming H. Revell, 1876), p. 158.

65. Arthur Darby Nock, *Conversion: The Old and the New in Religion from Alexander the Great to Augustine of Hippo* (Oxford: Clarendon Press, 1933), p. 7.

66. Thomas Chalmers, "The Expulsive Power of a New Affection," *Sermons and Discourses* (New York: Robert Carter, 1852), 2:271–78.

67. The words are those of historical theologian David F. Wells, *Turning to God: Biblical Conversion in the Modern World* (Grand Rapids: Baker Book House, 1989), p. 63.

68. See Billy Graham, *My Answer* (Garden City, N.Y.: Doubleday, 1960), p. 141.

69. Gordon W. Allport, *The Individual and His Religion* (New York: Macmillan, 1951), pp. 33–34.

70. Tim Stafford, "Franchising Hope," *Christianity Today*, 18 May 1992, p. 24.

71. Vernard Eller, *Christian Anarchy: Jesus' Primacy over the Powers* (Grand Rapids: Eerdmans, 1987), p. 183.

72. Edwin Diller Starbuck, "A Study of Conversion," *American Journal of Psychology* 8 (January 1897): 268–308.

73. John P. Kildahl, "Personality Correlates of Sudden Religious Converts Contrasted with Persons of Gradual Religious Development," Ph.D. diss., New York University, 1957 (Ann Arbor, Mich.: University Microfilms, 1963).

74. Erik H. Erikson, *Life History and the Historical Moment* (New York: Norton, 1975).

## Chapter 2 / Sinning and Suffering

1. See Maxwell Pierson Gaddis, *Brief Recollections of the late Rev. George W. Walker* (Cincinnati: Swormstedt and Poe, 1857), pp. 251–59. For the scope of the 1832 cholera epidemic and its impact on the life and career of Sylvester Graham, see chap. 6 in Stephen Nissenbaum, *Sex, Diet, and Debility in Jacksonian America: Sylvester Graham and Health Reform* (Westport, Conn.: Greenwood Press, 1980), pp. 86–104.

2. For an example of this view of the epidemic as an "afflictive dispensation of Divine Providence," although the author could not escape admitting that "many valuable lives also have been lost," see "Progress of the Indian Cholera," *Methodist Magazine and Quarterly Review* 14 (1832): 450–74. The yellow fever plague that devastated the South during the summer of 1878 was viewed by A. B. Leonard in "The Plague," *Christian Advocate*, 26 December 1878, p. 828, as a divine punishment of "national sins" like "irreligion, Sabbath desecration, dishonesty, party corruption, oppression of the poor freedman, intemperance, and hatred between the North and South." Admitting that the North was guilty of these sins as well as the South, Leonard went on to explain that the scourge fell upon the South because the North is guilty, "but not *equally* guilty."

3. Gaddis, *Brief Recollections*, p. 259.

4. "On Cholera — Its History, Cause, Etc.," *Methodist Quarterly Review* 4 (October 1850): 599–600.

5. This was the position of physician David Meredith Reese, *A Plain and Practical Treatise on the Epidemic Cholera, as it Prevailed in the City of New-York in the Summer of 1832: Including its Nature, Causes, Treatment, and Prevention* (New York: Conner and Cooke, 1833). See especially his appendix.

6. See Robert Claiborne, *God or Beast* (New York: W. W. Norton, 1974), p. 94.

7. Billy Graham, *World Aflame* (Garden City, N.Y.: Doubleday, 1965), chap. 7, pp. 65–79.

8. J. H. Fairchild, "The Nature of Sin," *Bibliotheca Sacra* 25 (January 1868): 30.

9. William H. Daniels, ed., *Moody: His Words, Work, and Workers* (New York: Nelson and Phillips, 1877), p. 256.

10. Bernard Ramm, *Offense to Reason: A Theology of Sin* (San Francisco: Harper and Row, 1985), p. 2.

11. W. M. Ferguson, *Methodism in Washington, District of Columbia* (Baltimore: Methodist Episcopal Book Depository, 1892), p. 64; Morton Thrift, *Memoir of the Rev. Jesse Lee with Extracts from His Journals* (New York: Bangs and Mason, 1823), p. 210. The Methodist opposition to dancing flew in the face of Wesley's early love of dancing with friends at Worcestershire and with his sisters on their visits to Wroot and Epworth. In 1872 the General Conference of the Methodist Episcopal Church denounced dancing as degrading and unchristian behavior. Those who refused to repent of this conduct were expelled from the church with the admonition, "Dancing wastes time, wastes health, scatters serious thought, compromises Christian character, leads to entangling association with frivolous minds and careless hearts."

12. W. D. Blanks, "Corrective Church Discipline in the Presbyterian Churches of the Nineteenth Century South," *Journal of Presbyterian History* 44 (June 1966): 102.

13. As quoted by J. Oliver Buswell, Jr., "The Origin and Nature of Sin," in Carl F. H. Henry, ed., *Basic Christian Doctrines* (New York: Holt, Rinehart and Winston, 1962), p. 104.

14. Henry Hayman, "The Economy of Pain," *Bibliotheca Sacra* 45 (July 1888): 486.

15. "Hints on Sin and Free Agency," *The Christian Spectator* 6 (April 1824): 180.

16. John Wesley, "Original Sin," in *Sermons*, ed. Albert C. Outler, vol. 2 of *The Works of John Wesley* (Nashville: Abingdon Press, 1985), p. 185.

17. O. D., "Sin Compared to Disease," *Monthly Religious Magazine* 2 (February 1845): 44, 37–45.

18. Lewis H. Steiner, "The Human Body and Disease, Considered from the Christian Standpoint," *Mercersburg Review* 11 (1859): 87; James T. Bixby, "The Scientific and Christian View of Illness," *New World* 8 (September 1899): 480.

19. Catherine Albanese, "Physical Religion: Natural Sin and Healing Grace in the Nineteenth Century," chap. 4 of her *Nature Religion in America: From the Algonkian Indians to the New Age* (Chicago: University of Chicago Press, 1990), pp. 120–22. See also Albanese, "Physic and Metaphysic in Nineteenth-Century America: Medical Sectarians and Religious Healing," *Church History* 55 (December 1986): 489–502; Albanese, "The Poetics of Healing: Root Metaphors and Rituals in Nineteenth-Century America," *Soundings* 63 (1980): 381–406.

20. Billy Graham, *My Answer* (Garden City, N.Y.: Doubleday, 1960), p. 140.

21. William G. T. Shedd, "The Atonement, A Satisfaction for the Ethical Nature of Both God and Man," in *Bibliotheca Sacra* 16 (1859): 749.

22. See Frederic Greeves, *The Meaning of Sin* (London: Epworth Press, 1956), p. 102.

23. Daniel E. Fountain, *Health, the Bible, and the Church: Biblical Perspectives on Health and Healing* (Wheaton, Ill.: Billy Graham Center, 1989), p. 58.

24. Henry Cowles, "Sin and Suffering in the Universe, as Related to the Power, Wisdom, and Love of God," *Bibliotheca Sacra*, 2d ser., 30 (October 1873): 732–33. For similar sensitivity to the suffering of animals who are not free moral agents, see Bixby, "The Scientific and Christian View of Illness," p. 473.

25. C. S. Lewis, *A Grief Observed* (1961; reprint New York: Seabury Press, 1973), pp. 35–36.

26. Peter DeVries, *The Blood of the Lamb* (Boston: Little, Brown, 1961), p. 238. For a discussion of DeVries, see also Ralph C. Wood, *The Comedy of Redemption: Christian Faith and Comic Vision in Four American Novelists* (Notre Dame: Notre Dame University Press, 1988), pp. 230–79.

27. Jennie Smith, *The Valley of Baca: A Record of Suffering and Triumph* (Cincinnati: Jennings and Pye, 1876), pp. 6–7.

28. John R. W. Stott, *What Christ Thinks of the Church* (Grand Rapids: Eerdmans, 1958), pp. 35, 50.

29. W. Somerset Maugham, *The Summing Up* (New York: Doubleday, 1938).

30. Patrick Fanning, *Visualization for Change* (Oakland, Calif.: New Harbinger, 1988), p. 279.

31. E. R. Eschbach, "The Meaning and Uses of Pain," *Reformed Church Review* 4th ser., 8 (January 1904): 70–80.

32. *Billy Graham Answers Your Questions* (Minneapolis: World Wide Publications, n.d.), p. 140.

33. Edna Hatlestad Hong, *Turn Over Any Stone* (Minneapolis: Augsburg Publishing House, 1970) and *Bright Valley of Love* (Minneapolis: Augsburg Publishing House, 1976).

34. George I. Chace, "Of the Moral Attributes of the Divine Being," *Bibliotheca Sacra* 2d ser., 7 (October 1850): 672. See also Thomas Munnell, "The Philosophy of Pain-Hell," *Christian Quarterly Review* 2 (1883): 97.

35. Woods Hutchinson, "The Value of Pain," *Monist* 7 (1897): 494–504; Benjamin W. Dwight, "The Doctrine of God's Providence, in Itself, and in Its Relations and Uses," *Bibliotheca Sacra*, 2d ser., 21 (July 1864): 625. See also Henry Hayman, "The Economy of Pain," pp. 585–86. Liberal evangelicals later in the century would begin to use evolutionary language: "the highest and best adaptation to the environment is that which utilizes pain as a protection." See Thomas C. Chamberlin, "The Problem of Suffering," *Biblical World* 8 (1896): 194. When joined with evolutionary

theory, pain so saves and preserves the organism that it almost loses any association with evil and becomes a supreme good.

36. Steiner, "The Human Body and Disease," p. 68.

37. Gaddis, *Brief Recollections,* p. 233.

38. "The Health of Clergymen," in the United Brethren publication *Religious Telescope,* 14 February 1849, p. 231.

39. Steiner, "The Human Body and Disease," p. 71.

40. L. B. Coles, *Philosophy of Health: Natural Principles of Health and Cure; or, Health and Cure Without Drugs: also, The Moral Bearings of Erroneous Appetites* (Boston: Ticknor, Reed and Fields, 1853).

41. William Andrus Alcott, *Letters to a Sister; or Woman's Mission* (Buffalo: George H. Derby, 1850), pp. 39, 42–43, 196.

42. See the headline in the "Health and Disease" section of *Christian Advocate,* 12 October 1882, p. 654.

43. Quoted by Sylvester Graham, *Lectures on the Science of Human Life* (Boston: Marsh, Capen, Lyon and Webb, 1839), 2:578–80; also see Arthur H. Grimshaw, *An Essay on the Physical and Moral Effects of the Use of Tobacco as a Luxury* (New York: William Harned, 1853).

44. These include James White and Ellen Gould White, James M. McLellan, J. H. Waggoner, Daniel T. Bourdeau, Joseph Bates, and others. F. Gerard Damsteegt has an excellent article on "Health Reform and the Bible in Early Sabbatarian Adventism" in *Adventist Heritage* 5 (Winter 1978): 13–21. See also William A. Alcott, *Tea and Coffee: Their Physical, Intellectual, and Moral Effects on the Human System* (Boston: George W. Light, 1839).

45. "Stimulants," *Christian Advocate,* 24 August 1882, p. 542; "The Abbe Moigno and Tobacco," *Christian Advocate,* 28 September 1882, p. 622. See also "Some of the Evils of Tobacco," *The Illustrated Christian Family Almanac for 1883* (Cleveland: Evangelical Association, 1883), p. 43; Cassandra Tate, "In the 1800s, Antismoking Was a Burning Issue," *Smithsonian* 20 (July 1989): 107–17.

46. Ralph Barns Grindrod, *Bacchus: An Essay on the Nature, Causes, Effects, and Cure of Intemperance* (London: J. Pasco, 1839); the first American edition of this 535-page tract was published in Hartford, Conn., by S. Andrus, 1851.

47. Frances E. Willard, *Woman and Temperance; or, The Work and Workers of the Woman's Christian Temperance Union* (Hartford, Conn.: Park Publishing, 1883; reprint, New York: Arno Press, 1972), pp. 147–48. Willard, *How to Win: A Book for Girls* (New York: Funk and Wagnalls, 1886), pp. 36–85.

48. Although the study finding a positive association between religious commitment and dietary adequacy is badly flawed — "healthful dietary behavior" is associated with "higher protein intake and meal regularity" — see the path-breaking attempt to study the connections between food and religion by William Alex McIntosh and Peggy A. Shifflett, "Dietary Behavior, Dietary Adequacy, and Religious Social Support: An Exploratory Study," *Review of Religious Research* 26 (1984): 158–75.

49. Willard, *How to Win,* p. 85.

50. *Harper's Weekly,* 22 January 1876, p. 74.

51. Steiner, "The Human Body and Disease," pp. 77–78.

52. See esp. chap. 3, "The Elimination of Pain," Donald De Marco, *The Anesthetic Society* (Front Royal, Va.: Christendom Publications, 1982), pp. 38–49.

53. As quoted in Gladys M. Hunt, "The Good of Suffering," *Christianity Today,* 24 May 1974, p. 36.

54. Christopher Lasch, "Engineering the Good Life: The Search for Perfection," *This World: A Journal of Religion and Public Life* (Summer 1989).

55. Gordon Allport, "Mental Health: A Generic Attitude," *Journal of Religion and Health* 4 (October 1964): 20.

56. Jennie Smith, *The Valley of Baca*, p. 6.

57. Sue V. Beeson, "The Gospel of Pain," *Journal of Speculative Philosophy* 16 (1882): 426–30.

58. See, e.g., the 15 December 1795 entry in *A Journal of the Travels of William Colbert, Methodist Preacher Thro' Parts of Maryland, Pennsylvania, New York, Delaware and Virginia in 1790 to 1838*, typescript of manuscript, Garrett-Evangelical Theological Seminary (1929), 2:71.

59. Stevenson to George Meredith, 5 September 1893, *The Letters of Robert Louis Stevenson to His Family and Friends*, ed. Sidney Calvin (New York: Charles Scribner's Sons, 1901), 2:362–63.

60. Robert Louis Stevenson, *Prayers Written at Vailima* (New York: Charles Scribner's Sons, 1912), pp. 1–2. In her introduction Mrs. Stevenson revealed, "With my husband, prayer, the direct appeal, was a necessity. When he was happy he felt impelled to offer thanks for that undeserved joy; when in sorrow, or pain, to call for strength to bear what must be borne" (viii).

61. Wayne E. Oates, *The Revelation of God in Human Suffering* (Philadelphia: Westminster Press, 1959), p. 45.

62. Jennie Smith, *The Valley of Baca*, pp. 11, 89; Smith, *From Baca to Beulah* (Cincinnati: Jennings and Pye, 1880), pp. 9, 75, 138; Smith, *Ramblings in Beulah Land, A Continuation of Experiences in the Life of Jennie Smith* (Philadelphia: Garrigues Brothers, 1886–87); S. L. W., *A Souvenir Affectionately Ascribed to Miss Jennie Smith* (Dayton: United Brethren Publishing House, 1885), p. 6. For similar annals of suffering, this time from Pennsylvania, see Mary Rankin, *Daughter of Affliction: A Memoir....*, 2d ed. (Dayton: United Brethren Printing Establishment, 1871).

63. *Charles Hodge*, ed. Mark Noll, p. 268.

64. Henry Hayman, "The Economy of Pain," *Bibliotheca Sacra* 45 (January 1888): 8–9; see also Stephen Olin, "Religious Training," *Methodist Quarterly Review* 31 (April 1849): 305.

65. Lyman Beecher Stowe, *Saints, Sinners, and Beechers* (Indianapolis: Ivor Nicholson and Watson, 1935), p. 353.

66. "Christian physicians and dentists, following the example of Christ, should care for HIV infected persons even at the risk of their own lives," according to a Christian Medical and Dental Society statement on "Acquired Immunodeficiency Syndrome" (adopted 29 April 1988).

67. The anthropologist, theologian, and missionary Aylward Shorter discusses this African perspective on AIDS in *Jesus and the Witchdoctor: An Approach to Healing and Wholeness* (Maryknoll, N.Y.: Orbis Books, 1985), pp. 5, 61–62.

68. "The Church's Response to AIDS," *Christianity Today*, 22 November 1985, pp. 50–52; "Responding to the AIDS Crisis," *Christianity Today*, 3 April 1987, pp. 34–36.

69. David L. Schiedermayer, "Choices in Plague Time," *Christianity Today*, 7 August 1987, p. 20. Sometimes the choice is like the old adage, "using a thorn to remove a thorn" or the Zulu proverb, "When a thorn is stuck in the foot, the whole body stoops to pick it out."

70. See the statements by the Seventh-day Adventists (1988), Southern Baptist Convention (1987), National Association of Evangelicals (1988), Conservative Baptist Association (1987), Independent Fundamental Churches (1988), International Pentecostal Church of Christ (1987), as reprinted in J. Gordon Melton, *The Churches Speak on AIDS* (Detroit: Gale Research, 1989).

71. *The Poetical Works of John and Charles Wesley* (London: Wesleyan Methodist Conference Office, 1868–72), 2:216.

## Chapter 3 / Weeping and Laughing

1. Historians have recently been challenged to study the art, literature, and customs of weeping. The first such summons actually came from Johan Huizinga, whose classic text *The Waning of the Middle Ages* (London: Edward Arnold, 1924) was partly inspired by his study of the weeping phenomenon in France and the Low Countries during the fourteenth and fifteenth centuries.

2. Chap. 6 of Ian D. Suttie, *The Origins of Love and Hate* (London: Kegan Paul, Trench, Trubner, 1948) is entitled "The 'Taboo' on Tenderness."

3. Syndicated columnist Jeff Greenfield, "That little bitty tear let down a lot of American women," *Dayton Daily News,* 4 October 1987.

4. Roy Porter, ed., *The Faber Book of Madness* (Boston: Faber and Faber, 1991), pp. 201–2, 531–34. See also Roy Porter, *A Social History of Madness* (New York: Weidenfeld and Nicolson, 1987), pp. 126–35.

5. Augustine, *Confessions,* 9.12.32–33.

6. William J. Kelley's editorial, "James Monroe Buckley," *Methodist Review* 103 (May–June 1920): 452.

7. M., "The Tear — Its Philosophy," *Quarterly Review of the Methodist Episcopal Church, South* 3 (October 1849): 620, 622.

8. Quoted in "NAE Excerpts," *Christianity Today,* 7 April 1989, p. 43.

9. See, e.g., B. W. Richardson, "The Physiology of Tears," *Christian Advocate,* 1 December 1892, p. 812.

10. William H. Frey and Muriel Langseth, *Crying: The Mystery of Tears* (Minneapolis: Winston Press, 1985).

11. David Thomas, *The Virginia Baptist; or, A View and a Defence of the Christian Religion as It is Professed by the Baptists of Virginia* (Baltimore: Enoch Story, 1774), p. 59. Thomas went on to argue that the weeping of "lively Christians" is "often with joy instead of sorrow."

12. John Atkinson, *The Garden of Sorrows; or, The Ministry of Tears* (New York: Carlton and Lanahan, 1868), p. 165. Atkinson was a deeply evangelical minister whose interests led him to complete the course at the medical department of the University of the City of New York prior to his writing of *The Garden of Sorrows.*

13. James K. Baxter, *Pig Island Letters* (London: Oxford University Press, 1966), p. 7.

14. Augustine, *Confessions and Enchiridion,* trans. and ed. Albert C. Outler (Philadelphia: Westminster Press, 1955), p. 198 [*Confessions,* 9.12.33].

15. As quoted in J. R. Dummelow, ed., *A Commentary on the Holy Bible* (New York: Macmillan, 1946), p. 351; *Mystic Treatises by Isaac of Nineveh,* trans. A. J. Wensinck (Wiesbaden: Martin Sändig, 1969), p. 95.

16. *The Ascetical Homilies of St. Isaac the Syrian* (Boston: Holy Transfiguration Monastery, 1984), p. 104. Sebastian Brock, *The Holy Spirit in the Syrian Baptismal Tradition* (Poona: Anita Printers, 1979), pp. 62–63; Constance Cavarnos, *St. Methodia of Kimolos* (Belmont, Mass.: Institute for Byzantine and Modern Greek Studies, 1987), p. 37.

17. Dylan Thomas, "In My Craft or Sullen Art," in *The Poems of Dylan Thomas,* ed. Daniel Jones (New York: New Directions, 1971), p. 202.

18. W. H. Davies, "Trails," *The Complete Poems of W. H. Davies* (Middletown, Conn.: Wesleyan University Press, 1965), p. 427.

19. Thanks to Donald Shelby for first pointing me to this illustration.

20. See Leonard Woods, *History of the Andover Theological Seminary* (Boston: James R. Osgood, 1885), pp. 163–65; see also Harriet Beecher Stowe, "New England Ministers," *Atlantic Monthly* 1 (February 1858): 489.

21. Evangelicals like to tell the Nietzsche criticism on themselves, and it appears in sermons and articles in a variety of guises. See, for example, Vernon C. Grounds,

"Soar with the Eagle, Sing with the Angels," *Christianity Today*, 27 August 1976, p. 10, where Nietzsche is quoted as saying "I would believe in their salvation if they looked a little more like people who have been saved."

22. See Karl A. Olsson, *Come to the Party* (Waco, Tex.: Word Books, 1972), p. 151. For Henry Fielding see *The History of Tom Jones* (New York: Modern Library, 1985), p. 361.

23. John Wesley, "[Letter] to Mrs. Susanna Wesley, May 28, 1725," in *Letters*, ed. Frank Baker, vol. 25 of *The Works of John Wesley* (Oxford: Clarendon Press, 1980), pp. 162–63.

24. As quoted in Robert C. Roberts, "Smiling with God: Reflections on Christianity and the Psychology of Humor," *Faith and Philosophy* 4 (April 1987): 168.

25. For the evangelical ban on dancing, see William E. Phipps, *Recovering Biblical Sensuousness* (Philadelphia: Westminster Press, 1975), pp. 32–38.

26. Quoted in Donald E. Demaray, *Laughter, Joy, and Healing* (Grand Rapids: Baker, 1986), p. 38.

27. William Tyndale, *A Pathway into the Holy Scripture*, in his *Doctrinal Treatises and Introductions to Different Portions of The Holy Scriptures*, ed. Henry Walter (Cambridge, Eng.: Cambridge University Press, 1848), p. 8.

28. Editorial in *Christian Oracle* 16 (11 May 1899): 5. The thrust of the article is to make Christian joy and laughter integral to a faith that believes in "eternal punishment" and to counter the teachings of George Elliott that "if many were to live eternally apart from God, thereby being punished,…the macerated form of St. Francis and the terrible denunciations of other esthetics are much more consistent with the Christian doctrine than is the 'rubicund jocularity' of some modern divines."

29. Anthony M. Ludovicki, *The Secret of Laughter* (London: Constable, 1932).

30. Roberts, "Smiling with God," 168–75.

31. See, as an example, Ben Patterson, "Heaven's Celebrity Roast," *Christianity Today*, 9 April 1990, pp. 21–22.

32. Sylvester Graham, *Lectures on the Science of Human Life* (Boston: Marsh, Capen, Lynn, and Webb, 1839), 2:659.

33. Mark Twain, quoted in Demaray, *Laughter, Joy, and Healing*, p. 25.

34. As quoted by Bill F. Fowler, "Hell-Fire and Folk Humor on the Frontier," in *Tire Shrinker to Dragster*, ed. William M. Hudson (Austin: Encino Press, 1968), p. 52.

35. M. C. Hazard, "Humor in the Bible," *Biblical World* 53 (September 1919): 514–19.

36. For Keeble's "ingenuous, dissembling and parabolic" style of humor, see Matthew C. Morrison, "Marshall Keeble's Eloquence of Disarming Humor," *Today's Speech* 17 (November 1969): 35–36.

37. C. W. Wilkinson, "Backwoods Humor," *Southwest Review* 24 (January 1939), p. 169, 179.

38. Charles A. Johnson, *The Frontier Camp Meeting* (Dallas: Southern Methodist University Press, 1955), p. 61. For a somewhat radical description of a "holy laugh" at an Alabama camp meeting see "The Captain Attends a Camp Meeting," in *Ring-Tailed Roarers: Tall Tales of the American Frontier, 1830-60*, ed. V. L. O. Chittick (Caldwell, Idaho: Caxton Printers, 1943), p. 237.

39. Abel Stevens, as quoted in William Henry Milburn, *Ten Years of Preacher Life* (New York: Derby and Johnson, 1859), pp. 360–61. Stevens goes on to say, "While they were as earnest as men about to meet death, and full of the tenderness which could 'weep with those who wept,' no men could better rejoice with those who rejoiced."

40. Doug Adams, *Humor in the American Pulpit: From George Whitefield through Henry Ward Beecher* (Aurora, Ill.: Sharing Company, 1975), pp. ix–xii, 1.

41. Fowler, "Hell-Fire and Folk Humor on the Frontier," p. 58.

42. Elizabeth Tokar, "Humorous Anecdotes Collected from a Methodist Minister," *Western Folklore* 26 (1967): 89–100.

43. Editorial, "Humor in the Pulpit," *Southern Methodist Review* 4 (March 1888): 112–15; W. A. Back, "Pulpit Pleasantry," *Quarterly Review of the Methodist Episcopal Church, South*, n.s. 9 (April 1891): 15–21. "It may be that the fathers were too solemn — that their solemnity amounted almost to sanctimoniousness, but are we not in danger of running to the other extreme?" (p. 18).

44. Webb B. Garrison, "Humor in the Pulpit," in *The Preacher and His Audience* (Westwood, N.J.: Fleming H. Revell, 1954), pp. 192–212.

45. Henry A. Reed, "Legatees and Legators of Laughter," *Methodist Review* 102 (September 1919): 733.

## Chapter 4 / Sleeping and Dreaming

1. John Milton, "Theme on Early Rising," in *Complete Prose Works of John Milton* (New Haven: Yale University Press, 1953), 1:1038–39.

2. *Petrarch's View of Human Life*, trans. Susannah Dobson (London: Printed for John Stockdale, 1791).

3. John Wesley, "On Redeeming the Time," *Sermons*, ed. Albert C. Outler, vol. 3 of *The Works of John Wesley* (Nashville: Abingdon Press, 1986), pp. 324–26.

4. See Urban Tigner Holmes, *Daily Living in the Twelfth Century, Based on the Observations of Alexander Neckam in London and Paris* (Madison: University of Wisconsin Press, 1952), pp. 134–35.

5. As reported in Peter Passell, "Sleep? Why There's No Money in It," *New York Times*, 2 August 1989, I,1:2.

6. Wesley, "On Redeeming the Time," p. 325.

7. See Charles F. Goss, "The Story of Dwight L. Moody's Life and Work," *Echoes from the Pulpit and Platform...[of] Dwight L. Moody* (Hartford, Conn.: A. D. Worthington, 1900), p. 82, where it is stated that Moody "did not need much sleep, and what he did need he could get at any time and under any circumstances."

8. Homer Rodeheaver, *Twenty Years with Billy Sunday* (Nashville: Cokesbury Press, 1936), p. 95.

9. Catharine E. Beecher and Harriet Beecher Stowe, *The American Woman's Home* (New York: J. B. Ford, 1870), pp. 194–95.

10. "Early Rising," *Religious Telescope*, 26 February 1845, p. 127.

11. "Hints on Sleep" [reprinted from *Water Cure Journal*], *Religious Telescope*, 14 February 1849, p. 230.

12. Donald F. Durnbaugh, "Work and Hope: The Spirituality of the Radical Pietist Communitarians," *Church History* 39 (1970): 72–90. The only more severe sleep diet I have encountered was that of Toussaint l'Overture, who reportedly slept only two hours a night. After noticing that most people around him were sleeping one-third of their lives away, he would only allow himself to go to sleep for one-twelfth of his life.

13. Robert Samuel Fletcher, *History of Oberlin College from Its Foundation through the Civil War* (Oberlin, Ohio: Oberlin College, 1943), p. 322.

14. Quoted in William E. Sangster, *The Pure in Heart* (New York: Abingdon Press, 1955), p. 173.

15. John Wesley to Sarah Wesley, 17 July 1781, in Luke Tyerman, *The Life and Times of John Wesley* (New York: Harper, 1872), 3:357.

16. *Chamfort Maxims: Anecdotes, Personalities, Letters, Historical Writings, etc.*, selected and trans. C. G. Pearson (Glastonbury, Eng.: Walton Press, 1973), p. 23; Nietzsche is quoted in Hilary Rubinstein, *Insomniacs of the World, Goodnight: A Bedside Book* (New York: Random House, 1974), p. 5.

17. "Early Rising," *Religious Telescope,* 23 January 1850, p. 201.

18. Rev. Dr. Belcher, "The Sunday Sickness," *Religious Telescope,* 16 June 1852, p. 165.

19. Nathan Bangs, "Influence of Private Character," *Ladies' Repository* (May 1848): 144.

20. *An Account of the Experience of Mrs. Hester Anne Rogers, written by herself. To Which is Added, Spiritual Letters; Calculated to Illustrate and Enforce Holiness of Heart...* (New York: S. and D. Forbes, 1830), pp. 49ff., 193.

21. Benjamin Franklin, *Poor Richard's Almanac,* emphasis added.

22. "Hints on Sleep," p. 230.

23. Shakespeare, *Macbeth,* 2.2.34–37.

24. In a sermon entitled "Gods Approbation of His Works," John Wesley said, "they that are before the throne of God serve him 'day and night'...that is, without any interval." *Sermons,* ed. Albert C. Outler, vol. 2 of *The Works of John Wesley* (Nashville: Abingdon Press, 1985), p. 292.

25. Many of these accounts can be found in Stephen Brook, ed., *The Oxford Book of Dreams* (New York: Oxford University Press, 1983).

26. James Stuart, *Three Years in North America* (New York: J. and J. Harper, 1833), 1:55–56; Michael Kammen, *Colonial New York: A History* (New York: Charles C. Scribner's Sons, 1975), p. 15.

27. For a typical sickbed dream sequence, see Maxwell Pierson Gaddis, *Brief Recollections of the Late George W. Walker* (Cincinnati: Swormstedt and Poe, 1857), pp. 345–46.

28. "Nearer, My God, to Thee," by Sarah F. Adams (1805–48) was based on the account of Jacob in Genesis 28:10–22.

29. Conclusion to Christine Downing, "Poetically Dwells Man on This Earth," *On Dreaming: An Encounter with Medard Boss,* ed. Charles Scott (Chico, Calif.: Scholars Press, 1982), p. 101. Reprinted from *Soundings* 60, no. 3 (Fall 1977): 329. From "In Memory of Sigmund Freud," *The Collected Poetry of W. H. Auden,* ed. Edward Mendelson (New York: Random House, 1945), p. 167.

30. Quoted in Brook, *The Oxford Book of Dreams,* p. 242.

31. John Opmeer, "Dreams and Visions: God's Picture Language," in *Those Controversial Gifts: Prophecy, Dreams, Visions, Tongues, Interpretation, Healing,* ed. George Mallone (Downers Grove, Ill.: InterVarsity Press, 1983), pp. 51–58.

32. *Memoirs of Rev. Charles G. Finney, written by Himself* (New York: Fleming H. Revell, 1876), pp. 19–21, 34, 37, 153, etc. See also the dream testimony of itinerant George Miller, who prepared the first *Discipline* of the Evangelical Association in 1809, as recounted in R. Yeakel, *Jacob Albright and his Co-Laborers* (Cleveland, Ohio: Evangelical Association Publishing House, 1883), pp. 239–51.

33. Horace Bushnell, *Nature and the Supernatural as Together Constituting the One System of God* (New York: Charles Scribner's Sons, 1901), pp. 465, 475–76, 484.

34. Abel Stevens, *Life and Times of Nathan Bangs, D.D.* (New York: Carlton and Porter, 1863), p. 82. This was but one of many dreams Bangs experienced during critical periods in his ministry. Other dreams recorded by Stevens include his commissioning to ministry (p. 61), his overcoming of severe spiritual doubts (p. 82) and discontentment (pp. 87–91), and his dealing with a difficult ministerial situation (pp. 184–85).

35. *Selected Shorter Writings of Benjamin B. Warfield,* ed. John E. Meeter (Grand Rapids: Baker Book House, 1973), 2:152–66, 159.

36. Benjamin Breckinridge Warfield, *The Inspiration and Authority of the Bible,* ed. Samuel G. Craig (Philadelphia: Presbyterian and Reformed Publishing Co., 1948), p. 83.

37. Tertullian, *A Treatise on the Soul,* chap. 47, in *Ante-Nicene Fathers,* ed. Alexander Roberts and James Davidson (Grand Rapids: Eerdmans, 1973), p. 226.

38. Dale W. Brown, *Flamed by the Spirit* (Elgin, Ill.: Brethren Press, 1978), p. 11.

39. See for example, David Wilkerson, *The Cross and the Switchblade* (New York: Bernard Geis Associates, 1963) and Demos Shakarian, *The Happiest People on Earth* (Old Tappan, N.J.: Chosen Books, 1975).

### Chapter 5 / Sexuality and Morality

1. Dorothy Bloch, *"So the Witch Won't Eat Me": Fantasy and the Child's Fear of Infanticide* (Boston: Houghton Mifflin, 1978).

2. As cited by Andrew Kimbrell, "Body Wars," *Utne Reader*, May/June 1992, p. 55.

3. Alan Dundes, "The Dead Baby Joke Cycle," *Western Folklore* 38 (July 1979): 154.

4. Rima D. Apple, *Mothers and Medicine: A Social History of Infant Feeding, 1890-1950* (Madison: University of Wisconsin Press, 1987).

5. Kristin Luker, *Abortion and the Politics of Motherhood* (Berkeley: University of California Press, 1984), pp. 193, 245.

6. Editorial, "Abortion and the Court," *Christianity Today*, 16 February 1973, p. 32. Harold Lindsell was the editor in 1973. See also Lindsell, *The World, The Flesh, and the Devil* (Minneapolis: World Wide Publications, 1973), 100–103.

7. Carl F. H. Henry, *Christian Countermoves in a Decadent Culture* (Portland, Ore.: Multnomah Press, 1986), pp. 57–58.

8. Michael J. Gorman, *Abortion and the Early Church: Christian, Jewish, and Pagan Attitudes in the Greco-Roman World* (New York: Paulist Press, 1982). For a different reading of the early church material, see Beverly Wildung Harrison, *Our Right to Choose: Toward a New Ethic of Abortion* (Boston: Beacon Press, 1983).

9. Ron Lee Davis with James D. Denney, *A Time for Compassion: A Call to Cherish and Protect Life* (Old Tappan, N.J.: Revell, 1986).

10. Janet Patterson and R. C. Patterson, *Abortion: The Trojan Horse* (Nashville: Thomas Nelson, 1974).

11. Dwight Hervey Small, *Christians Celebrate Your Sexuality: A Fresh, Positive Approach to Understanding and Fulfilling Sexuality* (Old Tappan, N.J.: Fleming H. Revell, 1974), p. 16.

12. James C. Hefley, *Sex, Sense, and Nonsense: What the Bible Does and Doesn't Say about Sex* (Elgin, Ill.: David C. Cook, 1972), p. 17.

13. See Philip Abbott, "Philosophers and the Abortion Question," *Political Theory* 6 (August 1978): 313–35.

14. C. Everett Koop and Francis A. Schaeffer, *Whatever Happened to the Human Race?* (Old Tappan, N.J.: Fleming H. Revell, 1979), pp. 50–51.

15. Peter Singer, *Practical Ethics* (New York: Cambridge University Press, 1979).

16. Richard John Neuhaus's pioneering article appeared as "Hyde and Hysteria," in *Christian Century*, 10–17 September 1980, pp. 849–52.

17. For evangelicalism as a family religion, see "On Family Religion," *Methodist Magazine* 4 (1821): 468–75; "Parental Duty and Responsibility," *Methodist Magazine* 5 (1822): 24–26, 62–67; Charles Franklin Thwing and Carrie E. Butler Thwing, *The Family: An Historical and Social Study* (Boston: Lee and Shepard, 1888), esp. pp. 99–100. See also Janet Fishburn, "The Family as a Means of Grace in American Theology," *Religious Education* 78 (1983): 90–102.

18. Samuel W. Cope, "Marriage and the Home," *Methodist Quarterly Review* 37 (July 1893): 264.

19. See Rev. Thomas Harmer's "Letter on Personal and Family Religion," dated 16 October 1778, *The Miscellaneous Works of the Rev. Thomas Harmer* (London, 1823), reprinted in *Methodist Magazine* 8 (1825): 86–89. Also see Jacob Moore, "An

Essay on the Obligation of Family Worship," *Methodist Magazine* 9 (1826): 254–57, 294–99.

20. Colleen McDannell, *The Christian Home in Victorian America, 1840-1900* (Bloomington: Indiana University Press, 1986). See also the excellent review essay by Robert L. Griswold, "The Christian Home in Victorian America, 1840-1900," *Hayes Historical Journal* 7 (Winter 1988): 61–65.

21. Peter Uhlenberg, "Reinforcing the Fragile Family," *Christianity Today,* 16 January 1987, pp. 31–33. Evangelical sensitivity to family issues is illustrated in the nineteenth century by "The Decadence of the American Family," *Christian Advocate,* 21 September 1882, p. 606; Richard Wheatley, "The Alleged Decay of the Family," *Methodist Review* 69 (November 1887): 858–82; and, more recently, by Rodney Clapp's interview with Robert Bellah in "Habits of the Hearth," *Christianity Today,* 3 February 1989, 20–24.

22. For evangelicals' covenantal theology of family, see Walter Wegner, "God's Pattern for the Family in the Old Testament," *Family Relationships and the Church: A Sociological, Historical, and Theological Study of Family Structures, Roles, and Relationships,* ed. Oscar E. Feucht (St. Louis: Concordia, 1970), pp. 25–56; Kenneth L. Gangel's series "Toward a Biblical Theology of Marriage and the Family," *Journal of Psychology and Theology* 5 (1977): 55–69, 150–62, 247–59, 318–31; Jack Balswick and Judith Balswick, "A Theological Basis for Family Relationships," *Journal of Psychology and Christianity* 6 (Fall 1987): 37–49.

23. John Modell, "Historical Reflections on American Marriage," in *Contemporary Marriage: Comparative Perspectives on a Changing Institution,* ed. Kingsley Davis (New York: Russell Sage, 1985), pp. 181–95.

24. Dwight Hervey Small, *The Right to Remarry* (Old Tappan, N.J.: Fleming H. Revell, 1975).

25. H. Wayne House, ed., *Divorce and Remarriage: Four Christian Views* (Downers Grove, Ill.: InterVarsity Press, 1990).

26. See Gary Richmond, *The Divorce Decision* (Waco, Tex.: Word Books, 1988); James E. Kilgore, *Try Marriage before Divorce* (Waco, Tex.: Word Books, 1978); E. Clinton Gardner, *Biblical Faith and Social Ethics* (New York: Harper and Row, 1960), p. 245; Anne Kristin Carroll, *From the Brink of Divorce: An Evangelical Marriage Counselor's Advice on How to Save Your Marriage* (Garden City, N.Y.: Doubleday, 1978).

27. Elizabeth Fox-Genovese, *Feminism without Illusions: A Critique of Individualism* (Chapel Hill: University of North Carolina Press, 1991). Feminists for Life (FFL) is a growing group that supports feminist issues but opposes abortion. See Kay Castonguay, "Feminists for Life," *Iris,* Spring/Summer 1990, pp. 49–52.

28. Quoted by Paul Ramsey in "Feticide/Infanticide upon Request," *Religion in Life* 39 (Summer 1970): 171.

29. Many blacks suspect abortion is another guise of genocide, which helps explain why blacks outside the evangelical tradition have been more prone than their white counterparts to speak out against abortion. See C. Eric Lincoln, "Why I Reversed My Stand on Laissez-Faire Abortion," *Christian Century,* 25 April 1973, pp. 477–79, where abortion is called "a retreat from responsibility which seems characteristic of our times" (p. 479). Robert McAfee Brown calls for a moratorium on "Abortion and the Holocaust" in *Christian Century,* 31 October 1984, pp. 1004–1005. For the reaction of Jewish leaders infuriated by John Cardinal O'Connor's analogy, see *Catholics United for Life Newsletter* (1984), p. 2. Also see James T. Burtchaell, *Rachel Weeping: The Case against Abortion* (San Francisco: Harper and Row, 1984), where many of the essays compare abortion with Auschwitz and the Holocaust.

30. Mary Ann Warren, "On the Moral and Legal Status of Abortion," in *The Monist* 57 (January 1973): 43–61. Michael Tooley, "Abortion and Infanticide," in *The Rights and Wrongs of Abortion,* ed. Marshall Cohen, Thomas Nagel, and Thomas

Scanlon (Princeton: Princeton University Press, 1974), p. 78. Judith Jarvis Thomson argues that the mother has the right to abort the fetus even if it is a human being; see "A Defense of Abortion," *Philosophy and Public Affairs* 1 (Fall 1971): 47–66. For L. W. Sumner's moderate position, see Sumner, *Abortion and Moral Theory* (Princeton: Princeton University Press, 1981). For Peter Singer, see "Conception and Misconception" in *TLS*, 30 October 1981, p. 1253.

31. Roger Rosenblatt, *Life Itself: Abortion in the American Mind* (New York: Random House, 1992), pp. 71, 9–10.

32. Quoted in William V. Rauscher, *Church and Frenzy* (New York: St. Martin's Press, 1980), p. 8.

33. Advocates of "reproductive choice" can be found in the evangelical community, but even here abortion is a right of last resort. See, for example, Virginia Ramey Mollenkott, "Reproductive Choice: Basic to Justice for Women," *Christian Scholars Review* 17 (March 1988): 286–93.

34. "As to whether or not the performance of an induced abortion is always sinful we are not agreed, but about the necessity and permissibility for it under certain circumstances we are in accord." From the evangelical statement, "A Protestant Affirmation on the Control of Human Reproduction," in *Birth Control and the Christian: A Protestant Symposium on the Control of Human Reproduction*, ed. Walter O. Spitzer and Carlyle L. Saylor (Wheaton, Ill.: Tyndale House, 1969), p. xxv.

35. John Jefferson Davis, *Evangelical Ethics: Issues Facing the Church Today* (Phillipsburg, N.J.: Presbyterian and Reformed Publishing, 1985), pp. 147, 155.

36. The Christian Medical and Dental Society's "Statement on Abortion," adopted 4 May 1985, reads in full:

I. We oppose the practice of abortion and urge the active development and employment of alternatives.
II. The practice of abortion is contrary to:
   A. The revealed, written Word of God
   B. Respect for the sanctity of human life
   C. Traditional, historical, and Judeo-Christian medical ethics.
III. We believe that Biblical Christianity affirms certain basic principles which dictate against interruption of human gestation; namely:
   A. The ultimate sovereignty of a loving God, the Creator of all life
   B. The great value of human life transcending that of the quality of life
   C. The moral responsibility of human sexuality.
IV. While we recognize the right of physicians and patients to follow the dictates of individual conscience before God, we affirm the final authority of Scripture which teaches the sanctity of human life.

37. According to Carl F. H. Henry, abortion can be justified in cases of danger to the mother, "extreme deformity," incest, and rape, but never "as a means of sexual gratification and of birth control." See Henry, *The Christian Mindset in a Secular Society* (Portland, Ore.: Multnomah Press, 1984), p. 103. Harold Lindsell would allow abortion "if the life of the mother is seriously imperiled," "if there are compelling psychiatric reasons" (e.g., rape), and sometimes in the case of "gross retardation or mongoloidism"; see *The World, The Flesh and The Devil*, pp. 101, 103.

38. Dorie Giles Williams, "Religion, Beliefs about Human Life, and the Abortion Decision," *Review of Religious Research* 24 (1982): 40–48; Richard J. Harris and Edgar W. Mills, "Religion, Values, and Attitudes toward Abortion," *Journal for the Scientific Study of Religion* 24 (1985): 137–54.

39. Helmut Thielicke, *The Ethics of Sex* (New York: Harper and Row, 1964), pp. 227–28, 235.

40. Harold B. Kuhn, "Abortion," in *Christian Ethics: An Inquiry into Christian*

*Ethics from a Biblical Theological Perspective,* ed. Leon O. Hynson and Lane A. Scott (Anderson, Ind.: Warner Press, 1983).

41. C. E. Cerling, Jr., "Abortion and Contraception in Scripture," *Christian Scholar's Review* 2 (Fall 1971): 57.

42. See Beverly A. McMillan, "I Changed My Mind about Abortion," *Good News* 17 (March–April 1984): 11.

43. John R. W. Stott, "Does Life Begin before Birth?" *Christianity Today,* 5 September 1980, pp. 50–51.

44. For the argument that "at the point of conception the one-celled human zygote is a person in the fullest theological sense," see John C. Rankin, "The Corporeal Reality of *Nepes* and the Status of the Unborn," *Journal of the Evangelical Theological Society* 31 (June 1988): 153–60.

45. Albert C. Outler, "The Beginnings of Personhood: Theological Considerations," *Perkins Journal* 27 (Fall 1973): 28–34, esp. 29.

46. Kenneth Kantzer, "The Origin of the Soul as Related to the Abortion Question" in Spitzer and Saylor, *Birth Control and the Christian,* p. 557.

47. "Endorsing Infanticide?" *Time,* 28 May 1973, p. 104.

48. Marjorie Reiley Maquire, "Personhood, Covenant, and Abortion," *American Journal of Theology and Philosophy* 6 (January 1985): 28–46.

49. John J. Davis, *Evangelical Ethics,* p. 170.

50. See the editorial, "Capable of Meaningful Life, Anyone?" *Christianity Today,* 29 March 1974, p. 29.

51. Dietrich Bonhoeffer, *Ethics* (New York: Macmillan, 1955), p. 131. Outler concludes with the same view of personhood. It is "a divine intention operating in a lifelong process that runs from nidification to death." See Outler, "The Beginnings of Personhood," p. 31.

52. Tertullian, *Apologeticum* 9.8.

53. For an articulate presentation of the prochoice, antiabortion position, see pastor-physician G. Timothy Johnson, "Abortion II," *Covenant Companion,* March 1989, p. 41.

54. Ian Gentles, "Good News for the Fetus: Two Fallacies in the Abortion Debate," *Policy Review* 40 (Spring 1987): 50–54.

55. J. W. Montgomery, "The Christian View of the Fetus," in Spitzer and Saylor, *Birth Control and the Christian,* pp. 83–86.

56. See W. Fred Graham, "A Tale of Two Documents: Presbyterians and Abortion," *Reformed Journal* 34 (November 1984): 7–9.

57. Richard Freund, "The Ethics of Abortion in Hellenistic Judaism," *Helios: Journal of the Classical Association of the Southwest* (1983): 125–37.

58. National Association of Evangelicals, "Statement on Abortion (1973)," as reported in J. Gordon Melton, *The Churches Speak on Abortion* (Detroit: Gale Research, 1989), p. 86.

59. Three of the four largest black Protestant denominations have issued antiabortion statements and resolutions.

60. Oliver O'Donovan, *The Christian and the Unborn Child* (Bramcote, Eng.: Grove Books, 1973).

61. Harrison, *Our Right to Choose,* p. 184.

62. Nancy Schrom Dye and Daniel Blake Smith, "Mother Love and Infant Death, 1750–1920," *Journal of American History* 73 (September 1986): 352.

63. Donald H. Parkerson and Jo Ann Parkerson, "'Fewer Children of Greater Spiritual Quality': Religion and the Decline of Fertility in Nineteenth-Century America," *Social Science History* 12 (Spring 1988): 49–70.

64. See Kathryn Kish Sklar, *Catharine Beecher: A Study in American Domesticity* (New Haven: Yale University Press, 1973), p. 208. For the appeal of hydropathic

living to women, see Susan E. Cayleff, "Gender, Ideology, and the Water-Cure Movement," in *Other Healers: Unorthodox Medicine in America,* ed. Norman Gevitz (Baltimore: Johns Hopkins University Press, 1988), pp. 82–98. Both John Lawson, a British adventurer whose account of travels in the Carolinas (*A New Voyage to Carolina* [London, 1709]) is particularly valuable for its description of the daily life and customs of the Indians, and Benjamin Franklin observed and wrote about the success Iroquois families and many southern woodland tribes had in limiting family size. See Wilbur R. Jacobs, "The Indian and the Frontier in American History — A Need for Revision," *Western Historical Quarterly* 4 (January 1973): 50.

65. John Ryle, "Libido and Libitum," *TLS,* 18 March 1983, p. 262.

66. Alan Graebner, "Birth Control and the Lutherans: The Missouri Synod as Case Study," in *Women in American Religion,* ed. Janet Wilson James (Philadelphia: University of Pennsylvania Press, 1980), pp. 229–52. See also Linda Gordon, *Woman's Body, Woman's Right: A Social History of Birth Control in America* (New York: Grossman, 1977), and James Reed, *From Private Vice to Public Virtue: The Birth Control Movement and American Society since 1830* (New York: Basic Books, 1978). See also Cerling, "Abortion and Contraception in Scripture," pp. 42–58.

67. See, for example, Mary Ann Mayo, *Caution: Sexual Choices May Be Hazardous to Your Health* (Grand Rapids: Zondervan, 1988).

68. Daniel O. Teasley, *Where Do They Come From? A Book for Children* (Anderson, Ind.: Gospel Trumpet Company, 1917), pp. 7, 11, 12.

69. James C. Hefley, *Sex, Sense, and Nonsense: What the Bible Does and Doesn't Say about Sex* (Elgin, Ill.: David C. Cook, 1971), pp. 84–85.

70. Cerling, "Abortion and Contraception in Scripture," p. 43.

71. Adam Clarke, whose commentaries were almost the "official" commentaries of evangelicalism throughout the nineteenth century, condemned "those addicted to this fascinating, unnatural and most destructive of crimes." See notes following commentary on Genesis 38:30 in "The First Book of Moses, Called Genesis," *The Holy Bible, Containing the Old and New Testament... With a Commentary and Critical notes...* by Adam Clarke (New York: Ezra Sargent, 1811), 1:Ddv.

72. Charlie W. Shedd, *The Stork Is Dead* (Waco, Tex.: Word Books, 1968), p. 73.

73. Some of both the earliest and the most recent studies confirm this observation. See Douglas E. P. Rosenau, "Sexuality and the Single Person," *Journal of Psychology and Christianity* 1 (Winter 1982): 30–36; Jean Wulf, David Prentice, Donna Hansum, Archie Ferrar, and Bernard Spilka, "Religiosity and Sexual Attitudes and Behavior among Evangelical Christian Singles," *Review of Religious Research* 26 (1984): 119–31.

74. See, for example, Letha Dawson Scanzoni and Nancy A. Hardesty, *All We're Meant to Be: Biblical Feminism for Today* (Nashville: Abingdon Press, 1986), p. 176.

75. Gary R. Collins, ed., *The Secrets of Our Sexuality: Role Liberation for the Christian* (Waco, Texas: Word Books, 1976), p. 114.

76. As quoted in Tom Minnery, "Homosexuals Can Change," *Christianity Today,* 6 February 1981, p. 37.

77. See Minnery, "Homosexuals Can Change," pp. 36–41. See also European psychotherapist Gerard Van den Aardweg, *Homosexuality and Hope: A Psychologist Talks about Treatment and Change* (Ann Arbor: Servant Books: 1985), where he argues that homosexuality is psychologically, not genetically, based and therefore can be successfully treated.

78. John White, *Eros Defiled: The Christian and Sexual Sin* (Downers Grove, Ill.: InterVarsity Press, 1977); David Field, *The Homosexual Way: A Christian Option?* (Downers Grove, Ill.: InterVarsity Press, 1979), p. 37; Frank York, "Is Homosexuality a Curable Illness?" *Focus on the Family* 2 (1988).

79. Alex Davidson, *The Returns of Love: Letters of a Christian Homosexual* (Downers Grove, Ill.: InterVarsity Press, 1971).

80. Letha Scanzoni and Virginia Ramey Mollenkott, *Is the Homosexual My Neighbor? Another Christian View* (San Francisco: Harper and Row, 1978). Ralph Blair is editor of *Review: A Quarterly of Evangelicals Concerned.*

81. Scott Reed with Paul Fromer, "Why Prolife Rhetoric Is Not Enough," *Christianity Today,* 20 May 1983, p. 19.

82. John J. Davis, *Evangelical Ethics,* pp. 49–50.

83. "A Protestant Affirmation on the Control of Human Reproduction," in Spitzer and Saylor, *Birth Control and the Christian,* pp. xxiii–xxxi, esp. xxv. See also John J. Davis, *Evangelical Ethics,* pp. 43–52.

84. David A. Fraser, "Sensuous Theology," *Reformed Journal,* February 1977, pp. 21, 22.

85. Fraser, "Sensuous Theology," p. 22.

86. Helmut Thielicke's helpful distinction between the primary and secondary purposes of marriage can be found in *The Ethics of Sex,* 204–5. For the view that homosexuals are engaging in acts that God forbids based on a doctrine of creation, see Field, *The Homosexual Way,* pp. 27–28.

87. See Lewis Penhall Bird's editorial introducing this special issue entitled "Evangelicalism and Issues in Sexuality," *Journal of Psychology and Christianity* 1 (Winter 1982): 2–3; see also Richard M. Ostrom, Robert E. Larzelere, and Steven K. Reed, "The Views of Selected Evangelical Christians on Sex Education," in the same issue, pp. 17–22.

88. Billy Sunday, "A Plain Talk to Women," in William T. Ellis, *"Billy" Sunday: The Man and His Message, with His Own Words Which Have Won Thousands for Christ* (Philadelphia: Winston, 1914), p. 227.

89. See John J. Davis, *Evangelical Ethics,* pp. 55–56.

90. The remarks of pediatrician Sidney Smith are quoted from "California Kids," in the evangelical youth ministries newsletter *Sources and Resources,* 15 August 1981.

91. The Christian Medical and Dental Society has cautiously stated that in vitro fertilization "may be morally justified when such a pregnancy takes place in the context of the marital bond"; laboratory research can be justified only "with the *explicit* intent of embryo transfer and eventual normal pregnancies"; clinical embryo transfer is morally viable only with the use of "gametes obtained from lawfully married couples." See the Christian Medical and Dental Society's "Statement on 'In Vitro Fertilization,'" adopted by the society's House of Delegates, 13 May 1983, available from the Christian Medical and Dental Society, Richardson, Texas.

92. Gilbert Meilaender, *The Limits of Love: Some Theological Explorations* (University Park: Pennsylvania State University Press, 1987), p. 46.

93. Thielicke, *Ethics of Sex,* pp. 248–68.

94. Thielicke, *Ethics of Sex,* pp. 262–63.

95. For a discussion of RU-486 see Lisa Sowle Cahill, "'Abortion Pill' RU 486: Ethics, Rhetoric, and Social Practice," *Hastings Center Report* 17 (October–November 1987): 5–8. See also the editorial by David Neff, "The Human Pesticide: Controversial Abortion Pills Are a Form of Chemical Warfare against Our Own Species," *Christianity Today,* 9 December 1988, pp. 16–17; Charles Colson, "Abortion Clinic Obsolescence," *Christianity Today,* 9 December 1988, p. 72; and an updated news item on the abortion pill, "Researchers Urge End of Ban on RU 486," by Kim A. Lawton, *Christianity Today,* 14 January 1991, pp. 60, 62.

96. George Grant, *The Quick and the Dead: RU-486 and the New Chemical Warfare against Your Family* (Wheaton, Ill.: Crossway, 1991).

97. Peter J. Leithart, "The RU-486 Icon," *First Things,* March 1992, p. 15.

98. Snorri Sturluson, *Heimskringla, Part Two: Sagas of the Norse Kings* (New York: Dutton, 1930), pp. 25–26.

99. "Statement on the Use of Fetal Tissue for Experimentation and Transplantation," resolution adopted 5 May 1989, Minneapolis, Minnesota, by the Christian Medical and Dental Society.

100. See "Curing or Killing," *Christianity Today*, 18 May 1992, pp. 40–41.

101. Sidney Callahan, "Value Choices in Abortion," in *Abortion: Understanding Differences*, ed. Sidney Callahan and Daniel Callahan (New York: Plenum Press, 1984), p. 326.

102. John J. Davis, *Evangelical Ethics*, p. 157.

103. Spencer Perkins, "The Prolife Credibility Gap," *Christianity Today*, 21 April 1989, p. 22.

104. For growing sensitivity to this issue, see Scott Reed, Paul Fromer, and Rodney Clapp, "If Not Abortion, What Then?" *Christianity Today*, 20 May 1983, pp. 14–23.

105. Jerry Falwell, *If I Should Die before I Wake* (Nashville: Thomas Nelson, 1986), pp. 10–12, 182. See also Falwell, *Listen America!* (Garden City, N.Y.: Doubleday, 1980), pp. 165–80.

106. Carol Jackson, "Can 'Adoption Not Abortion' Really Work?" *Good News*, March–April 1990, p. 30.

107. Bill J. Leonard, "The Rights of the 'Born,'" *Christian Century*, 6–13 January 1982, pp. 7–8.

108. "What Does It Mean to Be Pro-Life?" *Sojourners* 9 (November 1980). See also Donald Granberg, "What Does It Mean to Be 'Pro-Life'" in *Christian Century*, 12 May 1982, pp. 562–66.

109. For evangelical political activism, see Brenda D. Hofman, "Political Theology: The Role of Organized Religion in the Anti-Abortion Movement," *Journal of Church and State* 28 (Spring 1986): 225–47.

110. See Helen Rose Fuchs Ebaugh and C. Allen Haney, "Shifts in Abortion Attitudes, 1972–1978," *Journal of Marriage and the Family* 42 (August 1980): 491–99.

111. "Nor do I think the manner of destruction makes much difference," Gordon Zahn wrote in a letter to the editor of *Christianity and Crisis*. "If each of the millions of Holocaust victims had been individually immersed in a vat of acid (something akin to destruction of a human fetus by saline injection), it would have been no less a crime against humanity. The crime, as I see it, lies in the willful destruction of human lives at whatever stage to serve some socially or individually defined purpose" ("Abortion and 'Corruption,'" 26 May 1980, p. 166).

112. Bernard N. Nathanson's *Aborting America* (Garden City, N.Y.: Doubleday, 1979) had a tremendous impact because of the author's position as director of the world's busiest abortion clinic: New York's Center for Reproductive and Sexual Health. For Joseph Randall, formerly of the Atlanta Center for Reproductive Health, see *Fundamentalist Journal* 6 (April 1987): 61–62.

113. Kay Castonguay, "Planned Parenthood and Feminists for Life Argue the Abortion Issue," *Political Woman* 1 (Summer 1986): 11–15; Sidney Callahan, "Value Choices in Abortion," p. 296; and Mary Meehan, "More Trouble Than They're Worth? Children and Abortion," in Callahan and Callahan, *Abortion: Understanding Differences*, pp. 145–70.

114. David M. Feldman, *Marital Relations, Birth Control, and Abortion in Jewish Life* (1968; reprint New York: Schocken Books, 1974).

115. Mary Meehan, "The Other Right-to-Lifers," *Commonweal*, 18 January 1980, pp. 13–16.

116. See Milton C. Sernett, "The Rights of Personhood: The Dred Scott Case and the Question of Abortion," *Religion in Life* 49 (Winter 1980): 461–76; Sernett, "The Efficacy of Religious Participation in the National Debates over Abolitionism and

Abortion," *Journal of Religion* 64 (April 1984): 205–20. Also see Burtchaell, "Eliza and Lizzie Scott, and Infants Roe and Doe," *Rachel Weeping*, pp. 239–87.

117. Quoted in Donald De Marco, *The Anesthetic Society* (Front Royal, Va.: Christendom Publications, 1982), p. 94.

118. Vicki Kemper, "Abortion and the Front Lines," *Sojourners* 17 (November 1988): 5.

119. Paige Comstock Cunningham, "Reversing Roe vs Wade," *Christianity Today*, 20 September 1985, pp. 20–22.

120. William Lloyd Garrison, *The Liberator*, 1 January 1831, as quoted in John Bartlett, *Familiar Quotations*, 15th ed. (Boston: Little, Brown, 1980), p. 505.

121. Quoted in D. J. Enright, "The Conservative Contribution," *TLS*, 4 March 1983, p. 209.

122. Baruch A. Brody, *Abortion and the Sanctity of Human Life: A Philosophical View* (Cambridge, Mass.: MIT Press, 1975), p. 6.

123. Francis A. Schaeffer, *The Great Evangelical Disaster* (Westchester, Ill.: Crossway, 1984), pp. 102–3.

## Chapter 6 / Eating, Drinking, and Bathing

1. Judith Walzer Leavitt and Ronald L. Numbers, eds., *Sickness and Health in America*, 2d ed., rev. (Madison: University of Wisconsin Press, 1985), p. 9. For a graphic account of the filthy floors, damp and dirty beds, poorly prepared and cat-nibbled food encountered by itinerants, see Robert Boyd's *Personal Memoirs: Together with a Discussion upon the Hardships and Sufferings of Itinerant Life* (Cincinnati: Methodist Book Concern, 1862), pp. 184–96.

2. Patrick Süskind, *Perfume: The Story of a Murderer* (New York: A. A. Knopf, 1986), p. 3.

3. Sydney Howard Carney, "The Early Days of Medicine in America," *Munsey's Magazine* 28 (1902–06): 378.

4. Anti Bustle, "Reduce the Bustles or Enlarge the Doors," *Religious Telescope*, 21 May 1845, p. 175.

5. Robert Samuel Fletcher, *A History of Oberlin College from Its Foundation through the Civil War* (Oberlin, Ohio: Oberlin College, 1943), p. 317.

6. "Luxury and Disease," *The Camp Meeting With a Variety of Songs, Poetry, Prose, Anecdotes, Riddles, etc.* (Frederick-Town, Md., Printed for the Compilers, 1819), p. 31.

7. See Ronald L. Numbers, *Prophetess of Health: A Study of Ellen G. White* (New York: Harper and Row, 1976), pp. 48ff.

8. As quoted by Frances E. Willard, *How to Win: A Book for Girls* (New York: Funk and Wagnalls, 1886), p. 85.

9. Owsei Temkin, "An Historical Analysis of the Concept of Infection," in *Studies in Intellectual History* (Baltimore: Johns Hopkins University Press, 1953), pp. 142–43, 147.

10. "Influence of Cleanliness," *Religious Telescope*, 10 January 1849, p. 190. For Wesley see his 1791 sermon "On Dress" in *Sermons*, ed. Albert C. Outler, vol. 3 of *The Works of John Wesley* (Nashville: Abingdon Press, 1986), pp. 247–61. See also E. Brooks Holifield, *Health and Medicine in the Methodist Tradition* (New York: Crossroad, 1986). I obviously disagree with the downgrading of the role of religion in creating a culture of cleanliness that one finds in Richard L. Bushman and Claudia L. Bushman, "The Early History of Cleanliness in America," *Journal of American History* 74 (March 1988): 1213–38. Gentility can be upgraded as a major impetus toward cleanliness without making religion a minor force.

11. Benjamin Rush is quoted in Temkin, "An Historical Analysis of the Concept of Infection," p. 143. The Beecher advertisement, which appeared in the 1880s, is quoted in Bushman and Bushman, "The Early History of Cleanliness," p. 1218. See also Weldon S. Crowley, "Benjamin Rush: Religion and Social Activism," *Religion in Life* 43 (1974): 227–38.

12. James C. Whorton, "Christian Physiology: William Alcott's Prescription for the Millennium," *Bulletin of the History of Medicine* 49 (1975): 466–67.

13. Nettie M. Alderman, *Seventy Beautiful Years: A Tribute to the Memory of Carmi Alderman* (Ironton, Ohio: Register Publishing Company, 1900), p. 26.

14. Homer Rodeheaver, *Twenty Years with Billy Sunday* (Nashville: Cokesbury Press, 1936), p. 95.

15. Charles E. Rosenberg and Carroll Smith-Rosenberg, "Pietism and the Origins of the American Public Health Movement: A Note on John H. Griscom and Robert M. Hartley," in *Sickness and Health in America*, ed. Leavitt and Numbers, pp. 385–98.

16. *Annual Report of the Interments in the City and County of New York, for the Year 1842, with Remarks Thereon, And a Brief View of the Sanitary Condition of the City* (New York: James Van Norden, 1843), as quoted in Rosenberg and Smith-Rosenberg, "Pietism and the Origins of the American Public Health Movement," p. 388.

17. W. Lee Spottswood, *Brief Annals* (Harrisburg, Pa.: Methodist Episcopal Book Room, 1888), p. 188. Further examples of the filth and destitution evangelicals encountered when they went visiting can be found in Richard Wheatley, ed., *The Life and Letters of Mrs. Phoebe Palmer* (New York: Garland, 1984), pp. 211–12.

18. Samuel B. Halliday, *Lost and Found; or Life Among the Poor* (New York: Blakeman and Mason, 1859); Isaac Smithson Hartley, ed., *Memorial of Robert Milham Hartley* (Utica, N.Y., Curtis and Childs, 1882); Rosenberg and Smith-Rosenberg, "Pietism and the Origins of the American Public Health Movement," p. 389.

19. See, e.g., Ruth M. Alexander, "'We are Engaged as a Band of Sisters': Class and Domesticity in the Washingtonian Temperance Movement, 1840–1850," *Journal of American History* 75 (December 1988): 763–85.

20. Bill Wilson, *Alcoholics Anonymous Comes of Age* (New York: Harper, 1957), pp. 10–11, 59–64; Helen Smith Shoemaker, *I Stand by the Door: The Life of Sam Shoemaker* (New York: Harper and Row, 1967), pp. 189–93. See also John F. Woolverton, "Evangelical Protestantism and Alcoholism, 1933–1962: Episcopalian Samuel Shoemaker, The Oxford Group and Alcoholics Anonymous," *Historical Magazine of the Protestant Episcopal Church* 52 (March 1983): 53–65.

21. James C. Whorton, "Patient, Heal Thyself: Popular Health Reform Movement as Unorthodox Medicine," in *Other Healers: Unorthodox Medicine in America*, ed. Norman Gevitz (Baltimore: Johns Hopkins University Press, 1988), p. 56.

22. Quoted in George Griffenhagen, "Medicinal Liquor in the United States," *Pharmacy in History* 29 (1987): 29. For evangelicals' search for other substitutes (in this case horseradish) to the prescription "use a little brandy," even though "your creed will let you use it for medicine," see Alfred Brunson, *A Western Pioneer; or, Incidents of the Life and Times of Rev. Alfred Brunson* (Cincinnati: Hitchcock and Walden, 1872), 1:361.

23. As quoted in Betty A. O'Brien, "The Lord's Supper: Fruit of the Vine or the Cup of Devils?" *Methodist History* 31 (1993): 207–8.

24. I. D. Stewart, ed., *Minutes of General Conferences, 1827–1856* (Dover: Freewill Baptist Printing Establishment, 1859), 1:213.

25. Samuel Luckey, *The Lord's Supper* (New York: Carlton and Porter, 1859), pp. 237–38.

26. In *The Scriptural View of the Wine Question in a Letter to the Rev. Dr. Nott* (Leeds: Truth Seeker Office, 1849), pp. 49–50, Moses Stuart declared: "Whenever

the Scriptures speak of wine as a comfort, a blessing, or a libation to God…they mean…*only such wine as contained no alcohol that could have a mischievous tendency;* that wherein they denounce it, prohibit it, and connect it with drunkenness and reveling, they can mean *only alcoholic or intoxicating wine.*" The fullest discussion of the "two-wine" theory is in Edward H. Jewett, *The Two-Wine Theory Discussed by Two Hundred and Eighty-Six Clergymen on the Basis of "Communion Wine"* (New York: E. Steiger, 1888).

27. Moses Stuart, *Scriptural View of the Wine-Question* (New York: Leavitt, Trow, 1848). See also Eliphalet Nott, *Lectures on Temperance* (Albany, N.Y.: E. H. Pease, 1847).

28. See Alvah Hovey, "Patristic Testimony as to 'Wine Especially as Used in the Lord's Supper,'" *Baptist Quarterly Review* 10 (January 1988): 78–93; see also Moses Stuart, "What is the Duty of the Churches in Regard to the Use of Fermented (Alcoholic) Wine, in Celebrating the Lord's Supper?," *Methodist Magazine and Quarterly Review* 17 (1835): 426, 431, 438–39.

29. Daniel Dana, "Chapin's Essay on Sacramentary Use of Wine," *Literary and Theological Review* 2 (1835): 654–67.

30. William G. Schauffler, "What Wine Did Our Lord Jesus Christ Use at the Institution of the Eucharist?," *Biblical Repository and Quarterly Review* 8 (1836): 285–308; Thomas Laurie, "What Wine Shall We Use at the Lord's Supper?," *Bibliotheca Sacra* 26 (1869): 182.

31. Stuart, "What is the Duty of the Churches," p. 431.

32. See Howard Crosby, "Calm View of the Temperance Question," *Independent*, 20 January 1881; Dunlop Moore, "Sacramental Wine," *Presbyterian Review* 3 (January 1882): 78–107; and Horace Bumstead, "The Bible Sanction for Wine," *Bibliotheca Sacra* 38 (January 1881): 47–116.

33. Nathaniel Hewit, "The Wine Question," *Literary and Theological Review* 6 (June 1839): 216.

34. For the dispute over Delavan, see Betty O'Brien, "The Lord's Supper," p. 206. Also see "Wine at the Communion," *Watchman of the South*, 31 March 1842, p. 125; and 7 April 1842, p. 129.

35. See, e.g., William M. Thayer, *Communion Wine and Bible Temperance* (New York: National Temperance Society, 1878); J. B. Wakeley, *The American Temperance Cyclopaedia of History, Biography, Anecdote, and Illustration* (New York: National Temperance Society, 1875), p. 221; "Communion Wine," *Christian Advocate*, 19 August 1880, p. 537; and the review of Hugh Macmillan, *The Marriage in Cana of Galilee* (London: Macmillan, 1882) in *Methodist Quarterly Review* 65 (April 1883): 381.

36. *The Doctrines and Discipline of the Methodist Episcopal Church*, 1884, p. 226.

37. *Christian Advocate*, 8 September 1892, p. 607, Question 3688. As late as 5 April 1903, *Christian Advocate* estimated that while "very many churches" use grape juice, "the majority" still believe that Jesus had a reason for choosing the symbols of wine for one sacrament and water for the other (p. 590).

38. Amariah Brigham, *Observations on the Influence of Religion upon the Health and Physical Welfare of Mankind* (Boston: Marsh, Capen, and Lyon, 1835), pp. 121–22; *Christian Advocate*, 7 April 1881, 214; *Proceedings of the General Conference of the Evangelical Association*, 1899, p. 113.

39. Archibald A. Hodge, "The Results of the Discussion Conducted in the *Presbyterian Review* as to the Nature of Bible Wine and of the Wine Used by Christ in the Institution of the Lord's Supper," *Presbyterian Review* 3 (1883): 394–99. Also see Dunlop Moore, "Sacramental Wine," *Presbyterian Review* 3 (1883): 107.

40. P. Anstadt, "Communion Wine," *Lutheran Quarterly* 16 (January 1886): 6.

41. *Minutes of the South-East Indiana Conference of the Methodist Episcopal Church,* 1876, p. 27.

42. Norman Kerr, *Wines: Scriptural and Liturgical* (London: National Temperance Publication Depot, 1881), pp. 134–35.

43. Anstadt, "Communion Wine," pp. 41–42.

44. S. Sharp, "Fermented Wine for Communion," *Religious Telescope,* 29 June 1881, p. 627.

45. As quoted in William Chazanot, *Welch's Grape Juice: From Corporation to Co-Operation* (Syracuse: Syracuse University Press, 1977), p. 1.

46. Chazanot, *Welch's Grape Juice,* pp. 76–77.

47. John Ellis, *A Review of Rev. Edward H. Jewett's "Communion Wine"* (Mount Joy, Pa.: J. R. Hoffer, 1889), p. 24.

48. T. Grigg-Smith, *Intinction and the Administration of the Chalice* (Portsmouth, N.H.: Grosvenor Press, 1950), 13.

49. *New York Sun,* 6 January 1896.

50. *Union and Advertiser* 70 (11 June 1894): 9. See also the 16 July 1894 newspaper clipping about Dr. J. H. Robbins's proposal in Hingham, Massachusetts, in the "Scrapbook of Charles S. Forbes," Rochester Public Library.

51. *Union and Advertiser,* p. 9.

52. As quoted in the obituary for Charles Forbes in *New York Globe,* 3 October 1917. During plague years in the Middle Ages, specifically in the fourteenth century, records attest to the use of an early version of the "individual communion cup" for sick cases. They were called "pest chalices."

53. This is the suggestive analogy of Ottomar Rosenbach in *Physician versus Bacteriologist* (New York: Funk and Wagnalls, 1904), p. 247. Rosenbach lambastes modern "bacteriophobia" and its "inhuman," "antisocial," and "unchristian" tendencies, especially its "neglect of the laws of humanity and neighborly love" (p. 216).

54. "Scrapbook of Charles S. Forbes," 42–43; see also 28 April 1898 clipping on p. 40.

55. See, e.g., J. D. Kraut, "The Individual Communion Cup," *Lutheran Quarterly* 35 (October 1905): 588, 591; *Presbyterian* 64 (21 November 1894): 12–13; and more recently Reginald W. Dietz, "The Lord's Supper in American Lutheranism," in *Meaning and Practice of the Lord's Supper,* ed. Helmut T. Lehmann (Philadelphia: Muhlenberg Press, 1961), p. 162.

56. *Elmira Daily Advertiser,* 6 June 1898.

57. *Presbyterian* 64 (21 November 1894). See also *Christian Advocate,* 17 August 1893, p. 529.

58. *Evangelist* 66 (11 July 1895): 8. See also *Elmira Evening Star,* 11 June 1898, as clipped in the "Scrapbook of Charles S. Forbes," pp. 44–46.

59. *Evangelist,* p. 8.

60. *Christian Intelligencer,* 16 December 1896, p. 856; 23 December 1896, p. 884.

61. Kraut, "The Individual Communion Cup," p. 593.

62. "The Origin of the Individual Communion Cup," *Church Management* 12 (March 1931): 495.

63. *Christian Advocate,* 31 August 1899, p. 1374; 30 June 1898, p. 1045; 1 September 1898, p. 1407; 3 October 1907, p. 1588.

64. *Minutes of the General Assembly of the Presbyterian Church in the United States of America* (Philadelphia: MacCalla, 1896), pp. 47–48; *Digest of the Acts and Deliverances of the General Assembly of the Presbyterian Church in the United States of America* (Philadelphia: 1930), 1:825.

65. Felix L. Oswald, "Our National Health," *Chautauquan* 17 (1893), pp. 281–85.

66. M. O. Terry, "The Poisoned Chalice," *Physicians and Surgeons' Investigator*, 8 (15 June 1887): 163–65. In an article about Terry in his personal scrapbook, Charles Forbes crossed out words crediting Terry with "first physician" status in ringing the bell about the dangers of the common chalice. See the "Scrapbook of Charles S. Forbes," p. 2. Also see "The Danger of the Communion Cup," *Christian Advocate*, 11 October 1894, p. 666.

67. James M. Buckley, "A Misnomer," *Christian Advocate*, 6 June 1895, p. 353.

68. Reprinted in *Catalogue of Sanitary Communion Outfit Company* (Rochester, N.Y.: Burnett Printing, n.d.), p. 18.

69. See, e.g., Howard S. Anders, "Present Status of the Sanitary Movement for the Adoption of the Communion Cup," Address to the Pennsylvania State Medical Society, Chambersburg, Pennsylvania, 21 May 1895; reprinted from *Codex Medicus Philadelphiae*, October 1895.

70. "Report of Committee on Individual Communion Cups" (To Philadelphia's Fifth Baptist Church), 10 December 1897, as quoted in William H. Brackney, ed., *Baptist Life and Thought, 1600-1980* (Valley Forge: Judson Press, 1983), p. 279.

71. *Presbyterian* 64 (27 June 1894): 12.

72. *Christian Advocate*, 20 October 1898, p. 1699. Letter to G., June 1898, as clipped in the "Scrapbook of Charles S. Forbes," pp. 44–46.

73. Howard S. Anders, "Present Status of the Sanitary Movement for the Adoption of the Communion Cup." Reprinted from *Codex Medicus Philadelphiae*, October, 1895, 1.

74. *Evangelist* 66 (11 July 1895): 8.

75. *Christian Advocate*, 1 September 1898, p. 1408.

76. One reason for intinction's lack of appeal to evangelicals was its association with Roman Catholicism, as made explicit in *Churchman*, 15 September 1894. For the lay suggestion of intinction see M. O. Terry, "The Poisoned Chalice," *Physicians and Surgeons' Investigator* 8 (15 June 1887): 165.

77. E. W. Ryan, "Individual Communion Cups," *New York Evangelist*, 21 March 1895, p. 181.

78. *Christian Advocate*, 13 October 1898, p. 1645.

79. *Catalogue of Sanitary Communion Outfit Company* (Rochester, N.Y.: Barnett Printing, 1900), p. 9; *Western Christian Advocate*, 20 October 1895, p. 635; *Christian Advocate*, 17 October 1895, p. 674.

80. *Churchman*, 15 September 1894; *Christian Observer* 83 (4 December 1895): 10. James M. Buckley, editor of the *Christian Advocate*, did not mince words: "Considering the bribes and commissions offered to ministers for introducing the individual communion cups," he was surprised the movement had not spread faster; see *Christian Advocate*, 30 June 1898, pp. 1045 and 31 August 1899, p. 1374.

81. Anders, "Present Status of the Sanitary Movement," p. 3.

82. Mrs. C. H. Wetherbe, "Individual Christianity," *Christian Observer* 81 (10 October 1894): 5.

83. John W. Appel, "Individual Freedom," *Reformed Quarterly Review* 17 (October 1895): 410.

84. John H. Pitezel, "The Holy Communion in the Light of Methodist History and Usage," *Christian Advocate*, 27 June 1901, p. 1010.

85. W. C. Holliday, "The Common Cup, Or Individual Cups?," *New York*, 21 March 1895, pp. 180–81.

86. Joseph Pullman, "The Individual Cup and the Common Cup," *Christian Advocate*, 6 October 1898, pp. 1612–13. See editor Buckley's running exchange with Pullman, 13 October 1898, pp. 1645–46; 30 May 1901, pp. 851–52; 20 June 1901, pp. 967–68.

87. Bushman and Bushman, "The Early History of Cleanliness," pp. 1232–33.

88. Rev. S. S. Rahn, "That Individual Communion Cup," *Lutheran Quarterly* 29 (April 1899): 238.

89. G. D. Stahley, "A Common Cup, or Individual Cups," *Lutheran Quarterly* 29 (April 1899): 221–34.

90. Kraut, "The Individual Communion Cup," p. 592.

91. Obituary notice for Dr. Charles Forbes, *Rochester Democrat and Chronicle*, 5 October 1917.

92. See Bushman and Bushman, "The Early History of Cleanliness," pp. 1226–28.

93. S. S. Rahn used the "model gentleman" approach to justify the common cup. See Rahn, "That Individual Communion Cup," p. 240; see also physician G. D. Stahley, "A Common Cup, or Individual Cups."

94. Quoted in Buckley, "A Reply to a Defense of the Individual Cup" *Christian Advocate*, 13 October 1898, pp. 1645–46.

95. *Christian Observer* 83 (4 December 1895): 10.

96. Buckley, *Christian Advocate*, 1 September 1898, pp. 1046–48; 20 October 1898, p. 1686; 31 August 1899, p. 1374; 27 June 1901, p. 1008.

97. *Christian Observer* 83 (4 December 1895): 10; *Evangelist* 66 (11 July 1895): 8.

98. *Report of the Special Committee on the Use of Individual Communion Cups. Old South Church, Boston. October, 1896* (Boston, 1896), p. 4.

99. *Statement by A Member of the Special Committee on the Use of Individual Communion Cups. Old South Church, Boston* (Boston, 1896), pp. 5, 6, 8. The statement was signed by Henry D. Hyde on 11 November 1896.

100. This is the hymn Buckley quoted in "The Essential Significance and Use of the Holy Communion," *Christian Advocate*, 20 October 1898, p. 1685.

## Chapter 7 / Praying and Healing

1. Thomas F. Day, "A Great Man, A Boy, and a Catechism," undated typescript in Thomas F. Day Papers, San Francisco Theological Seminary Archives, as quoted in Douglas Firth Anderson, "Theological Controversy in the Far West: Presbyterians and Thomas F. Day, 1907–1912," unpublished manuscript.

2. The weeklies sampled by Betty O'Brien included the *Christian Advocate* editions of the Methodist Episcopal Church and Methodist Episcopal Church South, the Evangelical Association's *Der Christliche Botschafter* and *Evangelical Messenger*, the United Evangelical Church's *Evangelical*, and the United Brethren's *Religious Telescope*.

3. "'When Doctors Disagree,' Etc.," *Christian Advocate*, 24 August 1882, p. 529.

4. For example, Daniel Smith, "Review of Combe on Health," *Methodist Magazine and Quarterly Review* 22 (1840): 83–92.

5. Phillips Brooks, "The Beloved Physician," in *The Light of the World, and Other Sermons* (New York: E. P. Dutton, 1896), pp. 228–29.

6. Ezekiel Gilman Robinson, "The Place of Preaching in the Economy of Christianity," in *Lectures on Preaching Delivered to the Students of Theology at Yale College* (New York: Henry Holt, 1883), pp. 4–5.

7. William V. Kelley, "A Doctor's Confession," *Methodist Review* 90 (September 1908): 787.

8. John Gunn, *Domestic Medicine; or, Poor Man's Friend*, 13th ed. (Pittsburgh: J. Edwards and J. J. Newman, 1839), p. 520.

9. Rev. E. O. Haven, "The Medical Profession," *Methodist Quarterly Review* 47 (January 1865): 114.

10. E. Brooks Holifield, *Health and Medicine in the Methodist Tradition: Journey toward Wholeness* (New York: Crossroad, 1986).

11. An excellent treatment of evangelical programs of social welfare can be found in Norris Magnuson, *Salvation in the Slums: Evangelical Social Work, 1865-1920* (1977; reprint, Grand Rapids, Mich.: Baker Book House, 1990), esp. pp. 68–78.

12. Paul Starr, *The Social Transformation of American Medicine* (New York: Basic Books, 1982), pp. 170–71.

13. As quoted in Herbert A. Wisbey, *Soldiers without Swords: A History of the Salvation Army in the United States* (New York: Macmillan, 1956), p. 209.

14. United States Bureau of Census, *Benevolent Institutions, 1910* (Washington, D.C.: Government Printing Office, 1913), pp. 272–75.

15. David J. Wieand, "The Church and the Healing Arts," *Brethren Life and Thought* 4 (Summer 1959): 13.

16. John Harley Warner, *The Therapeutic Perspective: Medical Practice, Knowledge, and Identity in America, 1820-1885* (Cambridge, Mass.: Harvard University Press, 1986), p. 16.

17. William G. Rothstein, "The Botanical Movements and Orthodox Medicine," in *Other Healers: Unorthodox Medicine in America*, ed. Norman Gevitz (Baltimore: Johns Hopkins University Press, 1988), p. 36.

18. For an example of self-treatment of something as serious as a facial tumor, see Devereux Jarratt, *The Life of the Reverend Devereux Jarratt... Written by Himself, in a Series of Letters Addressed to the Rev. John Coleman* (Baltimore: Warner and Hanna, 1806), pp. 140 ff.

19. Charles Coleman Sellers, *Lorenzo Dow, The Bearer of the Word* (New York: Minton, Balch, 1928), pp. 202–203.

20. Mentioned in Morton T. Kelsey, *The Other Side of Silence: A Guide to Christian Meditation* (New York: Paulist Press, 1976), pp. 44–45.

21. Worthington Hooker, "The Mutual Influence of Mind and Body in Disease," *New Englander and Yale Review* (October 1845): 493–508.

22. J. E. P., "The Will as Medicine," *Christian Advocate*, 29 June 1882, p. 414. For physicians preparing medicine with prayer, see Maxwell Pierson Gaddis, *Brief Recollections of the Late Rev. George W. Walker*, (Cincinnati: Swormstedt and Poe, 1857), p. 222, where it was said of a certain Dr. John D. Elbert, "He even prepared his 'medicines' with prayer." See also an article in the *Episcopal Register* that offered "Hints to Physicians on the Value of Genuine and Heart-felt Piety," reprinted in *Christian Advocate*, 16 September 1826, p. 16.

23. Aylward Shorter, *Jesus and the Witchdoctor: An Approach to Healing and Wholeness* (Maryknoll, N.Y.: Orbis Books, 1985), pp. 133–34.

24. Lewis H. Steiner, "The Human Body and Disease," *Mercersburg Review* 11 (January 1859): 84.

25. Warner, *Therapeutic Perspective*, pp. 17, 15.

26. William Edward Biederwolf, *Whipping Post Theology, or Did Jesus Atone for Disease?* (Grand Rapids, Mich.: Eerdmans, 1934), p. 157.

27. Ivan Illich, *Limits to Medicine* (London: Marion Boyars, 1976), p. 116.

28. James Erwin, *Reminiscences of Early Circuit Life* (Toledo: Spear, Johnson, 1884), pp. 38–39.

29. For instances of clergy visitation and praying for the sick and dying in the nineteenth century, see Milton Bird, *The Life of Rev. Alexander Chapman* (Nashville: W. E. Dunaway, 1872), p. 186; Gaddis, *Brief Recollections*, pp. 268–69, 274; W. Lee Spottswood, *Brief Annals* (Harrisburg, Pa.: Methodist Episcopal Book Room, 1888), pp. 68–69; Thomas O. Summers, ed., *Biographical Sketches of Eminent Itinerant Ministers Distinguished... as Pioneers of Methodism Within the Bounds of the Methodist Episcopal Church, South* (Nashville: Southern Methodist Publishing House, 1859), pp. 194–95; Richard Beard, "An Account of Rev. William Harris," *Brief*

*Biographical Sketches of Some of the Early Ministers of the Cumberland Presbyterian Church*, 2d ser. (Nashville: Cumberland Presbyterian Board of Publication, 1874), pp. 138–39; James Robison, *Recollection of Rev. Samuel Clawson* (Pittsburgh: Charles A. Scott, 1885), pp. 146–47, 172–73; Henry Smith, *Recollections and Reflections of an Old Itinerant*, ed. George Peck (New York: Carlton and Phillips, 1854), pp. 168–69; J. P. Rodgers, *Life of Rev. James Needham, the Oldest Methodist Preacher* (Pilot Mountain, N.C.: Surry Printing House, 1899), p. 19.

30. Elnathan Corrington Gavitt, *Crumbs from My Saddle Bags, or, Reminiscences of Pioneer Life and Biographical Sketches* (Toledo: Blade Printing and Paper Co., 1884), pp. 173–74.

31. Erwin, *Reminiscences of Early Circuit Life*, pp. 341–42. An editorial in a United Brethren publication said that "it is the minister's business to propose prayer, as it is the physician's to administer medicinal remedies"; see "Visiting the Sick," *Religious Telescope*, 20 April 1881, p. 472.

32. One can see this beginning in chap. 11, "The Physician and the Sick Room," in Howard Henderson, *The Ethics and Etiquette of the Pulpit, Pew, Parish, Press and Platform* (Cincinnati: George P. Houston, 1892), pp. 73–79.

33. Mary Lamar Riley, "The 'Family Physician,'" Ph.D. diss., University of Chicago, 1985; Marshall Scott Legan, "Hydropathy, or the Water Cure," in *Pseudo-Science and Society in Nineteenth-Century America*, ed. Arthur Wrobel (Lexington: University Press of Kentucky, 1987), pp. 74–99.

34. For an example of how nasty the battle could get between allopathic and homeopathic physicians, see William E. Franklin, "The Trial of Thomas Blackwood: Presbyterians, Public Morals, and the Politics of Medicine on the Michigan Frontier," *American Presbyterian: Journal of Presbyterian History* 64 (Fall 1986): 167–74.

35. Judith Walzer Leavitt and Ronald L. Numbers, eds., *Sickness and Health in America: Readings in the History of Medicine and Public Health* (Madison: University of Wisconsin Press, 1978), pp. 5–6.

36. Walker Rumble, "Homeopathy in the Lehigh Valley," *Pennsylvania Magazine of History and Biography* 54 (October 1980): 485.

37. Jonathan Miller, *The Body in Question* (New York: Random House, 1978), p. 9.

38. See Vernon Coleman, *The Medicine Men* (London: Temple Smith, 1975): "Professor Henderson of Harvard has estimated that 1912 was the first year in human history when the random patient with the random disease consulting the random doctor had more than fifty-fifty chance of benefiting by the encounter" (pp. 9–10).

39. See "On the Progress of Medicine since 1803," *The Living Age* 236 (14 March 1903): 643.

40. Naomi Aronson, "The Discovery of Resistance: Historical Accounts and Scientific Careers," *Isis* 77 (December 1986): 630–46.

41. John N. Wilford, "Brilliant Loner Who Loves Genetics," *New York Times*, 11 October 1983, p. 22.

42. See John Wesley's denunciation of bloodletting and blistering as "extremely hurtful" in his letter to Mrs. Moon, 5 November 1762, *The Letters of the Rev. John Wesley*, ed. John Telford (London: Epworth Press, 1931), 4:195. For transfusions, see *Methodist Magazine* 10 (1827): 218–19.

43. Warner, *The Therapeutic Perspective*, p. 209. See also Warner's "Power, Conflict, and Identity in Mid-Nineteenth-Century American Medicine: Therapeutic Change at the Commercial Hospital in Cincinnati," *Journal of American History* 73 (March 1987): 934–56

44. Erwin, *Reminiscences of Early Circuit Life*, pp. 357, 361.

45. Alfred Brunson, *A Western Pioneer, or, Incidents of the Life and Times of Rev. Alfred Brunson...* (Cincinnati: Hitchcock and Walden, 1872), 1:272.

46. Samuel Thomson, *Learned Quackery Exposed; Or, Theory According to Art; As Exemplified in the Practice of the Fashionable Doctors of the Present Day* (n.p., 1809), p. 19.

47. Warner, *Therapeutic Perspective*, p. 117.

48. Ibid., pp. 117, 317. See also Leonard I. Sweet, *The Minister's Wife: Her Role in Nineteenth-Century American Evangelicalism* (Philadelphia: Temple University Press, 1983), pp. 184–211.

49. In one ad from 1882 issues of *Religious Telescope*, J. L. Stevens, M.D., guaranteed his remedy for cures from opium and morphine habits within ten to twenty days with, "No pay until cured."

50. William G. Rothstein, *American Physicians in the Nineteenth Century: From Sects to Science* (Baltimore: Johns Hopkins University Press, 1972), pp. 234–35; Joseph F. Kett, *The Formation of the American Medical Profession: The Role of Institutions, 1780–1860* (New Haven: Yale University Press, 1968), pp. 185–86; Paul Starr, *Social Transformation of American Medicine* (New York: Basic Books, 1982), p. 99.

51. According to Rumble, "Homeopathy in the Lehigh Valley," "By 1898…the 9,369 homeopathic physicians in the nation formed $12\frac{1}{2}$ percent of the whole" (p. 478).

52. James C. Whorton, "Patient, Heal Thyself: Popular Health Reform Movements as Unorthodox Medicine," in *Other Healers: Unorthodox Medicine in America*, ed. Norman Gevitz (Baltimore: Johns Hopkins University Press, 1988), p. 57.

53. Catherine L. Albanese, "Physical Religion: Natural Sin and Healing Grace in the Nineteenth Century," unpublished manuscript, p. 10.

54. Ronald G. Walters, *American Reformers, 1815–1860* (New York: Hill and Wang, 1978), pp. 145–72. For the way in which regular physicians used evangelical rhetoric to attack their "irregular," sectarian rivals, see Warner, *The Therapeutic Perspective*, pp. 20–21.

55. Warner, *The Therapeutic Perspective*, p. 62.

56. Robert Samuel Fletcher, *History of Oberlin College from Its Foundation through the Civil War* (Oberlin, Ohio: Oberlin College, 1943), pp. 319, 330.

57. William Alexander [aka Andrus] Alcott, *Lectures on Life and Health; or, The Laws and Means of Physical Culture* (Boston: Phillips, Sampson, 1853), pp. 26–27.

58. Alcott, as quoted in P. Gerard Damsteegt, "Health Reform and the Bible in Early Sabbatarian Adventism," *Adventist Heritage* 5 (Winter 1978): 13. See also James C. Whorton, "'Christian Physiology': William Alcott's Prescription for the Millennium," *Bulletin of the History of Medicine* 49 (Winter 1975): 466–81.

59. Albanese, "Physical Religion," p. 12.

60. C. S. Lewis, *Miracles: A Preliminary Study* (New York: Macmillan, 1947), p. 75.

61. Harry Houdini, *Miracle Mongers and Their Methods* (New York: E. P. Dutton, 1920), pp. v–vii.

62. Benjamin B. Warfield, *Counterfeit Miracles* (New York: Charles Scribner's Sons, 1918); John Calvin, *Institutes of the Christian Religion*, 4.19.19. Wesley is quoted in William Reddy's defense of faith cures entitled "Faith on the Earth," *Christian Advocate*, 12 October 1882, p. 643. See also the 19 October 1882 issue for a contrasting editorial (p. 657), and the article by Frank S. Townsend, "Faith-Cure," p. 660.

63. Warfield, *Counterfeit Miracles*, p. 6.

64. Harold John Ockenga, *Our Evangelical Faith* (Grand Rapids, Mich.: Zondervan Publishing House, 1946), pp. 40–41.

65. The comment was by Bishop Thomas Asbury Morris in "The Duty of Fasting," *Methodist Quarterly Review* 31 (1849): 212.

66. Bushnell, *Nature and the Supernatural as Together Constituting the One System of God* (New York: Charles Scribner's Sons, 1901), p. 485.

67. Ibid., p. 468.

68. Ibid., pp. 491, 448.

69. See Lewis B. Smedes, "What's Wrong with Celebrating a Miracle," *Reformed Journal* 39 (February 1989): 14, 21.

70. George I. Mavrodes, letter to the editor in *Reformed Journal* 39 (April 1989): 12.

71. Henry Stob, "Miracles," in Carl F. H. Henry, *Basic Christian Doctrines* (New York: Holt, Rinehart and Winston, 1962), pp. 82–83. Philosophical objections to miracles, as well as their theological rationale, are critiqued by Colin Brown, *That You May Believe: Miracles and Faith Then and Now* (Grand Rapids: Eerdmans, 1985). See also Colin Brown, "The Other Half of the Gospel?," *Christianity Today*, 21 April 1989, pp. 26–29.

72. Stob, "Miracles," p. 85.

73. See, e.g., James H. Smylie, "The Reformed Tradition," pp. 204–40; David Edwin Harrell, Jr., "The Disciples of Christ–Church of Christ Tradition," pp. 376–96; Gary B. Ferngren, "The Evangelical-Fundamentalist Tradition," pp. 486–513 in *Caring and Curing: Health and Medicine in the Western Religious Traditions*, ed. Ronald L. Numbers and Darrel W. Amundsen (New York: Macmillan, 1986).

74. Stob, "Miracles," pp. 84–85.

75. This is the position of William P. Harrison, "Mind and Faith Cures," *Southern Methodist Review* 25 (May 1887): 266.

76. Augustus H. Strong, *Systematic Theology* (Philadelphia: Judson Press, 1907), p. 133.

77. Harold Lindsell, *When You Pray* (Grand Rapids: Baker Book House, 1969), pp. 174–75, 91.

78. See Craig W. Ellison, ed., *Modifying Men: Implications and Ethics* (Washington: University Press of America, 1978).

79. See, e.g., John Scanzoni, "Evangelicals and Human Engineering Policy," in Ellison, *Modifying Men*, p. 248.

80. Gaddis, *Brief Recollections*, p. 323.

81. George Miller, *Kurze Beschreibung der Würkenden Gnade Gottes bey dem Erleuchteten evangelischen Prediger Jacob Albrecht* (Reading, Pa.: Johann Ritter, 1811), p. 25.

82. See S.'s call for fasting, which implies its slippage, "On the Duty of Self-Denial," *Methodist Magazine* 6 (1823): 257–60.

83. Quoted in Owen Chadwick, "The Religion of Samuel Johnson," *Yale University Library Gazette* 60 (April 1986): "Fast, that the body may be subject to the mind; / Eat, that the mind may use the body" (p. 125)

84. In *Experiments of Spiritual Life and Health*, ed. Winthrop S. Hudson (Philadelphia: Westminster Press, 1951), Roger Williams explains how "Prayer with Fasting is an Undoubted Means of Christian Health and Cheerfulness" (pp. 91–92).

85. Morris, "The Duty of Fasting," p. 214.

86. Johann Albrecht Bengel, *Gnomon of the New Testament* (Philadelphia: Perkinpine and Higgins, 1860), 2:723.

87. See item beginning "The Faith-Cure Camp-Meeting at Old Orchard Beach," *Christian Advocate*, 24 August 1882, p. 530; see also the item beginning "The following was telegraphed," *Christian Advocate* 18 May 1882, p. 306.

88. See John Q. Anderson, "Special Powers in Folk Cures and Remedies," pp. 163–74 in Wilson M. Hudson, ed., *Tire Shrinker to Dragster* (Austin: Encino Press, 1968).

89. "The Impropriety of Long Prayers," in *The American Baptist Magazine and Missionary Intelligence*, September 1818, pp. 399–401.

90. Donald E. Byrne, Jr., *No Foot of Land: Folklore of American Methodist Itinerants* (Metuchen, NJ.: Scarecrow Press, 1975), p. 155; quoting John Scarlett, *The Itinerant on Foot; or, Life-Scenes Recalled* (New York: W. C. Palmer, 1882), pp. 233–35.

91. R. Milton Winter, "Presbyterians and Prayers for the Sick: Changing Patterns of Pastoral Ministry," *American Presbyterians: Journal of Presbyterian History* 64 (Fall 1986): 141.

92. See *An Account of the Experience of Hester Anne Rogers...* (New York: B. Waugh and T. Mason, 1832), pp. 30–32.

93. See Finney's "Prevailing Prayer" and "The Prayer of Faith" lectures in *Lectures on Revivals of Religion* (New York: Revell, 1868), pp. 48–66, 67–82.

94. See Harrison, "Mind and Faith Cures," p. 263.

95. In this study, Dr. Randolph C. Byrd randomly assigned half of 393 patients to an "experimental" group prayed over by three to seven evangelical Christians and the other half to a control group that received no prayers. Statistics demonstrated that the two patient groups were equally sick when they entered the hospital but that the patients prayed for had fewer complications during their stay. "Positive Therapeutic Effects of Intercessory Prayer in a Coronary Care Unit Population," *Southern Medical Journal* 81 (July 1988): 326–29.

96. Adoniram Judson Gordon, *The Ministry of Healing, or Miracles of Cure in All Ages,* 3d ed., rev. (Chicago: Fleming H. Revell, 1882), p. 143.

97. Len G. Broughton, *Religion and Health* (New York: Fleming H. Revell, 1909), p. 16.

98. Donald Dayton, "The Rise of the Evangelical Healing Movement in Nineteenth-Century America," *Pneuma: Journal for the Society of Pentecostal Studies* 4 (Spring 1982): 18.

99. Townsend, "Faith Cure," p. 660.

100. Jeff Kirby, "The Recovery of Healing Gifts," in *Those Controversial Gifts: Prophecy, Dreams, Visions, Tongues, Interpretation, Healing,* ed. George Mallone (Downers Grove, Ill.: InterVarsity Press, 1983), p. 102.

101. Rodney Clapp, "Faith Healing: A Look at What's Happening," *Christianity Today,* 16 December 1983, p. 13.

102. Alfred T. Schofield, *A Study of Healing* (New York: Fleming H. Revell, 1899), pp. 117–18.

103. W. B. Carman, "Spiritual Therapeutics," *Physician's and Surgeon's Investigator* 8 (15 November 1887): 335.

104. See Harrison, "Faith-Cure in the Light of Scripture," *Quarterly Review of the Methodist Episcopal Church, South* 28, n.s. 5 (January 1889): 402.

105. Quoted in Schofield, *A Study of Faith Healing,* p. 11.

106. "It is as much God's will to heal the body as it is to heal the soul"; F. F. Bosworth, *Christ the Healer: Messages on Divine Healing* (Miami Beach: F. F. Bosworth, 1948), p. 13.

107. See, e.g., C. E. Putnam, *Modern Religio-Healing: Man's Theories or God's Word* (Chicago: C. E. Putnam, 1924).

108. See Walter Moxon, "Faith Healing," *Contemporary Review* 48 (1885): 707–22.

109. See Clapp, "Faith Healing," *Christianity Today,* 16 December 1983, p. 13.

110. See Bruce Barron's analysis of this in *The Health and Wealth Gospel* (Downers Grove, Ill.: InterVarsity Press, 1987).

## Chapter 8 / Aging and Saging

1. Diane Apostolis Cappadona, "The Spirit and the Vision: The Influence of Romantic Evangelicalism on Nineteenth-Century American Art," Ph.D. diss., George Washington University, 1988, pp. 66–67.

2. Thomas Cole Sketchbook, Papers in the New York State Library, Box 6, folder 3, microfilm. Subsequent references in the text to the sketchbook notes are to these papers.

3. Cole, Sketchbook, ibid., and *Catalogue. The Voyage of Life! A Series of Allegorical Pictures,* in Box 6, folder 5, entitled "Exhibition Catalogs, Notes, Expense Accounts."

4. Thomas R. Cole, *The Journey of Life: A Cultural History of Aging in America* (New York: Cambridge University Press, 1992), p. 124.

5. David O. Moberg, "What the Graying of America Means to the Local Church," *Christianity Today,* 20 November 1981, p. 30. "More older Americans are members of religious organizations than of all other voluntary associations combined."

6. For the concept of the third age, and its theological implications, see "Aged to Perfection — The Third Age," in *Homiletics* 4 (January–March 1992): 43–46.

7. Gerald J. Gruman, "Cultural Origins of Present-day 'Ageism': The Modernization of the Life Cycle," in *Aging and the Elderly: Humanistic Perspectives in Gerontology,* ed. Stuart F. Spicker, Kathleen M. Woodward, and David D. Van Tassel (Atlantic Highlands, N.J.: Humanities Press, 1978), pp. 359–87. For Bradbury, see *Dandelion Wine* (1957; reprint New York: Bantam, 1959).

8. William R. Manchester, *The Glory and the Dream: A Narrative History of America, 1932–1972* (Boston: Little, Brown, 1974), p. 63.

9. Thomas R. Cole, "Past Meridian: Aging and the Northern Middle Class, 1830–1930," Ph.D. diss., University of Michigan, 1980 (Ann Arbor: UMI, 1988), p. 3. This dissertation was revised and published as *The Journey of Life.*

10. David Hackett Fischer, *Growing Old in America,* rev. ed. (New York: Oxford University Press, 1978), pp. 26–76; Cole, "The 'Enlightened' View of Aging: Victorian Morality in a New Key," in *What Does It Mean to Grow Old? Reflections from the Humanities,* ed. Thomas R. Cole and Sally A. Gadow (Durham: Duke University Press, 1986), p. 120; see also Cole, "Past Meridian," pp. 22–55.

11. Cole revises Fischer's perspectives on venerating the aged, evaluating them more as a "ritualistic form of compensation for the renunciations of intergenerational transmission" than a literal practice. See Cole, "Past Meridian," pp. 7, 9.

12. Cole, "Past Meridian," pp. 15–16.

13. Jean Abernethy, *Old Is Not a Four-Letter Word: New Moods and Meanings in Aging* (Nashville: Abingdon Press, 1975).

14. George A. Beard, *Legal Responsibilities in Old Age…* (New York: Russells' American Steam Printing House, 1876), p. 21.

15. See Gustavus Emanuel Hiller, *The Christian Family* (Cincinnati: Jennings and Graham, 1907), pp. 131–32.

16. S. D. Gordon and Mary Kilgore Gordon, *Quiet Talks on Home Ideals* (New York: Fleming H. Revell, 1909), pp. 177–78.

17. Philip Greven, *Spare the Child: The Religious Roots of Punishment and the Psychological Impact of Physical Abuse* (New York: Knopf, 1991).

18. See, e.g., the Southern Baptist *Evelyn Duball's Handbook for Parents* (Nashville: Broadman Press, 1974), p. 116, where spanking is denounced because "it doesn't work." Also see "Why Christians Spank," Grant Wacker's favorable review of Philip Greven's book *Spare the Child,* in *Christianity Today,* 9 March 1992, pp. 40–42.

19. I depend heavily here on a sensitive study by Carol J. Boggs, "An Analysis

of Selected Christian Child Rearing Manuals," *Family Relations* 32 (January 1983): 73–80.

20. James Dobson, *Dare to Discipline* (Wheaton, Ill.: Tyndale House, 1970), p. 173.

21. Donald Joy, *Parents, Kids, and Sexual Integrity: Equipping Your Child For Healthy Relationships* (Dallas: Word Books, 1988), p. 94.

22. Cole, "Past Meridian," pp. 56–94.

23. For the doctrine of usefulness, see Leonard I. Sweet, *The Minister's Wife: Her Role in Nineteenth-Century American Evangelicalism* (Philadelphia: Temple University Press, 1983), pp. 87–94.

24. *Memoirs of Rev. Charles G. Finney* (New York: Fleming H. Revell, 1876), p. 112.

25. For veneration as one of the ideological "casualties of democratic individualism," see Cole, "The Ideology of Old Age and Death in American History," *American Quarterly* 31 (Summer 1979): 223–31.

26. Cole, "Past Meridian," p. 234. See also Stephen Nissenbaum, *Sex, Diet, and Debility in Jacksonian America: Sylvester Graham and Health Reform* (Westport, Conn.: Greenwood Press, 1980).

27. Charles W. Hodell, "Browning's Vision of Old Age," *Methodist Review* 83 (January 1901): 99–104.

28. Paul Neff Garber, *The Romance of American Methodism* (Greensboro, N.C.: Piedmont Press, 1931), p. 104.

29. Charles S. Porter, *"Abandonment of God Deprecated by the Aged." Sermon: Delivered in the First Presbyterian Church, Utica, New York* (Utica: R. Northway, 1842), pp. 15–16.

30. J. Wilbur Chapman, *The Life and Work of Dwight L. Moody: Presented to the Christian World as a Tribute to the Memory of the Greatest Apostle of the Age* (Philadelphia: J. C. Winston, 1900), pp. 264, 265; Dwight L. Moody, *Weighed and Wanting: Addresses on the Ten Commandments* (Chicago: Fleming H. Revell, 1898), p. 71.

31. Cole, "Past Meridian," p. 125; see also pp. 219, 234.

32. For the lament "I have outlived my generation," see Thomas S. Hinde, "Our Duty Toward the Aged," *Methodist Magazine and Quarterly Review* 15 (1833): 105.

33. *The Diary of Isaac Backus*, vol. 3, ed. William G. McLoughlin (Providence: Brown University Press, 1979).

34. See also Carole Haber, *Beyond Sixty-five: The Dilemmas of Old Age in America's Past* (New York: Cambridge University Press, 1983).

35. Richard B. Calhoun, *In Search of the New Old: Redefining Old Age in America, 1945-1970* (New York: Elsevier, 1978).

36. Billy Graham, *My Answer* (Garden City, N.Y.: Doubleday, 1960), pp. 187, 190.

37. Quoted in Milton Leon Barron, *The Aging American: An Introduction to Social Gerontology and Geriatrics* (New York: Thomas Y. Crowell, 1961), p. 231. For this view's continuing prevalence in evangelical circles (e.g., "65 Is a Lousy Age"), see Bill Stephens, comp., *The Issues We Face...and Some Biblical Answers* (Nashville: Broadman Press, 1974), pp. 89–97.

38. Abraham Heschel, "To Grow in Wisdom," *Christian Ministry* 44 (March 1971): 31–37.

39. Cole, "The 'Enlightened' View of Aging," pp. 117, 124; Cole, "Past Meridian," p. 4.

40. Cole, "The 'Enlightened' View," p. 129.

41. William L. Hendricks, *A Theology for Aging* (Nashville: Broadman Press, 1986).

42. Eugene C. Bianchi, *Aging as a Spiritual Journey* (New York: Crossroad, 1984), p. 2.

43. Quoted in Eugene W. Brice, "Growing Older," *Pulpit Digest,* May/June 1983, p. 65.

44. Erik H. Erikson, *The Life Cycle Completed: A Review* (New York: W. W. Norton, 1982). See also Erik H. Erikson, Joan M. Erikson, and Helen Q. Kivnick, *Vital Involvement in Old Age* (New York: W. W. Norton, 1982).

## Chapter 9 / Deathbeds and Graveyards

1. For the importance of sickroom protocols, see "The Sick-Room," *Christian Advocate,* 10 January 1878, p. 30, but most particularly James Parkinson's health guide *Medical Admonitions to Families: Respecting the Preservation of Health, and the Treatment of the Sick* (Portsmouth, N.H.: Charles Peirce, 1803). Also see W. Worthington Hooker, "The Mutual Influence of Mind and Body in Disease," *New Englander and Yale Review* 3 (October 1845): 499.

2. Daniel Parish Kidder, ed., *The Dying Hours of Good and Bad Men Contrasted* (New York: Carlton and Phillips, 1853), pp. 82–84.

3. Kidder, *The Dying Hours,* p. 73.

4. Ibid., pp. 4, 65, 84, 109.

5. A. Gregory Schneider, "The Ritual of Happy Dying among Early American Methodists," *Church History* 56 (1987): 348–63.

6. Kidder, *The Dying Hours,* p. 34.

7. Schneider, "The Ritual of Happy Dying," pp. 353–54.

8. Irene Quenzler Brown, "Death, Friendship, and Female Identity during New England's Second Great Awakening," *Journal of Family History* 12 (October 1987): 367–87, esp. 377, 380, 381.

9. Stephen L. Stillman, "A Death Bed Scene," *Methodist Magazine and Quarterly Review* 13 (1831): 419.

10. Erich Fromm, *Escape from Freedom* (New York: Rinehart, 1941), pp. 245–46.

11. H. Paul Santmire, "Nothing More Beautiful than Death?," *Christian Century,* 14 December 1983, pp. 1154–58; Ron Rosenbaum, "Turn On, Tune In, Drop Dead," *Harper's,* July 1982, pp. 32–42; Robert L. Gram, "The Myth of Meaningful Death," *Church Herald,* 19 March 1982; Paul Ramsey, "The Indignity of 'Death with Dignity,'" *Hastings Center Studies* 2 (May 1974): 47–62. See also Michael Ignatieff, "Modern Dying," *New Republic,* 26 December 1988, pp. 28–33.

12. "Layman," "Thoughts on the Origin of Natural Death," *Quarterly Review of the Methodist Episcopal Church, South* 3 (October 1849): 561, 562. The reaction to this anonymous article was immediate and intense. See, e.g., "Western," "Thoughts on Natural Death," *Quarterly Review of the Methodist Episcopal Church, South* 4 (April 1850): 243–64, and Layman's rejoinder, "Additional Thoughts on the Origin of Natural Death," ibid., 4 (October 1850): 602–36.

13. David E. Stannard, *The Puritan Way of Death* (New York: Oxford University Press, 1977), p. 171.

14. Philippe Ariès, *The Hour of Our Death,* trans. Helen Weaver (New York: Knopf, 1981).

15. Elsewhere, Wiesel has written: "And so if the first death in history enters our collective memory as a murder, it means that death itself is an injustice. Perhaps Cain killed in protest against death." See Elie Wiesel, *Messengers of God: Biblical Portraits and Legends* (New York: Random House, 1976), p. 60

16. Elisabeth Kübler-Ross, *Living with Death and Dying* (New York: Macmillan, 1982), p. 169.

17. John Atkinson, *The Garden of Sorrows; or, The Ministry of Tears* (New York: Carlton and Lanahan, 1868), p. 125.

18. Henry Ward Beecher, *Star Papers; or, Experiences of Art and Nature* (New York: J. C. Derby, 1855), p. 125, 123.

19. R. D. Blackmore, "Dominus Illuminatio Mea," in *The Oxford Book of English Verse*, ed. Arthur Quiller-Couch (New York: Oxford University Press, 1900), p. 862.

20. R. Maurice Boyd, *A Lover's Quarrel with the World* (Burlington, Ont.: Welch Publishing, 1985; reprint, Philadelphia: Westminster Press, 1988), p. 142.

21. Charles Wesley, "A Funeral Hymn," *Hymns and Sacred Poems*, published by John and Charles Wesley (Bristol, Eng., 1742), in *The Poetical Works of John and Charles Wesley*, collected and arranged by G. Osborn (London: Wesleyan Methodist Conference Office, 1869), 2:184.

22. *The Complete Poems of Emily Dickinson*, ed. Thomas H. Johnson (Boston: Little, Brown, 1960), p. 690 (no. 1691).

23. Charles Wesley, "A Funeral Hymn," 2:184.

24. *Billy Graham Answers Your Questions* (Minneapolis: World Wide Publications, n.d.), p. 137.

25. Carl F. H. Henry, *The Christian Mindset in a Secular Society: Promoting Evangelical Renewal and National Righteousness* (Portland, Ore.: Multnomah Press, 1984), p. 38.

26. *The Journal of the Rev. John Wesley*, ed. Nehemiah Curnock (London: Epworth Press, 1938), 8:35.

27. Henry Moore, *The Life of the Rev. John Wesley* (New York: N. Bangs and J. Emory, for the Methodist Episcopal Church, 1825), 2:317.

28. "But be alive — this only matters, / Alive, to the end of ends alive!" Boris Pasternak, "Fame," in *Poems*, 2d ed., rev., trans. Eugene M. Kayden (Yellow Springs, Ohio: Antioch University Press, 1964), p. 235.

29. E. Stanley Jones, *The Divine Yes* (Nashville: Abingdon Press, 1975).

30. *Søren Kierkegaard's Journals and Papers*, ed. and trans. Howard V. Hong and Edna H. Hong (Bloomington: Indiana University Press, 1976), 6:315 (no. 6617).

31. See Don Lewis, *Religious Superstition through the Ages* (London: Mowbrays, 1975), p. 139.

32. "Always to Care, Never to Kill: A Declaration on Euthanasia," *Wall Street Journal*, 27 November 1991. See also Hessel Bouma III, Douglas Diekema, Edward Langerak, Theodore Rottman, and Allen Verhey, *Christian Faith, Health, and Medical Practice* (Grand Rapids, Mich.: Eerdmans, 1989), pp. 290–303.

33. "Cessation of useless means in truly terminal cases should in no way be confused with euthanasia...the deliberate choice of death as a moral end." John Jefferson Davis, *Evangelical Ethics: Issues Facing the Church Today* (Phillipsburg, N.J.: Presbyterian and Reformed Publishing, 1985), p. 186. See also Gerald A. Larue, *Euthanasia and Religion* (Los Angeles: Hemlock Society, 1985), pp. 101–2, 120–22.

34. On 29 April 1988, the Christian Medical and Dental Society adopted a statement on euthanasia that avows their opposition to "active intervention with the intent to produce death for the relief of suffering, economic considerations or convenience of patient, family, or society." They do not, however, oppose the "withdrawal or failure to institute artificial means of life support" to those whose "death appears imminent beyond reasonable hope of recovery."

35. See the discussion in Bouma et al., *Christian Faith, Health, and Medical Practice*, pp. 48–51.

36. As quoted in James W. Angell, *Learning to Manage Our Fears* (Nashville: Abingdon Press, 1981), p. 24.

37. Quoted in Joseph Bayly, "Is It Life or Death That is Prolonged?," *Christianity Today*, 5 February 1982, p. 30.

38. Davis, *Evangelical Ethics*, pp. 191–92.

39. See Norman Geisler, *Ethics: Issues and Alternatives* (Grand Rapids, Mich.: Zondervan, 1971), p. 235. See also Davis, *Evangelical Ethics*, p. 191.

40. Douglas K. Stuart, "'Mercy Killing' — Is It Biblical?," *Christianity Today,* 27 February 1976, pp. 9–11.

41. Antony Flew, "The Principle of Euthanasia," in *Euthanasia and the Right to Death,* ed. A. B. Downing (London: Peter Owen, 1969), pp. 46–47. See also Millard J. Erickson and Ines E. Bowers, "Euthanasia and Christian Ethics," *Journal of the Evangelical Theological Society* 19 (1976): 15–24, esp. p. 22.

42. Davis, *Evangelical Ethics,* p. 192.

43. Lewis B. Smedes, "Morality and Suicide," *Reformed Journal,* January 1983, p. 10.

44. Erickson and Bowers, "Euthanasia and Christian Ethics," p. 18.

45. See, e.g., William E. Phipps, "Christian Perspectives on Suicide," *Christian Century,* 30 October 1985, pp. 970–73; see also Wallace Gray, "Can Suicide Ever Be Christian?," *Circuit Rider,* May 1984, p. 3.

46. Thomas D. Kennedy, "Suicide and the Silence of Scriptures," *Christianity Today,* 20 March 1987, pp. 22–23.

47. William Sims Bainbridge, "The Religious Ecology of Deviance," *American Sociological Review* 54 (April 1989): 288–95.

48. This same thought is expressed in Cowper's hymn "God Moves in a Mysterious Way": "The bud may have a bitter taste, / But sweet will be the flow'r."

49. See James W. Fraser, *Cremation: Is It Christian?* (Neptune, NJ.: Loizeaux Brothers, 1965). Fraser is a minority voice today.

50. Howard Henderson, *The Ethics and Etiquette of the Pulpit, Pew, Parish, Press and Platform. A Manual of Manners for Ministers and Members* (Cincinnati: George P. Houston, 1892), pp. 79, 84.

51. John Jefferson Davis, *What about Cremation? A Christian Perspective* (Winona Lake, Ind.: BMH Books, 1989). Also see Paul E. Irion, *Cremation* (Philadelphia: Fortress Press, 1968).

52. John Wesley, *Explanatory Notes upon the New Testament* (London: Epworth Press, 1950), p. 739.

53. Charles Wesley, "On the Death of Samuel Hitchens," *Hymns and Sacred Poems* (Bristol, Eng., 1749), in *The Poetical Works of John and Charles Wesley,* 3:214.

54. C. S. Lewis, *The Chronicles of Narnia* (New York: Macmillan, 1956), 7:184.

# Index of Bible References

# General Index

*General Index*